W9-AAN-963

WITHDRAWN

Child Abuse
SOURCEBOOK

Fourth Edition

Health Reference Series

Fourth Edition

Child Abuse
SOURCEBOOK

*Basic Consumer Health Information about Child Neglect
and the Physical, Sexual, and Emotional Abuse of Children,
including Abusive Head Trauma, Bullying, Munchausen
by Proxy Syndrome, Statutory Rape, Incest, Educational
Neglect, Exploitation, and the Long-Term Consequences of
Child Maltreatment, Featuring Facts about Risk Factors,
Prevention Initiatives, Reporting Requirements, Legal
Interventions, Child Protective Services, and
Therapy Options*

*Along with Information for Parents, Foster Parents, and
Adult Survivors of Child Abuse, a Glossary of Related Terms,
and Directories of Additional Resources*

OMNIGRAPHICS

615 Griswold, Ste. 901, Detroit, MI 48226

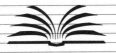
Batavia Public Library
Batavia, Illinois

Bibliographic Note

Because this page cannot legibly accommodate all the copyright notices, the Bibliographic Note portion of the Preface constitutes an extension of the copyright notice.

* * *

Omnigraphics, Inc.
Editorial Services provided by Omnigraphics, Inc.,
a division of Relevant Information, LLC

Keith Jones, *Managing Editor*

* * *

Copyright © 2016 Relevant Information, LLC
ISBN 978-0-7808-1524-7
E-ISBN 978-0-7808-1525-4

Library of Congress Cataloging-in-Publication Data

Names: Omnigraphics, Inc., issuing body.

Title: Child abuse sourcebook: basic consumer health information about child neglect and the physical, sexual, and emotional abuse of children, including abusive head trauma, bullying, munchausen syndrome by proxy, statutory rape, incest, educational neglect, exploitation, and the long-term consequences of child maltreatment, featuring facts about risk factors, prevention initiatives, reporting requirements, legal interventions, child protective services, and therapy options; along with information for parents, foster parents, and adult survivors of child abuse, a glossary of related terms, and directories of additional resources.

Description: Fourth edition. | Detroit, MI: Omnigraphics, [2016] | Series: Health reference series | Includes bibliographical references and index.

Identifiers: LCCN 2016018968 (print) | LCCN 2016025719 (ebook) | ISBN 9780780815247 (hardcover: alk. paper) | ISBN 9780780815254 (ebook) | ISBN 9780780815254 (eBook)

Subjects: LCSH: Child abuse--United States. | Child abuse--United States--Prevention. | Abused children--United States.

Classification: LCC HV6626.52 .C557 2016 (print) | LCC HV6626.52 (ebook) | DDC 362.76--dc23

LC record available at https://lccn.loc.gov/2016018968

Electronic or mechanical reproduction, including photography, recording, or any other information storage and retrieval system for the purpose of resale is strictly prohibited without permission in writing from the publisher.

The information in this publication was compiled from the sources cited and from other sources considered reliable. While every possible effort has been made to ensure reliability, the publisher will not assume liability for damages caused by inaccuracies in the data, and makes no warranty, express or implied, on the accuracy of the information contained herein.

∞

This book is printed on acid-free paper meeting the ANSI Z39.48 Standard. The infinity symbol that appears above indicates that the paper in this book meets that standard.

Printed in the United States

Table of Contents

Part II: Physical and Sexual Abuse of Children

Part III: Child Neglect and Emotional Abuse

Part V: Child Abuse Preventions, Interventions, and Treatments

Part VI: Parenting Issues and Child Abuse Risks

Part VII: Additional Help and Information

Preface

About This Book

According to data from the most recent Child Maltreatment report published by the U.S. Department of Health and Human Services (HHS), a total of 1,546 fatalities were reported across 50 states. Based on these data, a nationally estimated 1,580 children died from abuse and neglect. This translates to a rate of 2.13 deaths per 100,000 children. Nearly three-quarters of these fatalities involved children who were younger than 3 years old. Child maltreatment can create visible welts, bruises, and broken bones, or it can be invisible, producing deep emotional scars and life-long mental health challenges. Children who have been the victims of abuse or neglect can experience difficulty with social interaction, physical injuries, and even death.

Child Abuse Sourcebook, Fourth Edition, provides updated information about child neglect and the physical, emotional, and sexual abuse of children, including facts about severe punishment, abusive head trauma, Munchausen by proxy syndrome, rape, incest, exploitation, medical neglect, educational neglect, bullying, and aggression through technology. The book explains the differences between situations that require legal intervention and those considered to be parental choices, even when controversial. Facts about child protective services and interventions by the court system are also included. Parenting issues that may relate to child abuse risks, including domestic violence, postpartum depression, military service, substance abuse, and disciplinary strategies, are addressed, and information for adult survivors of child abuse is provided. The volume concludes with a glossary, a state-by-state list of contact information for reporting suspected child maltreatment, and a directory of resources for finding additional help and information.

How to Use This Book

This book is divided into parts and chapters. Parts focus on broad areas of interest. Chapters are devoted to single topics within a part.

Part I: Child Maltreatment explains the types of intentional actions that U.S. state laws typically recognize as forms of abuse. These include physical abuse, sexual abuse and exploitation, emotional abuse, neglect, and abandonment. Related issues, including bullying and exposure to violence, are also explored. The part concludes with a discussion of long term consequences of physical, psychological, behavioral and economic abuse.

Part II: Physical and Sexual Abuse of Children concerns itself with modes of maltreatment that result from physical actions, including physical abuse, abusive head trauma (shaken baby syndrome), and Munchausen by proxy syndrome. It reports on the physical and behavioral indicators of sexual abuse and provides facts about incest and abuse in dating relationships. It also discusses statutory rape laws and extraterritorial sexual exploitation of children.

Part III: Child Neglect and Emotional Abuse provides information about forms of abuse that are generally less visible than physical abuse. These can result from the failure of a parent or guardian to take appropriate action on a child's behalf—such as neglecting a child's healthcare—or other behaviors that negatively impact a child's mental development or psychological well-being. The part also discusses a wide range of other topics related to neglect and abuse including, technology and abuse, sexual exploitation of children, international parental kidnapping, and maltreatment of disabled children.

Part IV: Adult Survivors of Child Abuse explains the long-term consequences of experiencing maltreatment during childhood, and it discusses the outcomes that may emerge in adulthood. Mental health issues related to the vestiges of child abuse are also addressed. Early life stress and adult chronic fatigue syndrome (CFS) are also discussed, as well as the reactions to trauma by survivors of childhood abuse.

Part V: Child Abuse Preventions, Interventions, and Treatments reports on various strategies, laws, and regulations intended to reduce the incidence of child abuse. It presents various child abuse prevention strategies and initiatives, and explains how child protective services can intervene in suspected abuse cases. It also discusses therapy options for children and adults who have been impacted by abuse.

Part VI: Parenting Issues and Child Abuse Risks describes some of the most common family challenges that place children in dangerous situations, including domestic violence, mental health issues, parental substance abuse, and inappropriate forms of discipline. It provides tips for improving parenting skills and also offers suggestions for foster and adoptive parents.

Part VII: Additional Help and Information includes a glossary of terms related to child abuse and child protective services, a state-by-state list of contact information for reporting suspected child maltreatment, and a directory of organizations involved in efforts to end child abuse and heal its effects.

Bibliographic Note

This volume contains documents and excerpts from publications issued by the following U.S. government agencies: Centers for Disease Control and Prevention (CDC); Child Welfare Information Gateway; Federal Bureau of Investigation (FBI); National Human Genome Research Institute (NHGRI); National Institute of Child Health and Human Development (NICHD); National Institute of Justice (NIJ); National Institute of Mental Health (NIMH); National Institute on Drug Abuse (NIDA); National Institutes of Health (NIH); Office of Juvenile Justice and Delinquency Prevention (OJJDP); Office of the Assistant Secretary for Planning and Evaluation (ASPE); Stopbullying.gov; Substance Abuse and Mental Health Services Administration (SAMHSA); U.S. Agency for International Development (USAID); U.S. Department of Education (ED); U.S. Department of Health and Human Services (HHS); U.S. Department of Justice (DOJ); U.S. Department of Labor (DOL); U.S. Department of State (DOS); and U.S. Department of Veterans Affair (VA).

In addition, this volume contains copyrighted documents from the following organization: The Nemours Foundation

It may also contain original material produced by Omnigraphics, Inc. and reviewed by legal consultant.

About the Health Reference Series

The *Health Reference Series* is designed to provide basic medical information for patients, families, caregivers, and the general public. Each volume takes a particular topic and provides comprehensive coverage. This is especially important for people who may be dealing with a newly diagnosed disease or a chronic disorder in themselves or in a family member. People looking for preventive guidance, information about disease warning signs, medical statistics, and risk factors for health problems will also find answers to their questions in the *Health Reference Series*. The *Series*, however, is not intended to serve as a tool for diagnosing illness, in prescribing treatments, or as a substitute for the physician/patient relationship. All people concerned about medical symptoms or the possibility of disease are encouraged to seek professional care from an appropriate health care provider.

A Note about Spelling and Style

Health Reference Series editors use *Stedman's Medical Dictionary* as an authority for questions related to the spelling of medical terms and the *Chicago Manual of Style* for questions related to grammatical structures, punctuation, and other editorial concerns. Consistent adherence is not always possible, however, because the individual volumes within the *Series* include many documents from a wide variety of different producers, and the editor's primary goal is to present material from each source as accurately as is possible. This sometimes means that information in different chapters or sections may follow other guidelines and alternate spelling authorities.

Legal Review

Legal consultation services for *Child Abuse Sourcebook*, Fourth Edition, provided by:

K. Karthikeyan, MA, BL

Our Advisory Board

We would like to thank the following board members for providing initial guidance on the development of this series:

- Dr. Lynda Baker, Associate Professor of Library and Information Science, Wayne State University, Detroit, MI

- Nancy Bulgarelli, William Beaumont Hospital Library, Royal Oak, MI
- Karen Imarisio, Bloomfield Township Public Library, Bloomfield Township, MI
- Karen Morgan, Mardigian Library, University of Michigan-Dearborn, Dearborn, MI
- Rosemary Orlando, St. Clair Shores Public Library, St. Clair Shores, MI

Health Reference Series *Update Policy*

The inaugural book in the *Health Reference Series* was the first edition of *Cancer Sourcebook* published in 1989. Since then, the *Series* has been enthusiastically received by librarians and in the medical community. In order to maintain the standard of providing high-quality health information for the layperson the editorial staff at Omnigraphics felt it was necessary to implement a policy of updating volumes when warranted.

Medical researchers have been making tremendous strides, and it is the purpose of the *Health Reference Series* to stay current with the most recent advances. Each decision to update a volume is made on an individual basis. Some of the considerations include how much new information is available and the feedback we receive from people who use the books. If there is a topic you would like to see added to the update list, or an area of medical concern you feel has not been adequately addressed, please write to:

Managing Editor
Health Reference Series
Omnigraphics, Inc.
615 Griswold, Ste. 901
Detroit, MI 48226

Part One

Child Maltreatment

Chapter 1

Defining Child Maltreatment

Understanding Child Abuse and Neglect

When children are nurtured, they can grow up to be happy and healthy adults. But when they lack an attachment to a caring adult, receive inconsistent nurturing, or experience harsh discipline, the consequences can affect their lifelong health, well-being, and relationships with others.

This chapter provides information to help service providers and others concerned about the health and well-being of children to understand child abuse and neglect, its effects, and what each of us can do to address it when it occurs.

This chapter contains text excerpted from the following sources: Text under the heading "Understanding Child Abuse and Neglect" is excerpted from "Building Community Building Hope," Child Welfare Information Gateway, U.S. Department of Health and Human Services (HHS), 2016; Text under the heading "How Is Child Abuse and Neglect Defined in Federal Law?" is excerpted from "What Is Child Abuse and Neglect? Recognizing the Signs and Symptoms," Child Welfare Information Gateway, U.S. Department of Health and Human Services (HHS), July 2013; Text under the heading "State Definitions of Child Abuse and Neglect" is excerpted from "State Definitions of Child Abuse and Neglect," Child Welfare Information Gateway, U.S. Department of Health and Human Services (HHS), December 18, 2010. Reviewed May 2016; Text under the heading "Why Does Child Abuse Occur?" is excerpted from "Building Community Building Hope," Child Welfare Information Gateway, U.S. Department of Health and Human Services (HHS), 2016.

What Is Child Abuse and Neglect?

Child abuse or neglect often takes place in the home at the hands of a person the child knows well—a parent, relative, babysitter, or friend of the family. There are four major types of child maltreatment. Although any of the forms may be found separately, they often occur together. Each State is responsible for establishing its own definitions of child abuse and neglect that meet Federal minimum standards. Most include the following:

- **Neglect** is failure to provide for a child's basic needs.

- **Physical abuse** is physical injury as a result of hitting, kicking, shaking, burning, or otherwise harming a child.

- **Sexual abuse** is any situation where a child is used for sexual gratification. This may include indecent exposure, fondling, rape, or commercial exploitation through prostitution or the production of pornographic materials.

- **Emotional abuse** is any pattern of behavior that impairs a child's emotional development or sense of self-worth, including constant criticism, threats, and rejection.

How Is Child Abuse and Neglect Defined in Federal Law?

Federal legislation lays the groundwork for State laws on child maltreatment by identifying a minimum set of acts or behaviors that define child abuse and neglect. The Federal Child Abuse Prevention and Treatment Act (CAPTA), (42 U.S.C.A. §5106g), as amended and reauthorized by the CAPTA Reauthorization Act of 2010, defines child abuse and neglect as, at minimum:

"Any recent act or failure to act on the part of a parent or caretaker which results in death, serious physical or emotional harm, sexual abuse or exploitation; or an act or failure to act which presents an imminent risk of serious harm."

Most Federal and State child protection laws primarily refer to cases of harm to a child caused by parents or other caregivers; they generally do not include harm caused by other people, such as acquaintances or strangers. Some State laws also include a child's witnessing of domestic violence as a form of abuse or neglect.

State Definitions of Child Abuse and Neglect

While Federal legislation sets minimum standards for States that accept Federal funding, each State is responsible for defining child maltreatment in State law. Definitions of child abuse and neglect are typically located in two places within each State's statutory code:

- Civil statutes provide definitions of child maltreatment to guide individuals who are mandated to identify and report suspected child abuse and determine the grounds for intervention by State child protection agencies and civil courts. Locate definitions for your State by conducting a State Statutes Search on the Information Gateway website.

- Criminal statutes define those forms of child maltreatment that can subject an offender to arrest and prosecution in criminal courts.

Many States recognize four major types of maltreatment in their definitions, including neglect, physical abuse, sexual abuse, and emotional abuse or neglect.

Why Does Child Abuse Occur?

Child abuse and neglect affect children of every age, race, and income level. However, research has identified many factors relating to the child, family, community, and society that are associated with an increased risk of child abuse and neglect. Studies also have shown that when multiple risk factors are present, the risk is greater. Some of the most common risk factors include the following:

- **Immaturity.** Young parents may lack experience with children or be unprepared for the responsibility of raising a child.

- **Unrealistic expectations.** A lack of knowledge about normal child development or behavior may result in frustration and, ultimately, abusive discipline.

- **Stress.** Families struggling with poverty, unstable housing, divorce, or unemployment may be at greater risk.

- **Substance use.** The effects of substance use, as well as time, energy, and money spent obtaining drugs or alcohol, significantly impair parents' abilities to care for their children.

- **Intergenerational trauma.** Parents' own experiences of childhood trauma impact their relationships with their children.

- **Isolation.** Effective parenting is more difficult when parents lack a supportive partner, family, or community.

These circumstances, combined with the inherent challenges of raising children, can result in otherwise well-intentioned parents causing their children harm or neglecting their needs. On the other hand, evidence shows that the great majority of families who experience these circumstances will not abuse or neglect their children. Protective factors, such as the ones discussed in this guide, act as buffers to help many families who are under stress parent effectively.

How Many Children Are Abused and Neglected in the United States?

In Federal fiscal year (FFY) 2014, the most recent year for which national child maltreatment statistics are available, about 3.6 million reports (allegations of maltreatment) were made to child protective services concerning the safety and well-being of approximately 6.6 million children.

As a result of these reports, a nationally estimated 702,000 (unique count) children were found to be victims of child abuse or neglect. (Unique count is defined as counting each child only once regardless of the number of reports of abuse and neglect.) Of these children, three quarters (75.0 percent) were neglected, 17.0 percent were physically abused, and fewer than 10 percent (8.3 percent) were sexually abused.

Child deaths are the most tragic results of maltreatment. In FFY 2014, an estimated 1,580 children died due to abuse or neglect. Of the children who died, 72.3 percent suffered neglect and 41.3 percent suffered physical abuse either exclusively or in combination with another maltreatment type.

What Are the Consequences?

Child maltreatment is a traumatic experience, and the impact on survivors can be profound. Traumatic events, whether isolated (e.g., a single incident of sexual abuse) or ongoing (e.g., chronic emotional abuse or neglect), overwhelm children's ability to cope and elicit powerful physical and emotional responses. These responses continue even when the danger has passed, often until treatment is received. Traumatic events may impair a child's ability to trust others, sense of personal safety, and effectiveness in navigating life changes. Research shows that child maltreatment, like other trauma, is associated with poor health and mental health outcomes in children and families, and those negative effects can last a lifetime.

The trauma of child abuse or neglect has been associated with increased risk of:

- Depression and suicide attempts
- Substance abuse
- Developmental disabilities and learning problems
- Social problems with other children and with adults
- Teen pregnancy
- Lack of success in school
- Chronic illnesses, including heart disease, cancer, and lung disease, among others

In addition to the impact on the child and family, child abuse and neglect affects the community as a whole—including medical and mental health, law enforcement, judicial, public social services, and nonprofit agencies—as they respond to incidents and support victims. One analysis of the immediate and long-term economic impact of child abuse and neglect suggests that child maltreatment costs the nation approximately $220 million every day, or $80 billion per year.

Chapter 2

Child Abuse and Neglect Fatalities

Introduction to Child Abuse and Neglect Fatalities

Despite the efforts of the child protection system, child maltreatment fatalities remain a serious problem. Although the untimely deaths of children due to illness and accidents are closely monitored, deaths that result from physical assault or severe neglect can be more difficult to track. The circumstances surrounding a child's death, its investigation, and communication across all the disciplines involved complicate data collection.

How Many Children Die Each Year From Child Abuse or Neglect?

According to data from the National Child Abuse and Neglect Data System (NCANDS), 50 States reported a total of 1,484 fatalities. Based on these data, **a nationally estimated 1,520 children died from abuse and neglect in 2013.** This translates to a rate of 2.04 children per 100,000 children in the general population and an average of four children dying every day from abuse or neglect. This rate decreased

---

This chapter includes text excerpted from "Child Abuse and Neglect Fatalities 2013: Statistics and Interventions," U.S. Department of Health and Human Services (HHS), April 2015.

slightly from FFY 2012 and showed a 12.7-percent decrease from 2009. NCANDS defines "child fatality" as the death of a child caused by an injury resulting from abuse or neglect or where abuse or neglect was a contributing factor.

The number and rate of fatalities have fluctuated during the past 5 years. The national estimate is influenced by which States report data as well as by the U.S. Census Bureau's child population estimates. Some States that reported an increase in child fatalities between 2010 and 2012 attributed it to improvements in reporting after the passage of the Child and Family Services Improvement and Innovation Act.

Most data on child fatalities come from State child welfare agencies. However, States may also draw on other data sources, including health departments, vital statistics departments, medical examiners' offices, law enforcement, and fatality review teams. This coordination of data collection contributes to better estimates.

Many researchers and practitioners believe that child fatalities due to abuse and neglect are still underreported. One report on national child abuse and neglect deaths in the United States estimates that approximately 50 percent of deaths reported as "unintentional injury deaths" are reclassified after further investigation by medical and forensic experts as deaths due to maltreatment. It is often more difficult to establish whether a fatality was caused by neglect than it is to establish a physical abuse fatality. The different agencies that come into contact with a case of a possible child neglect fatality may have differing definitions of what constitutes neglect, and these definitions may be influenced by the laws, regulations, and standards of each agency.

Issues affecting the accuracy and consistency of child fatality data include:

- Variation among reporting requirements and definitions of child abuse and neglect and other terms

- Variation in death investigation systems and training

- Variation in State child fatality review and reporting processes

- The length of time (up to a year in some cases) it may take to establish abuse or neglect as the cause of death

- Inaccurate determination of the manner and cause of death, resulting in the miscoding of death certificates; this includes deaths labeled as accidents, sudden infant death syndrome (SIDS), or "manner undetermined" that would have been attributed to abuse or neglect if more comprehensive investigations had been conducted

- Limited coding options for child deaths, especially those due to neglect or negligence, when using the International Classification of Diseases to code death certificates

- The ease with which the circumstances surrounding many child maltreatment deaths can be concealed or rendered unclear

- Lack of coordination or cooperation among different agencies and jurisdictions

A report by the U.S. Government Accountability Office that assessed NCANDS data, surveys and interviews with State child welfare administrators and practitioners, and site visit reports to three States suggests that facilitating the sharing of information and increased cooperation among Federal, State, and local agencies would provide a more accurate count of maltreatment deaths. A study of child fatalities in three States found that combining at least two data sources resulted in the identification of more than 90 percent of child fatalities ascertained as due to child maltreatment.

What Groups of Children Are Most Vulnerable?

Research indicates that very young children (ages 4 and younger) are the most frequent victims of child fatalities. NCANDS data for 2013 demonstrated that children younger than 1 year accounted for 46.5 percent of fatalities; children younger than 3 years accounted for almost three-fourths (73.9 percent) of fatalities. These children are the most vulnerable for many reasons, including their dependency, small size, and inability to defend themselves.

How Do These Deaths Occur?

Fatal child abuse may involve repeated abuse over a period of time (e.g., battered child syndrome), or it may involve a single, impulsive incident (e.g., drowning, suffocating, or shaking a baby). In cases of fatal neglect, the child's death results not from anything the caregiver does, but from a caregiver's failure to act. The neglect may be chronic (e.g., extended malnourishment) or acute (e.g., an infant who drowns after being left unsupervised in the bathtub).

In 2013, 71.4 percent of children who died from child maltreatment suffered neglect either alone or in combination with another maltreatment type, and 46.8 percent suffered physical abuse either alone or in combination with other maltreatment. Medical neglect either alone or in combination was reported in 8.6 percent of fatalities.

Who Are the Perpetrators?

No matter how the fatal abuse occurs, one fact of great concern is that the perpetrators are, by definition, individuals responsible for the care and supervision of their victims. In 2013, parents, acting alone or with another parent, were responsible for 78.9 percent of child abuse or neglect fatalities. More than one-quarter (27.7 percent) were perpetrated by the mother acting alone, 12.4 percent were perpetrated by the father acting alone, and 24.6 percent were perpetrated by the mother and father acting together. Nonparents (including kin and child care providers, among others) were responsible for 17.0 percent of child fatalities, and child fatalities with unknown perpetrator relationship data accounted for 4.2 percent of the total.

There is no single profile of a perpetrator of fatal child abuse, although certain characteristics reappear in many studies. Frequently, the perpetrator is a young adult in his or her mid-20s, without a high school diploma, living at or below the poverty level, depressed, and who may have difficulty coping with stressful situations. Fathers and mothers' boyfriends are most often the perpetrators in abuse deaths; mothers are more often at fault in neglect fatalities.

How Do Communities Respond to Child Fatalities?

The response to the problem of child abuse and neglect fatalities is often hampered by inconsistencies, including:

- Underreporting of the number of children who die each year as a result of abuse and neglect

- Lack of consistent standards for child autopsies or death investigations

- The varying roles of Child Protective Services (CPS) agencies in investigation in different jurisdictions

- Uncoordinated, non-multidisciplinary investigations

- Medical examiners or elected coroners who do not have specific child abuse and neglect training

To address some of these inconsistencies, multidisciplinary and multiagency child fatality review teams have emerged to provide a coordinated approach to understanding child deaths, including deaths caused by religion-based medical neglect. Federal legislation further supported the development of these teams in an amendment to the 1992 reauthorization of the Child Abuse Prevention and Treatment Act (CAPTA), which required States to include information on child death review (CDR) in their program plans. Many States received initial funding for these teams through the Children's Justice Act, from grants awarded by the Administration on Children, Youth and Families in the U.S. Department of Health and Human Services (HHS).

Child fatality review teams, which exist at a State, local, or State/local level in the District of Columbia and in every State, are composed of prosecutors, coroners or medical examiners, law enforcement personnel, CPS workers, public health-care providers, and others. Child fatality review teams respond to the issue of child deaths through improved interagency communication, identification of gaps in community child protection systems, and the acquisition of comprehensive data that can guide agency policy and practice as well as prevention efforts.

The teams review cases of child deaths and facilitate appropriate follow-up. Follow-up may include ensuring that services are provided for surviving family members, providing information to assist in the prosecution of perpetrators, and developing recommendations to improve child protection and community support systems.

Recent data show that 49 States have a case-reporting tool for CDR; however, there had been little consistency among the types of information compiled. This contributed to gaps in the understanding of infant and child mortality as a national problem. In response, the National Center for the Review and Prevention of Child Deaths, in cooperation with 30 State CDR leaders and advocates, developed a web-based CDR Case Reporting System for State and local teams to use to collect data and analyze and report on their findings. As of February 2015, 43 States were using the standardized system, and 3 more were considering adopting the system. As more States use the system and the numbers of reviews entered into it increase, a more representative and accurate view of how and why children die from abuse and neglect will emerge. The ultimate goal is to use the data to advocate for actions to prevent child deaths and to keep children healthy, safe, and protected.

Since its 1996 reauthorization, CAPTA has required States that receive CAPTA funding to set up citizen review panels. These panels of volunteers conduct reviews of CPS agencies in their States, including policies and procedures related to child fatalities and investigations. As of December 2013, 17 State CDR boards serve additional roles as the citizen review panels for child fatalities.

How Can These Fatalities Be Prevented?

When addressing the issue of child maltreatment, and especially child fatalities, prevention is a recurring theme. The prevention strategies and initiatives discussed below offer a variety of approaches.

Child Fatality Review Teams

Well-designed, properly organized child fatality review teams appear to offer hope for defining the underlying nature and scope of fatalities due to child abuse and neglect. The child fatality review process helps identify risk factors that may assist prevention professionals, such as those engaged in home visiting and parenting education, to prevent future deaths. In addition, teams are demonstrating effectiveness in translating review findings into action by partnering with child welfare and other child health and safety groups. In some States, review team annual reports have led to State legislation, policy changes, or prevention programs. Findings associated with these reviews have identified decreases in child fatalities.

Data Collection and Analysis

Some States have begun to integrate other data with CPS data to help identify high-risk families and provide prevention services before maltreatment happens. Integrating data from birth certificates, emergency room visits, and other social services sectors with CPS data and then analyzing those data for trends in risk may also help child welfare professionals make better-informed decisions about prevention. Users of the CDR Case Reporting System can record their recommendations for prevention efforts. Examples of recommendations include improved multiagency coordination policies for death investigations; improvements in CPS intake, referral, and case-management procedures; intensive home visiting; worker training; and improved judicial practices.

A Public Health Approach

A number of experts have championed a public health approach to addressing child maltreatment fatalities, which focuses on improving the health and well-being of individuals and communities before child maltreatment happens. Specifically, a public health approach involves defining the problem, identifying risk and protective factors, understanding consequences, and developing prevention strategies. And, true to its name, a public health approach involves the entire community in preventing child maltreatment and ensuring that parents have the support and services they need before abuse and neglect can occur.

Improved Training

Several recent articles have noted the need for better training for child welfare workers in identifying potentially fatal situations. Current child welfare training curricula do not always address child maltreatment fatalities; in fact, a recent study of preservice child welfare training curricula in 20 States found that only 10 States even mentioned child maltreatment fatalities, and only 1 State included a full section on the topic. Given the complex nature of child maltreatment, training needs to go beyond the use of tools and assessments to include good critical thinking and decision-making skills.

Federal Initiatives

The Federal Government has a long history of promoting prevention. The first National Child Abuse Prevention Week, declared by Congress in 1982, was replaced the following year with the first National Child Abuse Prevention Month. Other activities followed, including a 1991 initiative by Louis W. Sullivan, M.D., the Secretary of HHS, designed to raise awareness and promote coordination of prevention and treatment. In 2003, the Office on Child Abuse and Neglect, within the Children's Bureau, Administration for Children and Families, HHS, launched a child abuse prevention initiative that included an opportunity for individuals and organizations across the country to work together. This ongoing initiative also includes the publication of an annual resource guide. Increasingly, this effort focuses on promoting protective factors that enhance the capacity of parents, caregivers, and communities to protect, nurture, and promote the healthy development of children.

In early 2013, Congress passed H.R. 6655, which establishes the Commission to Eliminate Child Abuse and Neglect Fatalities. The Commission will develop recommendations for a national strategy to reduce fatalities resulting from child abuse and neglect, specifically:

- The Commission is tasked with studying the use of funding under titles IV-B, IV-E, and XX (SSBG) of the Social Security Act to reduce fatalities from child abuse and neglect.

15

- A report to the President and Congress with the Commission's findings and recommendations is due within 2 years.

- Federal agencies must develop a plan to address the Commission's recommendations within 6 months after the report is submitted to the President and Congress.

- $2 million is authorized out of the TANF contingency fund for the Commission for FY 2013 and 2014.

Summary

While the exact number of children affected is uncertain, child fatalities due to abuse and neglect remain a serious problem in the United States. Fatalities disproportionately affect young children and most often are caused by one or both of the child's parents. Child fatality review teams appear to be among the most promising current approaches to accurately count, respond to, and prevent child abuse and neglect fatalities, as well as other preventable deaths.

Chapter 3

Child Abuse Statistics

Child Maltreatment

- The national estimates of children who received an investigation or alternative response increased 7.4 percent from 2010 (3,023,000) to 2014 (3,248,000).

- The number and rate of victims of maltreatment have fluctuated during the past 5 years. Comparing the national estimate of victims from 2010 (698,000) to 2014 (702,000) show an increase of less than 1 percent.

- Three-quarters (75.0%) of victims were neglected, 17.0 percent were physically abused, and8.3 percent were sexually abused.

- For 2014, a nationally estimated 1,580 children died of abuse and neglect at a rate of 2.13 per100,000 children in the national population.

Deaths from Child Maltreatment

Child fatalities are the most tragic consequence of maltreatment. For FFY 2014, 50 states reported 1,546 fatalities. Based on these data, a nationally estimated 1,580 children died from abuse and neglect. According to the analyses performed on the child fatalities for whom case-level data were obtained:

_____

This chapter includes text excerpted from "Child Maltreatment," U.S. Department of Health and Human Services (HHS), 2015.

- The national rate of child fatalities was 2.13 deaths per 100,000 children.

- Nearly three-quarters (70.7%) of all child fatalities were younger than 3 years old.

- Boys had a higher child fatality rate than girls at 2.48 boys per 100,000 boys in the population.

- Girls died of abuse and neglect at a rate of 1.82 per 100,000 girls in the population.

- Almost 90 percent (88.4%) of child fatalities were comprised of White (43.0%), African-American (30.3%), and Hispanic (15.1%) victims.

- Four-fifths (79.3%) of child fatalities involved at least one parent.

Characteristics of Victims

- The youngest children are the most vulnerable to maltreatment. In FFY 2014, 52 states reported that more than one-quarter (27.4%) of victims were younger than 3 years. The victimization rate was highest for children younger than 1 year (24.4 per 1,000 children in the population of the same age). Victims who were 1, 2, or 3 years old had victimization rates of 12.3, 11.6, and 11.0 victims per 1,000 children of those respective ages in the population. In general, the rate of victimization decreased with age.

- The majority of victims (percentages not shown) were of three races or ethnicities—White (44.0%), Hispanic (22.7%), and African-American (21.4%). African-American children had the highest rate of victimization at 15.3 per 1,000 children in the population of the same race or ethnicity and American-Indian or Alaska Native children had the second highest rate at 13.4 per 1,000 children. Hispanic and White children had lower rates of victimization at 8.8 and 8.4 per 1,000 children in the population of the same race or ethnicity.

- The victimization rate among children younger than age 18 was higher among girls overall, though sex patterns differ by age group. Boys in the age groups of <1 and 1–5 have consistently higher rates than girls in the same two age groups. Girls in the age groups 6–10 and 11–17 have consistently higher rates than boys in the same age group, especially for girls ages 11–17. The victimization rates for these older girls are 35 percent higher than the rates for older boys. The rates of both boys and girls in the age group of <1 have been increasing for several years.

Characteristics of Perpetrators

- Victim data were analyzed by relationship of victims to their perpetrators. A victim may have been maltreated multiple times by the same perpetrator or by different combinations of perpetrators (e.g., mother alone, mother and nonparent(s), mother and father). In addition, a perpetrator who maltreats multiple children may have different relationships with the victims (parent, neighbor, etc.). This analysis counts every combination of relationships for each victim in each report and, therefore, the percentages total more than 100.0 percent. For FFY 2014, one or both parents maltreated 91.6 percent of victims. The parent(s) could have acted together, acted alone, or acted with up to two other people to maltreat the child. A perpetrator who was not the child's parent maltreated nearly 13 percent (12.6%) of victims. The largest categories in the nonparent group were male relative, male partner of parent, and "other."

Chapter 4

When Children Are Exposed to Violence

Children's Exposure to Violence

The association between delinquency and victimization is a common focus in juvenile justice research. Some observers have found that victimization and delinquency largely overlap, with most victims engaging in delinquency and most delinquents being victimized at some point in their lives. The literature in the bullying and peer victimization field paints a different picture. It points to three distinct groups of children: in addition to the children who are both victims and offenders (often referred to as bully-victims or, as in this chapter delinquent-victims), a second group are primarily victims and a third group are primarily offenders. One may explain the contrast in this way: many studies have relied simply on measures of association between delinquency and victimization (e.g., correlation or regression analyses).

When researchers look beyond the association between delinquency and victimization (even when that association is strong), they are likely to find groups of children who are primarily victims or primarily offenders. Research has not fully explored how large these groups are and how their characteristics and experiences differ.

This chapter includes text excerpted from "Children's Exposure to Violence and the Intersection Between Delinquency and Victimization," Office of Juvenile Justice and Delinquency Prevention (OJJDP), U.S. Department of Justice (DOJ), October 2013.

21

Defining Delinquents, Victims, and Delinquent Victims in the NatSCEV Study Group

The National Survey of Children's Exposure to Violence (NatSCEV) is a national study that is both large and comprehensive in its assessment of victimization and delinquency. Thus, it provides a look at how victimization and delinquency converge or diverge among youth of different ages.

Using the interview data from NatSCEV, the research team categorized adolescents ages 10 to 17 into one of four groups: those youth who were primarily delinquents and not victims (primarily delinquents), those who were primarily victims and not delinquents (primarily victims), those who were both delinquents and victims (delinquent-victims), and those who were neither victims nor delinquents. The criteria for defining these groups are based on work done in an earlier study and take into account that many children have minor victimizations and that they engage in different kinds of delinquency, including violent delinquency, property delinquency, and forms of mild delinquency, such as skipping school or getting drunk.

In the interest of clarity, the researchers defined the subgroups in terms of key characteristics that the literature on victimization and delinquency suggests.

Definition of Victimized versus Nonvictimized Youth

From previous analyses, the researchers determined that one of the best measures of victimization intensity is the number of types of victimization per respondent based on the screening categories that the Juvenile Victimization Questionnaire (JVQ) uses. Although simply adding up the number of different types of victimization (including parental abuse, sex offenses, property offenses, and peer victimizations) does not take into account repeated victimizations of the same type, analyses have suggested that factoring in repeated victimizations and other measures of victimization severity does not produce substantively different results in identifying highly victimized youth.

For the purposes of this study, the researchers defined victimized youth as those who suffered three or more victimizations in the past year. They chose this number because the mean number of types of victimization in the past year per respondent in the NatSCEV study was 2.68 and because the JVQ and NatSCEV include many common kinds of victimizations, such as being hit by a sibling or having property stolen. Consequently, the researchers categorized non-/low-victimized youth as those who suffered two victimizations or fewer in the past year.

Definition of Delinquent versus Nondelinquent Youth

Based on the literature on delinquency, the researchers considered it important to distinguish among types of delinquent behavior. The researchers clearly delineated the study's delinquency measures into the following types: those that involved violent behavior (assaults and carrying weapons), those that involved property delinquency (breaking something, stealing from a store), those that involved drug and alcohol use (drinking, smoking marijuana), and those that involved minor delinquency (truancy, cheating on tests). Violent behavior and property delinquency are categorized as separate types, and for the most part delinquency involving substance use or minor forms of rule violating is categorized as mild delinquency.

As with victimized youth, some categories of delinquent youth are defined as those who committed more delinquent acts than the past-year mean (i.e., two or more types of delinquent acts within the past year). Given the inclusion of relatively minor and perhaps normative delinquent acts in the Frequency of Delinquency Behavior, the researchers decided that defining those who committed fewer than the mean number of delinquent acts in the past year as non-delinquent would adequately identify youth with no or only minor delinquency.

Categories of Delinquent-Victims

The researchers first defined three groups of youth who fell into the delinquent-victim overlap category. They defined "Violent Delinquent-Victims," consistent with descriptions from other studies of victimization and delinquency, as youth who in the past year engaged in violent, interpersonal acts or carried weapons and who experienced three or more violent victimizations in the past year. As suggested in the trauma response literature, the research team termed the second defined group as "Delinquent Sex/Maltreatment Victims," who had experienced sexual victimization or a form of child maltreatment and had engaged in two or more delinquent acts in the past year. They defined the third group, "Property Delinquent-Victims," as delinquent and highly victimized youth whose delinquencies were related solely to property crime and who had three or more victimizations of any type in the past year.

Categories of Primarily Delinquent Youth

In contrast to these three groups of delinquent-victims, the study also categorized some youth as primarily delinquent. These were youth who had rates of victimization below the mean of three in the past year, but who had engaged in violent (youth categorized as "Assaulters") or property delinquency (youth categorized as "Property Delinquents"), which were the most serious and least frequent delinquencies.

Categories of Youth Who Are Primarily Victims

The researchers defined two groups who were primarily victims but not delinquents. These were the "Mild Delinquency Victims," who had greater than mean levels of victimization (three or more victimizations within the past year) but no property or violent delinquency, and "Nondelinquent Sex/Maltreatment Victims," who had experienced a sexual victimization or a form of child maltreatment but had committed fewer than two delinquent acts in the past year. This last group was distinguished as a separate category because the victimization literature suggests special seriousness for youth who experience even one incident of sexual victimization or child maltreatment, which are also acts that lead to the involvement of child protective services or police referrals.

The grouping criteria illustrate, to some degree, the intricacy of establishing these categories given the complexity of victimization and delinquent behavior. As such, the categorizing approach examines both the number of types of behavior (above or below the mean for victimization and delinquency) and the type of delinquency or victimization (e.g., violent, property, sexual, or maltreatment). As a result, some youth may fit into more than one of the established categories. To keep the groups mutually exclusive, the researchers established a hierarchy for categorizing individuals who fell into more than one typology group (e.g., a youth who committed a violent act or carried a weapon within the previous year and had been sexually victimized in addition to undergoing three or more violent victimizations, and who therefore would fall into both the violent delinquent-victim and delinquent sex/maltreatment victim typology groups). The hierarchy is as follows, from the most severe to the least severe combination of delinquency and victimization: violent delinquent-victims, delinquent sex/ maltreatment victims, assaulters, nondelinquent sex/maltreatment victims, property delinquent-victims, property delinquents, mild delinquency victims, and mild delinquency non-/low-victimized youth (note that assaulters and nondelinquent sex/maltreatment victims, although they are categorized as primarily delinquent and primarily victims, respectively, are regarded as higher in the hierarchy than property delinquent-victims). This ordering was presented in the original typology using the Developmental Victimization Survey (DVS) data, which established this order according to which group of individuals was most similar based on their demographic characteristics. For consistency, the ordering remained the same for the purposes of this analysis based on the NatSCEV data.

Findings by Gender and Typology Group for Delinquents, Victims, and Delinquent-Victims

Victimization and Delinquency Patterns Among Boys

Among boys overall, the primarily delinquent group comprised 20.8 percent of the total sample. Boys who were primarily victims with little or no delinquency comprised 17.9 percent of the total sample, and the group who were both victimized and delinquent comprised 18.1 percent. Substantial percentages of all three groups were evident throughout the developmental course for boys ages 10 to 17. However, the proportion of boys in the primarily victim group differed between ages 12 and 13 (declining from 27.8 percent to 15.5 percent). At ages 13 and 14, the proportion of boys in the delinquent-victim group increased from 14.7 percent to 28.2 percent and was elevated through age 17.

The boys in the delinquent-victim group had considerably more victimization than the boys who were primarily victims, disclosing 6.3 and 4.5 different kinds of victimization in the past year, respectively. This delinquent-victim group had a greater percentage of victims than the primarily victim group in every category of victimization except for bullying victimization. These boys had particularly greater percentages of sexual victimization (which includes sexual harassment) (40 percent for delinquent-victim boys versus 13 percent for primarily victim boys), witnessing family violence (26 percent for delinquent-victim boys versus 12 percent for primarily victim boys), and Internet victimization (14 percent for delinquent-victim boys versus 1 percent for primarily victim boys). The primarily victim group of boys had a greater percentage of victims than the delinquent-victim group in only one victimization category—bullying victimization (58 percent versus 40 percent).

The boys in the delinquent-victim group were also more delinquent than the primarily delinquent group (3.9 and 2.7 delinquent activities in the past year, respectively), which may be in part a function of the definitional criteria that set a higher threshold of delinquent activities for delinquent-victim boys than for primarily delinquent boys. The elevation of their drugs/minor delinquency score was particularly large (1.4 for delinquent-victims versus 0.8 for the primarily delinquent group).

Victimization and Delinquency Patterns among Girls

Girls had different patterns in both typology groups and age of changes in victimization and delinquency. Except for the group of girls who were neither victims nor delinquents (52.5 percent), the largest group of girls was the primarily victim group (21.2 percent). The primarily delinquent group (13 percent) and delinquent-victim group (13.3 percent) were smaller than the comparable groups among boys, reflecting that girls tend to engage in less delinquency than boys. A rise in both delinquency and victimization for girls appeared particularly notable between ages 11 and 12; as girls got older, the victimization component remained stable and then rose, while the delinquency component rose and then fell.

The patterns of victimization and delinquency for girls are generally similar to those for boys in terms of both the number and types of victimizations and delinquent acts. The delinquent-victim girls were more victimized than the primarily victim girls, disclosing 6.4 and 4.2 different victimizations in the past year, respectively. (This is not a function of the definitional criteria that set a higher threshold of victimizations for delinquent-victim girls than for primarily victim girls.) The delinquent-victim girls had greater percentages of victimization in every category of victimization except bullying victimization. Their victimization rates were particularly higher for sexual victimization, for which the rate among delinquent-victim girls (58 percent) was more than twice that among the primarily victim girls (27 percent); and Internet victimization, for which the rate among delinquent-victim girls was more than four times higher than among the primarily victim girls (33 percent versus 7 percent) and much higher than the equivalent rate among delinquent-victim boys (14 percent).

Delinquent-victim girls were also more delinquent than the primarily delinquent girls (3.3 and 2.0 delinquent activities in the past year, respectively). As with the boys, their drugs/minor delinquency scores were particularly elevated (1.7 for delinquent-victim girls versus 0.6 for primarily delinquent girls).

Implications for Adolescent Development and for Intervention by Practitioners

Age Onset of Increasing Risk for Victimization and Delinquency

Delinquency and victimization are widespread among youth ages 10 to 17, and they are statistically associated. However, in addition to those who experience both, it is possible to identify large groups within this age range who are victimized but not delinquent as well as those who are delinquent but experienced few types of victimization.

The relative sizes of these various groups appear to change as children age; they also differ by gender. The delinquent-victim group among boys is larger overall and increases substantially between ages 13 and 14. This may reflect an increase in delinquent activities around the time they enter high school among those who had previously been primarily victims. The high school environment may expose them to older delinquent role models and present them with conditions of more independence and less supervision than middle school.

For girls, the pattern change appears to occur earlier (between ages 11 and 12) and is associated with an increase in both victimization and delinquency, but particularly victimization. This is likely related to the onset of pubertal changes in girls and shows up in the data as a particularly marked increase in sexual harassment.

Increased Risk of Both Delinquency and Victimization for Delinquent-Victims

For both genders, the data reveal worrying facts about the group who are both victimized and delinquent. This group manifests higher levels of both victimization and delinquency than either the primarily victim or primarily delinquent group. This group also has more additional adversities, lower levels of social support, and higher rates of mental health symptoms. This is consistent with observations from the bullying literature that the so-called "bully-victims" are often the most distressed children. Improving strategies for identifying and helping this group of children is an obvious priority.

Timing of Interventions to Reduce Victimization and Delinquency

The current study is not longitudinal, and so it is limited in the inferences that can be made about how to identify children who are on track to become distressed delinquent-victims. This group does not appear to be discernible on the basis of demographic, family, or school variables collected in this study. The age comparisons suggest that victims who have additional adversities and higher levels of victimization and mental health symptoms may also be those at greatest risk of moving into delinquent activities. Targeting prevention at highly victimized youth with mental health symptoms may be important.

The study points clearly to the importance of early intervention. For girls, a large jump in victimization and delinquency occurs between ages 11 and 12; for boys, the delinquent-victim group increases between ages 13 and 14. This strongly suggests that delinquency and victimization prevention efforts need to be marshaled around or before the fifth grade, and they need to include components that minimize sexual aggression and harassment.

The transition to high school may also be a crucial juncture, especially for boys. Further study may better determine how children at this juncture both are targeted as victims and initiate multiple delinquent activities. Better early-warning systems may identify students who need special guidance and education from early in their high school careers.

Chapter 5

Child Exploitation

Chapter Contents

Section 5.1

Child Labor – A Form of Child Exploitation

This section includes text excerpted from "What are
Child Labor and Forced Labor?" U.S. Department of
Labor (DOL), December 14, 2012. Reviewed May 2016.

What is Child Labor?

A **child** or **children** are minors under the age of 18 years.

Child labor includes those children (minors under age 18) working
in the worst forms of child labor (WFCL) as outlined in International
Labor Organization (ILO) Convention 182 and children engaged in
work that is exploitative and/or interferes with their ability to participate in and complete required years of schooling, in line with ILO
Convention 138. ILO Convention 182 defines the WFCL as:

1. all forms of slavery or practices similar to slavery, such as the
    sale and trafficking of children, debt bondage and serfdom and
    forced or compulsory labor, including forced or compulsory
    recruitment of children for use in armed conflict;

2. the use, procuring or offering of a child for prostitution, the
    production of pornography or for pornographic performances;

3. the use, procuring or offering of a child for illicit activities,
    in particular for the production and trafficking of drugs as
    defined in the relevant international treaties; and

4. work which, by its nature or the circumstances in which it is
    carried out, is likely to harm the health, safety or morals of
    children.

According to ILO Convention 182, hazardous work "shall be determined by national laws or regulations or by the competent authority,
after consultation with the organizations of employers and workers
concerned, taking into consideration relevant international standards..." As this suggests, forms of work identified as "hazardous"
for children may vary from country to country. ILO Recommendation

No. 190, which accompanies ILO Convention 182, gives additional guidance on identifying "hazardous work." ILO Recommendation No. 190 states in Section II, Paragraph 3 that "[i]n determining the types of work referred to under Article 3(d) of the Convention, and in identifying where they exist, consideration should be given, inter alia to:

1. work which exposes children to physical, psychological, or sexual abuse;

2. work underground, underwater, at dangerous heights or in confined spaces;

3. work with dangerous machinery, equipment and tools, or which involves the manual handling or transport of heavy loads;

4. work in an unhealthy environment which may, for example, expose children to hazardous substances, agents or processes, or to temperatures, noise levels, or vibrations damaging to their health;

5. work under particularly difficult conditions such as work for long hours or during the night or work where the child is unreasonably confined to the premises of the employer."

Child labor spans nearly every sector and kind of work. Children harvest cotton in Uzbekistan, work as domestic servants in Haiti and mine diamonds in the Central African Republic. It is important to recognize that not all work performed by children is exploitative. Children of legal working age who perform work that does not hinder their mental, physical or emotional development can be an asset to their families' welfare and their nations' economic development. Activities that would qualify as non-exploitative under these international standards include performing household chores, assisting parents in a family business outside of school hours, and working in non-hazardous activities after school or during vacations to earn extra income.

Drivers of Child Labor

Children enter the labor force due to both supply factors and industry demand for cheap, unskilled labor, among other factors. Poverty is the most salient source of pressure leading to the supply of child labor. Production processes that require an abundance of unskilled labor or that require certain physical attributes—small stature, agility and so on—can also create demand for child labor. In addition, price pressures encourage suppliers, especially at points upstream in the supply chain, to find the cheapest labor. Children may be the only workers willing to work for these wages, or adults may find that these wage levels do not allow them to meet basic needs and they must put their children to work to supplement family income. These fundamental supply and demand factors are often reinforced by factors such as a lack of adequate access to education, inadequate employment potential for those who do receive education, exclusionary social attitudes based on caste or ethnicity, gender and cultural attitudes about work and education.

Section 5.2

Vulnerable Children and Child Labor

This section includes text excerpted from "What is Modern Slavery?"
U.S. Department of State, June 16, 2010. Reviewed May 2016.

Victims of Human Trafficking

Over the past 15 years, "trafficking in persons" and "human trafficking" have been used as umbrella terms for activities involved when someone obtains or holds a person in compelled service.

The U.S. government considers trafficking in persons to include all of the criminal conduct involved in forced labor and sex trafficking, essentially the conduct involved in reducing or holding someone in compelled service. Under the Trafficking Victims Protection Act as amended (TVPA) and consistent with the United Nations Protocol to Prevent, Suppress and Punish Trafficking in Persons, Especially Women and Children (Palermo Protocol), individuals may be trafficking victims regardless of whether they once consented, participated in a crime as a direct result of being trafficked, were transported into the exploitative situation, or were simply born into a state of servitude.

Despite a term that seems to connote movement, at the heart of the phenomenon of trafficking in persons are the many forms of enslavement, not the activities involved in international transportation.

Forced Child Labor

Most international organizations and national laws recognize that children may legally engage in certain forms of work. There is a growing consensus, however, that the worst forms of child labor should be eradicated. The sale and trafficking of children and their entrapment in bonded and forced labor are among these worst forms of child labor. A child can be a victim of human trafficking regardless of the location of that exploitation. Indicators of forced labor of a child include situations in which the child appears to be in the custody of a non-family member who has the child perform work that financially benefits someone outside the child's family and does not offer the child the option of leaving. Anti-trafficking responses should supplement, not replace, traditional actions against child labor, such as remediation and education. However, when children are enslaved, their abusers should not escape criminal punishment by virtue of longstanding patters of limited responses to child labor practices rather than more effective law enforcement action.

Child Soldiers

Child soldiering can be a manifestation of human trafficking where it involves the unlawful recruitment or use of children—through force, fraud, or coercion—as combatants, or for labor or sexual exploitation by armed forces. Perpetrators may be government forces, paramilitary organizations, or rebel groups. Many children are forcibly abducted to be used as combatants. Others are made unlawfully to work as porters, cooks, guards, servants, messengers, or spies. Young girls can be forced to marry or have sex with male combatants. Both male and female child soldiers are often sexually abused and are at high risk of contracting sexually transmitted diseases.

Child Sex Trafficking

According to UNICEF, as many as two million children are subjected to prostitution in the global commercial sex trade. International covenants and protocols obligate criminalization of the commercial sexual exploitation of children. The use of children in the commercial sex trade is prohibited under both U.S. law and the Palermo Protocol as well as by legislation in countries around the world. There can be no exceptions and no cultural or socioeconomic rationalizations preventing the rescue of children from sexual servitude. Sex trafficking has devastating consequences for minors, including long-lasting physical and psychological trauma, disease (including HIV/AIDS), drug addiction, unintended pregnancy, malnutrition, social ostracism, and death.

Section 5.3

Ending Child Labor

This section includes text excerpted from "Ending Child Labor,"
U.S. Agency for International Development (USAID), June 12, 2014.

Global social movements have proven we can end child labor. Civil-society organizations in over 100 countries on every continent launched a Global March against Child Labor in 1998. The march crossed 103 countries and culminated in a conference at the International Labor Organization (ILO) in Geneva in June 1998 where activists called on governments, international organizations, companies and civil society to come together to end child labor.

The ILO launched the World Day against Child Labor in 2002. Each year on June 12, the day brings together governments, employers' and workers' organizations, civil society and millions of people from around the world to highlight the plight of child laborers and what can be done to help them.

The movement is succeeding in its ambitious goals. In the late 1990s, the estimated number of children in various forms of child labor was nearly 250 million. Today, that figure has dropped to 168 million. The decline has particularly benefitted girls; total child labor among girls has fallen by 40 percent since 2000, compared to a drop of 25 percent for boys.

Child labor is defined as work that is hazardous to a child's health, education, or physical or mental development. Too often, it traps children in a cycle of poverty. Too many children in the world still work instead of going to school. For example, an estimated 98 million children worldwide work in agriculture. Children harvest tobacco, cocoa, rubber and other global commodities. Children also work in dangerous industries like shipbreaking in Pakistan and Bangladesh, and in services such as construction and restaurant work. However, the U.S.

Government has made a substantial contribution to ending this vicious cycle for tens of millions of children.

What Have We Learned about What Works?

Social mobilization and awareness-raising: Like so many of the world's 'wicked' problems, addressing child labor requires a concerted effort by multiple stakeholders acting together. Work to promote awareness of child labor among citizens and consumers in developed countries, and among families and communities in developing countries where children are at risk, has proven to be an important part of the solution. U.S. Government agencies, in particular the U.S. Department of Labor, have produced important reports documenting the issues thoroughly. Recognizing that raising public awareness also requires compelling photo and video documentation, in the mid-2000s USAID supported the creation of a photo and video repository, in particular to document conditions faced by girls. This material was ultimately turned into a film, Stolen Childhoods. The film documented not only the problem but examples of what interventions could help working children—such as a new USAID-supported schoolhouse in communities of coffee pickers in Kenya, creating opportunities for children who had been working on coffee farms to attend school for the first time.

Another very important part of the solution is *mobilizing communities* and empowering them to work at a grassroots level on practical solutions to address root causes of child labor. For example, through our Global Labor Program, USAID has helped workers in the rubber sector in Liberia to organize, mobilize and negotiate with their employer to end exploitative wage practices that compelled rubber tappers to bring their children to work. In the early 2000s, the problem of child labor on the world's largest rubber plantation in Liberia came to light. Adult tappers were compelled to bring their entire families to work with them just to meet their daily quotas. Following the exposure of this problem, a transnational campaign emerged, linking civil-society organizations and trade unions in Liberia with consumer, labor and human rights groups in the United States. Through USAID's Global Labor Program, the Solidarity Center was able to work directly with rubber workers in Liberia and assist them to organize, join unions and negotiate better wages and working conditions for themselves and their families. Today, thanks to the combination of effective awareness-raising, campaigning in the United States and the work of trade unions in Liberia to negotiate a collective bargaining agreement, there is a school on the rubber plantation where all children attend school while their parents, the adult workers, are paid a living wage.

Businesses are also an important part of the solution to the child labor problem. Awareness-raising campaigns have succeeded in flagging this as a business issue for many companies worldwide in many industries, and those companies and industries are working on innovative new approaches to ensuring their supply chains do not exploit workers. Goodweave is one of the best-known examples of a program effectively addressing child labor in a sector where it was endemic, the carpet-weaving sector in India. Goodweave is a certification system that works with retailers, rug importers and exporters, and looms to ensure that child labor is not used in carpet production. The program is active in the 'carpet belt' of India and Nepal, and recently extended into Afghanistan. The program provides educational transition programs and works with schools to ensure that children that are found working receive the assistance and support they need to go to school. By building awareness about the widespread use of child labor in the rug industry and creating an effective market-based solution, Good-Weave is ending child labor one rug at a time. Since 1995, 11 million child labor free carpets bearing the GoodWeave label have been sold worldwide, and the number of 'carpet kids' has dropped from 1 million to 250,000. GoodWeave's work in Afghanistan is supported by the U.S. Department of Labor.

Finally, *governments* also have a very critical role to play in addressing child labor, through their role in establishing laws and policies to protect children, and equally important, their role in *ensuring that all children have access to basic education.* USAID's Education Strategy is working to increase access to education for all children worldwide, and in particular for children in crisis and conflict environments. To achieve these goals, USAID is committed to working closely with host country governments and civil society to contribute to shared goals. For example, we are supporting a multi-million dollar initiative in Haiti, *Room to Learn*, that is working to provide universal, compulsory access to education in Haiti. USAID works closely with the Government of Haiti to build up the education system and provide safe, equitable education to children. USAID and the Government of Haiti are planning to work together to offer schooling to working children. Last March, USAID Assistant Administrator Eric Postel visited Haiti to set priorities for the design of the program. Postel visited an evening school for working children with former Minister of Education Vanneur Pierre. A study commissioned by the USAID/Haiti's education office estimated more than 24,000 children work as domestic servants. Most of them are teenage girls whose education level is low. The Room to Learn project will work with the Haitian Ministry to offer improved services for these girls.

As we learn more and more about the root causes of child labor, we also are moving further back toward addressing those causes and preventing child labor from taking place at all. We now know that poverty and shocks play a significant role in driving children into work, and also in driving adults into forced and trafficked labor. Development assistance will have a very significant role to play in addressing these issues. With more support for social protection programs that have been proven to play an effective role in helping poor families cope with various types of shocks, we can keep even more children in school and continue to ensure children receive other basic protections.

Support for the World Day grows every year and today we look forward to even wider support from governments, employers' and workers' organizations, NGOs and civil society, international and regional organizations and active citizens worldwide. You can add your voice to the millions worldwide that will celebrate our continued progress toward ending child labor.

Chapter 6

Sexual Exploitation of Children

Sex Trafficking

The Office of Juvenile Justice and Delinquency Prevention (OJJDP) states that "commercial sexual exploitation of children (CSEC) involves crimes of a sexual nature committed against juvenile victims for financial or other economic reasons". Commercial sexual exploitation of children is a both a domestic and international problem. One count estimates sex trafficking to victimize more than 200,000 children in the United States annually. An additional 244,000–360,000 children in the United States are at risk each year of being trafficked and sexually exploited. In the United States, children are most likely to be sexually exploited by their families or family friends for monetary gain. Commercial sexual exploitation manifests in numerous forms, such as brothels, sex trafficking, mail order brides, sex tourism, pornography, prostitution, stripping, lap dancing, and phone sex companies. The most common forms of child commercial sexual exploitation are sex trafficking, child pornography, and child sex tourism. One source

---

This chapter contains text excerpted from the following sources: Text under the heading "Sex Trafficking" is excerpted from "Commercial Sexual Exploitation of Children/Sex Trafficking," Office of Juvenile Justice and Delinquency Prevention (OJJDP), 2015; Text under the heading "The Prostitution of Children" is excerpted from "The Prostitution of Children," U.S. Department of Justice (DOJ), June 3, 2015.

39

estimates a child sex trafficker can make as much as much as $650,000 annually exploiting four children Exact estimates of prevalence and monetary gain, however, vary extensively because true numbers and figures remain unknown due to a lack of awareness about the issue, general underreporting of the crime, and the difficulties associated with identifying victims and perpetrators.

The Prostitution of Children

It is illegal to lure, transport, or obtain a child to engage in prostitution or any illegal sexual activity. Children involved in this form of commercial sexual exploitation are victims. Offenders of this crime, also commonly referred to as traffickers or pimps, recruit, entice, or capture children in order to sell them for sex in exchange for cash, goods, or in– kind favors. Under federal law, the prostitution of children is considered a form of human trafficking, also referred to as sex trafficking. Sex trafficking is a lucrative industry, and criminals traffic children just as they would traffic drugs or other illegal substances. This is a serious crime under federal law, and convicted offenders face serve statutory penalties.

International Sex Trafficking of Minors

One form of sex trafficking involves the cross border transportation of children. In these situations, traffickers recruit and transfer children across international borders in order to sexually exploit them in another country. The traffickers can be individuals working alone, organized crime groups, enterprises, or networks of criminals working together to traffic children into prostitution across country lines.

This form of sex trafficking is a problem in the United States, and recovered victims originate from all over the world, including less-developed areas, such as South and Southeast Asia, Central America, and South America, to more developed areas, such as Western Europe. Once in the United States, a child may be trafficked to any or multiple states within the country. These victims are often trafficked far from home, and thrown into unfamiliar locations and culture. They may be given a false passport or other documentation to conceal their age and true identity. They may also struggle with the English language. All these factors make it extremely difficult for these children to come forward to law enforcement.

In addition, many foreign victims originate from nations that suffer from poverty, turbulent politics and unstable economics. Children from these countries are seen as easy targets by traffickers because they face problems of illiteracy, limited employment opportunities, and bleak financial circumstances in their home country. It is not uncommon for a foreign victim to be coerced by a trafficker under false pretenses. The child is told that a better life or job opportunity awaits them in the United States. However, once in the United States they are introduced into a life of prostitution controlled by traffickers.

Domestic Sex Trafficking of Minors

The United States not only faces a problem of foreign victims trafficked into the country, but there is also a homegrown problem of American children being recruited and exploited for commercial sex. Under federal law, a child does not need to cross international or even state borders to be considered a victim of commercial sexual exploitation, and unfortunately, American children are falling victim to this crime within the United States.

Pimps and traffickers sexually exploit children through street prostitution, and in adult night clubs, illegal brothels, sex parties, motel rooms, hotel rooms, and other locations throughout the United States. Many recovered American victims are street children, a population of runaway or throwaway youth who often come from low income families, and may suffer from physical abuse, sexual abuse and family abandonment issues. This population is seen as an easy target by pimps because the children are generally vulnerable, without dependable guardians, and suffer from low self-esteem. Victims of the prostitution of children, however, come from all backgrounds in terms of class, race, and geography (i.e. urban, suburban, and rural settings).

Often in domestic sex trafficking situations, pimps will make the child victim feel dependent on prostitution for life necessities and survival. For example, a pimp will lure a child with food, clothes, attention, friendship, love, and a seemingly safe place to stay. After cultivating a relationship with a child and engendering a false sense of trust, the pimp will begin engaging the child in prostitution. It is also common for pimps to isolate victims by moving them far away from friends and family, altering their physical appearances, or continuously moving victims to new locations. In many cases, victims become so hardened by the environment in which they must learn to survive that they are incapable of leaving the situation on their own.

Child Victims of Prostitution

The term prostitution can delude or confuse one's understanding of this form of child sexual exploitation. It is important to emphasize that the children involved are victims. Pimps and traffickers manipulate children by using physical, emotional, and psychological abuse to keep them trapped in a life of prostitution. It is not uncommon for traffickers to beat, rape, or torture their victims. Some traffickers also use drugs and alcohol to control them.

Technological advances, in particular the Internet, have facilitated the commercial sexual exploitation of children by providing a convenient worldwide marketing channel. Individuals can now use websites to advertise, schedule, and purchase sexual encounters with minors. The Internet and web-enabled cell phones also allow pimps and traffickers to reach a larger clientele base than in the past, which may expose victims to greater risks and dangers.

In addition, many child victims suffer from physical ailments, including tuberculosis, infections, drug addition, malnutrition, and physical injuries resulting from violence inflicted upon them. Venereal diseases also run rampant. Children may also suffer from short–term and long–term psychological effects such as depression, low self-esteem, and feelings of hopelessness.

Chapter 7

Sibling Abuse

Prevalence of Sibling Abuse

The term "siblings" generally refers to biological brothers and sisters—children who share the same two parents—but in a broader sense it may also refer to any children who are part of a family unit. These include half siblings, who share one common parent, and step siblings, who are not biologically related but who become part of a family as a result of marriage or partnership between their parents. Studies have shown that the risk of sexual abuse is usually more common between step siblings, but accurate statistics are difficult to compile about abuse between related individuals because of the powerful societal taboo against incest, which causes it to go underreported due to embarrassment, fear, denial, or lack of understanding.

Defining Sibling Abuse

When a child is victimized by a sibling, it is termed sibling abuse. Physical aggression—pushing, shoving, or more serious acts of violence—as well as bullying or harassment, are examples of sibling abuse. Unless serious physical harm takes place, parents may ignore this behavior, believing it to be normal childhood activity. But sibling abuse can have severe consequences for survivors, often troubling them well into adulthood.

"Sibling Abuse," © 2016 Omnigraphics, Inc. Reviewed May 2016.

Classification of Sibling Abuse

Sibling abuse is a fairly broad term that can be classified into three types:

- Physical sibling abuse
- Emotional or psychological sibling abuse
- Sexual sibling abuse

Physical sibling abuse. This is a very common form of sibling abuse, as arguments can often lead to physical fighting, pinching, slapping, or hair pulling. These conflicts may become abusive in the course of time and may escalate into violence or serious injury. Weapons, if used, may result in fatal consequences. What begins as sibling rivalry, if not checked, may end up in tragedy within the family. One of the characteristic features of physical sibling abuse is that the perpetrator of the abuse is usually bigger and/or stronger than the victim, although this is not always the case. Physical sibling abuse is not gender- specific, and therefore children of either sex may be the abusers.

Emotional/psychological sibling abuse. Physical sibling abuse is often quite evident, making it somewhat easier to take steps to protect the victim. However, emotional or psychological sibling abuse can be harder to detect. It is also very difficult to measure the impact of this form of sibling abuse. Quarrels between the adults in the family or acts of bullying at school can leave a deep impression upon the young mind. A child may also be emotionally abused by acts like belittling, demeaning, frightening, humiliating, name- calling, or threatening. Survivors of such abuse may become emotionally closed off, withdrawing from social contact and preferring to be alone. They tend to underperform both at school and at home and to become aggressive in other areas of their lives. Identifying emotional abuse early can help head off future problems.

Sexual sibling abuse. Many types of sexual contact or related activity between siblings can be termed sexual sibling abuse. This can include such acts as using sexually toned language, exposing genitals to another sibling, inappropriate touching, deliberate exposure to pornography, and sexual assaults or rape. Sexual sibling abuse can occur between full siblings, half siblings, or step siblings, although it is generally more common in the case of a half sibling or step sibling. The general belief is that boys tend to be the perpetrators, but there are also considerable evidences of girls being abusers.

Physical sibling abuse. This is a very common form of sibling abuse, as arguments can often lead to physical fighting, pinching, slapping, or hair pulling. These conflicts may become abusive in the course of time and may escalate into violence or serious injury. Weapons, if used, may result in fatal consequences. What begins as sibling rivalry, if not checked, may end up in tragedy within the family. One of the characteristic features of physical sibling abuse is that the perpetrator of the abuse is usually bigger and/or stronger than the victim, although this is not always the case. Physical sibling abuse is not gender- specific, and therefore children of either sex may be the abusers.

Emotional/psychological sibling abuse. Physical sibling abuse is often quite evident, making it somewhat easier to take steps to protect the victim. However, emotional or psychological sibling abuse can be harder to detect. It is also very difficult to measure the impact of this form of sibling abuse. Quarrels between the adults in the family or acts of bullying at school can leave a deep impression upon the young mind. A child may also be emotionally abused by acts like belittling, demeaning, frightening, humiliating, name- calling, or threatening. Survivors of such abuse may become emotionally closed off, withdrawing from social contact and preferring to be alone. They tend to underperform both at school and at home and to become aggressive in other areas of their lives. Identifying emotional abuse early can help head off future problems.

Sexual sibling abuse. Many types of sexual contact or related activity between siblings can be termed sexual sibling abuse. This can include such acts as using sexually toned language, exposing genitals to another sibling, inappropriate touching, deliberate exposure to pornography, and sexual assaults or rape. Sexual sibling abuse can occur between full siblings, half siblings, or step siblings, although it is generally more common in the case of a half sibling or step sibling. The general belief is that boys tend to be the perpetrators, but there are also considerable evidences of girls being abusers.

Risk Factors for Sibling Abuse

There are several factors that may be increase the likelihood of sibling abuse, and it vital that parents understand the root cause behind such behavior. Some factors that researchers have identified include:

• Parents away absent from the home for long periods of time

• Lack of emotional attachment between parents and children

- Parents allowing sibling rivalry and fights to go unchecked
- Parents' inability to teach their children to deal with conflicts in a healthy manner.
- Parents not intervening when children are involved in violent acts
- Parents creating a competitive environment by favoritism or frequently comparing siblings to each other
- Denial of the problem's existence, both by parents and children
- Overburdening children by giving responsibilities beyond their ability
- Exposure to violence from different environments, such as home, media, and school
- Parents failing to teach their children about sexuality and their personal safety
- Children who witness to, or are victims of, sexual abuse
- Early access to pornography

Detecting Sibling Abuse

Sibling abuse may often be difficult to detect, especially when both parents are busy with their professional lives. Parents need to be alert to identify this behavior and take necessary action as early as possible. One symptom of sibling abuse is when one child is almost always the aggressor, while the other tends to be the victim. Other signs of sibling abuse include:

- A child avoids his or her sibling
- Noticeable changes in behavior, eating habits, and sleep patterns
- Frequent nightmares
- A child stages abuse staging it in a play or reveals it in a story
- A child acts out in an inappropriate sexual manner
- Increase in the intensity of animosity between the siblings

Safeguarding Children from Sibling Abuse

Some steps that parents can take to help safeguard children from sibling abuse include:

- Discourage rivalry between siblings

- Establish rules that will bar children from indulging in emotional abuse of their siblings, and stick to them so that children realize their importance

- Give responsibilities to children based on their abilities, rather than overburdening them with tasks for which they are unprepared

- Talk to children on a regular basis to gain their trust and encourage them ask to for help from parents when they need it

- Learn the art of mediating conflicts.

- Teach children to that any kind of unwanted physical contact is inappropriate and should be reported to an adult

- Build a healthy environment for sharing and talking about sexual issues.

- Be aware of children's media preferences to identify inappropriate videos, games, music, etc.

Dealing with Sibling Abuse

Acts like biting, hitting, or physical torture of a child by his or her sibling should not be taken lightly. Parents need to intervene and take necessary actions, including:

- Separate the siblings whenever they indulge in any kind of violence

- When the situation is under control, discuss the behavior with all the members of the family, as well as the children involved

- Listen patiently to understand the children's feelings

- Restate what they say to clarify your understanding is concerning the problem

- Encourage the children to work together

- Do not ignore, blame, or punish the child, but take a neutral stand and avoid favoritism

- Be sure the children know the family rules, as well as the consequences of failing to follow them

- Teach the children anger management techniques

- Follow up by observing future behavior carefully

- Seek professional help if the parents feel that things are beyond their control

Sibling Abuse and Its Impact in Later Life

Events or incidents of sibling abuse that take place during childhood may have long-term psychological effects whose impact may not be revealed until a later stage of life. Researchers have found these effects may include:

- Alcohol and drug addiction

- Anxiety

- Depression

- Eating disorders

- Lack of trust

- Low self-esteem

Conclusion

Children who have been victims of sibling abuse tend to have feelings of insecurity and a poor self-image well into adulthood. As much as physical abuse, emotional sibling abuse has a long-lasting impact. And the effects of this behavior do not only affect the victim. The abuser, too, has the potential to indulge in abusive relationships throughout his or her adulthood, making intervention critical for both individuals.

References

1. "Sibling Abuse Help Guide." LeavingAbuse. August 23, 2015.

2. Boyse RN, Kyla. "Sibling Abuse." University of Michigan Health System, November 2012.

Chapter 8

Bullying

What Is Bullying?

Bullying is when a person or a group shows unwanted aggression to another person who is not a sibling or a current dating partner. Cyberbullying (or "electronic aggression") is bullying that is done electronically, including through the Internet, e-mail, or mobile devices, among others.

Bullying can be:

- **Physical**: punching, beating, kicking, or pushing; stealing, hiding, or damaging another person's belongings; forcing someone to do things against his or her will

- **Verbal**: teasing, calling names, or insulting another person; threatening another person with physical harm; spreading rumors or untrue statements about another person

- **Relational**: refusing to talk to someone or making them feel left out; encouraging other individuals to bully someone

To be considered bullying, the behavior in question must be aggressive. The behavior must also involve an imbalance of power (e.g., physical strength, popularity, access to embarrassing details about a person)

This chapter includes text excerpted from "Bullying: Condition Information," National Institute of Child Health and Human Development (NICHD), January 28, 2014.

and be repetitive, meaning that it happens more than once or is highly likely to be repeated.

Bullying also includes cyberbullying and workplace bullying.

- **Cyberbullying** has increased with the increased use of the social media sites, the Internet, e-mail, and mobile devices. Unlike more traditional bullying, cyberbullying can be more anonymous and can occur nearly constantly. A person can be cyberbullied day or night, such as when they are checking their email, using Facebook or another social network site, or even when they are using a mobile phone.

- **Workplace bullying** refers to adult behavior that is repeatedly aggressive and involves the use of power over another person at the workplace. Certain laws apply to adults in the workplace to help prevent such violence.

What Are Common Signs of Being Bullied?

Signs of bullying include:

- Depression, loneliness, or anxiety
- Low self-esteem
- Headaches, stomach aches, tiredness, or poor eating habits
- Missing school, disliking school, or having poorer school performance than previously
- Self-destructive behaviors, such as running away from home or inflicting harm on oneself
- Thinking about suicide or attempting to commit suicide
- Unexplained injuries
- Lost or destroyed clothing, books, electronics, or jewelry
- Difficulty sleeping or frequent nightmares
- Sudden loss of friends or avoidance of social situations

How Does Bullying Affect Health and Well-Being?

Bullying can lead to physical injury, social problems, emotional problems, and even death. Children and adolescents who are bullied are at increased risk for mental health problems, including depression, anxiety, headaches, and problems adjusting to school. Bullying also can cause long-term damage to self-esteem.

Children and adolescents who are bullies are at increased risk for substance use, academic problems, and violence to others later in life.

Children or adolescents who are both bullies and victims suffer the most serious effects of bullying and are at greater risk for mental and behavioral problems than those who are only bullied or who are only bullies.

National Institute of Child Health and Human Development (NICHD) research studies show that anyone involved with bullying—those who bully others, those who are bullied, and those who bully and are bullied—are at increased risk for depression.

NICHD-funded research studies also found that unlike traditional forms of bullying, youth who are bullied electronically—such as by computer or cell phone—are at higher risk for depression than the youth who bully them. Even more surprising, the same studies found that cyber victims were at higher risk for depression than were cyber-bullies or bully-victims (i.e., those who both bully others and are bullied themselves), which was not found in any other form of bullying.

What Are Risk Factors for Being Bullied?

Children who are at risk of being bullied have one or more risk factors:

- Are seen as different from their peers (e.g., overweight, under-weight, wear their hair differently, wear different clothing or wear glasses, or come from a different race/ethnicity)

- Are seen as weak or not able to defend themselves

- Are depressed, anxious, or have low self-esteem

- Have few friends or are less popular

- Do not socialize well with others

- Suffer from an intellectual or developmental disability

What Can Be Done to Help Someone Who Is Being Bullied?

Support a child who is being bullied:

- You can listen to the child and let him or her know you are available to talk or even help. A child who is being bullied may struggle talking about it. Consider letting the child know there are other people who can talk with him or her about bullying.

In addition, you might consider referring the child to a school counselor, psychologist, or other mental health specialist.

- Give the child advice about what he or she can do. You might want to include role-playing and acting out a bullying incident as you guide the child so that the child knows what to do in a real situation.

Follow up with the child to show that you are committed to helping put a stop to the bullying.

Address the bullying behavior:

- Make sure a child whom you suspect or know is bullying knows what the problem behavior is and why it is not acceptable.

Table 8.1. Help for Prevention Against Bullying

The problem	What you can do
A crime has occurred or someone is at immediate risk of harm.	Call 911.
Someone is feeling hopeless, helpless, or thinking of suicide.	Contact the National Suicide Prevention Lifeline online or at 1-800-273-TALK (8255). This toll-free call goes to the nearest crisis center in a national network. These centers provide crisis counseling and mental health referrals.
Someone is acting differently, such as sad or anxious, having trouble completing tasks, or not taking care of themselves.	Find a local counselor or other mental health services.
A child is being bullied in school.	Contact the: Teacher School counselor School coach School principal School superintendent or Board of Education
Child is being bullied after school on the playground or in the neighborhood	Neighborhood watch Playground security Team coach Local precinct/community police
The child's school is not addressing the bullying	Contact the: School superintendent Local Board of Education or State Department of Education

- Show kids that bullying is taken seriously. If you know someone is being a bully to someone else, tell the bully that bullying will not be tolerated. It is important, however, to demonstrate good behavior when speaking with a bully so that you serve as a role model of good interpersonal behavior.

If you feel that you have taken all possible steps to prevent bullying and nothing has worked, or someone is in immediate danger, there are other ways for you to help.

Are There Laws Against Bullying?

Adults and children have the right not to be bullied or harassed by their peers, school staff, co-workers, or other people.

State and local lawmakers have taken steps to prevent bullying. In addition to state laws, federal laws also prohibit bullying. Title IX is a federal law that prohibits discrimination based on sex—including harassment and bullying—in schools that receive federal funding.

There are also laws to protect children from disability harassment, which includes bullying behavior toward persons with disabilities. Disability harassment violates the Individuals with Disabilities Education Act (IDEA). Under the Section 504 and Title II of IDEA, disability harassment in schools is defined as "intimidation or abusive behavior toward a student based on disability that creates a hostile environment by interfering with or denying a student's participation in or receipt of benefits, services, or opportunities in the institution's program. Harassing conduct may take many forms, including verbal acts and name-calling, as well as nonverbal behavior, such as graphic and written statements, or conduct that is physically threatening, harmful, or humiliating."

Are Certain Groups of Children or Adolescents More at Risk for Being Bullied?

Children or adolescents who are at higher risk of being bullied include:

- Those who are, or who are perceived to be, lesbian, gay, bisexual, or transgender
- Those with disabilities or other special needs
- Certain racial, ethnic, or national origin groups
- Certain religious or faith groups

Chapter 9

Long-Term Effects and Consequences of Child Abuse and Neglect

Chapter Contents

Section 9.1

Effects of Child Maltreatment on Brain Development

This section includes text excerpted from "Understanding the Effects of Maltreatment on Brain Development," Child Welfare Information Gateway, U.S. Department of Health and Human Services (HHS), April 2015.

In recent years, there has been a surge of research into early brain development. Neuroimaging technologies, such as magnetic resonance imaging (MRI), provide increased insight about how the brain develops and how early experiences affect that development.

One area that has been receiving increasing research attention involves the effects of abuse and neglect on the developing brain, especially during infancy and early childhood. Much of this research is providing biological explanations for what practitioners have long been describing in psychological, emotional, and behavioral terms. There is now scientific evidence of altered brain functioning as a result of early abuse and neglect. This emerging body of knowledge has many implications for the prevention and treatment of child abuse and neglect.

This section provides basic information on typical brain development and the potential effects of abuse and neglect on that development. The information is designed to help professionals understand the emotional, mental, and behavioral impact of early abuse and neglect in children who come to the attention of the child welfare system.

How the Brain Develops

What we have learned about the process of brain development helps us understand more about the roles both genetics and the environment play in our development. It appears that genetics predispose us to develop in certain ways, but our experiences, including our interactions with other people, have a significant impact on how our predispositions are expressed. In fact, research now shows that many capacities thought to be fixed at birth are actually dependent on a sequence of experiences combined with heredity. Both factors are essential for optimum development of the human brain.

Early Brain Development

The raw material of the brain is the nerve cell, called the neuron. During fetal development, neurons are created and migrate to form the various parts of the brain. As neurons migrate, they also differentiate, or specialize, to govern specific functions in the body in response to chemical signals. This process of development occurs sequentially from the "bottom up," that is, from areas of the brain controlling the most primitive functions of the body (e.g., heart rate, breathing) to the most sophisticated functions (e.g., complex thought). The first areas of the brain to fully develop are the brainstem and midbrain; they govern the bodily functions necessary for life, called the autonomic functions. At birth, these lower portions of the nervous system are very well developed, whereas the higher regions (the limbic system and cerebral cortex) are still rather primitive. Higher function brain regions involved in regulating emotions, language, and abstract thought grow rapidly in the first 3 years of life.

The Growing Child's Brain

Brain development, or learning, is actually the process of creating, strengthening, and discarding connections among the neurons; these connections are called synapses. Synapses organize the brain by forming pathways that connect the parts of the brain governing everything we do—from breathing and sleeping to thinking and feeling. This is the essence of postnatal brain development, because at birth, very few synapses have been formed. The synapses present at birth are primarily those that govern our bodily functions such as heart rate, breathing, eating, and sleeping.

The development of synapses occurs at an astounding rate during a child's early years in response to that child's experiences. At its peak, the cerebral cortex of a healthy toddler may create 2 million synapses per second. By the time children are 2 years old, their brains have approximately 100 trillion synapses, many more than they will ever need. Based on the child's experiences, some synapses are strengthened and remain intact, but many are gradually discarded. This process of synapse elimination—or pruning—is a normal part of development. By the time children reach adolescence, about half of their synapses have been discarded, leaving the number they will have for most of the rest of their lives.

Another important process that takes place in the developing brain is myelination. Myelin is the white fatty tissue that forms a sheath to insulate mature brain cells, thus ensuring clear transmission of neurotransmitters across synapses. Young children process information slowly because their brain cells lack the myelin necessary for fast, clear nerve impulse transmission. Like other neuronal growth processes, myelination begins in the primary motor and sensory areas (the brain stem and cortex) and gradually progresses to the higher-order regions that control thought, memories, and feelings. Also, like other neuronal growth processes, a child's experiences affect the rate and growth of myelination, which continues into young adulthood.

By 3 years of age, a baby's brain has reached almost 90 percent of its adult size. The growth in each region of the brain largely depends on receiving stimulation, which spurs activity in that region. This stimulation provides the foundation for learning.

Adolescent Brain Development

Studies using MRI techniques show that the brain continues to grow and develop into young adulthood (at least to the mid twenties). White matter, or brain tissue, volume has been shown to increase in adults as old as 32. Right before puberty, adolescent brains experience a growth spurt that occurs mainly in the frontal lobe, which is the area that governs planning, impulse control, and reasoning. During the teenage years, the brain goes through a process of pruning synapses—somewhat like the infant and toddler brain— and also sees an increase in white matter and changes to neurotransmitter systems. As the teenager grows into young adulthood, the brain develops more myelin to insulate the nerve fibers and speed neural processing, and this myelination occurs last in the frontal lobe. MRI comparisons between the brains of teenagers and the brains of young adults have shown that most of the brain areas were the same—that is, the teenage brain had reached maturity in the areas that govern such abilities as speech and sensory capabilities. The major difference was the immaturity of the teenage brain in the frontal lobe and in the myelination of that area.

Normal puberty and adolescence lead to the maturation of a physical body, but the brain lags behind in development, especially in the areas that allow teenagers to reason and think logically. Most teenagers act impulsively at times, using a lower area of their brains— their "gut reaction"—because their frontal lobes are not yet mature.

Impulsive behavior, poor decisions, and increased risk-taking are all part of the normal teenage experience. Another change that happens during adolescence is the growth and transformation of the limbic system, which is responsible for our emotions. Teenagers may rely on their more primitive limbic system in interpreting emotions and reacting since they lack the more mature cortex that can override the limbic response.

Plasticity—The Influence of Environment

Researchers use the term plasticity to describe the brain's ability to change in response to repeated stimulation. The extent of a brain's plasticity is dependent on the stage of development and the particular brain system or region affected. For instance, the lower parts of the brain, which control basic functions such as breathing and heart rate, are less flexible, or plastic, than the higher functioning cortex, which controls thoughts and feelings. While cortex plasticity decreases as a child gets older, some degree of plasticity remains. In fact, this brain plasticity is what allows us to keep learning into adulthood and throughout our lives. The developing brain's ongoing adaptations are the result of both genetics and experience. Our brains prepare us to expect certain experiences by forming the pathways needed to respond to those experiences. For example, our brains are "wired" to respond to the sound of speech; when babies hear people speaking, the neural systems in their brains responsible for speech and language receive the necessary stimulation to organize and function. The more babies are exposed to people speaking, the stronger their related synapses become. If the appropriate exposure does not happen, the pathways developed in anticipation may be discarded. This is sometimes referred to as the concept of "use it or lose it." It is through these processes of creating, strengthening, and discarding synapses that our brains adapt to our unique environment.

The ability to adapt to our environment is a part of normal development. Children growing up in cold climates, on rural farms, or in large sibling groups learn how to function in those environments. Regardless of the general environment, though, all children need stimulation and nurturance for healthy development. If these are lacking (e.g., if a child's caretakers are indifferent, hostile, depressed, or cognitively impaired), the child's brain development may be impaired. Because the brain adapts to its environment, it will adapt to a negative environment just as readily as it will adapt to a positive one.

59

Sensitive Periods

Researchers believe that there are sensitive periods for development of certain capabilities. These refer to windows of time in the developmental process when certain parts of the brain may be most susceptible to particular experiences. Animal studies have shed light on sensitive periods, showing, for example, that animals that are artificially blinded during the sensitive period for developing vision may never develop the capability to see, even if the blinding mechanism is later removed.

It is more difficult to study human sensitive periods, but we know that, if certain synapses and neuronal pathways are not repeatedly activated, they may be discarded, and their capabilities may diminish. For example, infants have a genetic predisposition to form strong attachments to their primary caregivers, but they may not be able to achieve strong attachments, or trusting, durable bonds if they are in a severely neglectful situation with little one-on-one caregiver contact. Children from Romanian institutions who had been severely neglected had a much better attachment response if they were placed in foster care—and thus received more stable parenting—before they were 24 months old. This indicates that there is a sensitive period for attachment, but it is likely that there is a general sensitive period rather than a true cut-off point for recovery.

While sensitive periods exist for development and learning, we also know that the plasticity of the brain often allows children to recover from missing certain experiences. Both children and adults may be able to make up for missed experiences later in life, but it is likely to be more difficult. This is especially true if a young child was deprived of certain stimulation, which resulted in the pruning of synapses (neuronal connections) relevant to that stimulation and the loss of neuronal pathways. As children progress through each developmental stage, they will learn and master each step more easily if their brains have built an efficient network of pathways to support optimal functioning.

Memories

The organizing framework for children's development is based on the creation of memories. When repeated experiences strengthen a neuronal pathway, the pathway becomes encoded, and it eventually becomes a memory. Children learn to put one foot in front of the other to walk. They learn words to express themselves. And they learn that a smile usually brings a smile in return. At some point, they no longer have to think much about these processes—their brains manage these experiences with little effort because the memories that have been created allow for a smooth, efficient flow of information.

The creation of memories is part of our adaptation to our environment. Our brains attempt to understand the world around us and fashion our interactions with that world in a way that promotes our survival and, hopefully, our growth, but if the early environment is abusive or neglectful, our brains may create memories of these experiences that adversely color our view of the world throughout our life.

Babies are born with the capacity for implicit memory, which means that they can perceive their environment and recall it in certain unconscious ways. For instance, they recognize their mother's voice from an unconscious memory. These early implicit memories may have a significant impact on a child's subsequent attachment relationships.

In contrast, explicit memory, which develops around age 2, refers to conscious memories and is tied to language development. Explicit memory allows children to talk about themselves in the past and future or in different places or circumstances through the process of conscious recollection.

Sometimes, children who have been abused or suffered other trauma may not retain or be able to access explicit memories of their experiences; however, they may retain implicit memories of the physical or emotional sensations, and these implicit memories may produce flashbacks, nightmares, or other uncontrollable reactions. This may be the case with very young children or infants who suffer abuse or neglect.

Responding to Stress

We all experience different types of stress throughout our lives. The type of stress and the timing of that stress determine whether and how there is an impact on the brain. The National Scientific Council on the Developing Child outlines three classifications of stress:

1. **Positive stress** is moderate, brief, and generally a normal part of life (e.g., entering a new child care setting). Learning to adjust to this type of stress is an essential component of healthy development.

2. **Tolerable stress** includes events that have the potential to alter the developing brain negatively, but which occur infrequently and give the brain time to recover (e.g., the death of a loved one).

3. **Toxic stress** includes strong, frequent, and prolonged activation of the body's stress response system (e.g., chronic neglect).

Healthy responses to typical life stressors (i.e., positive and tolerable stress events) are very complex and may change depending on individual and environmental characteristics, such as genetics, the presence of a sensitive and responsive caregiver, and past experiences. A healthy stress response involves a variety of hormone and neurochemical systems throughout the body, including the sympathetic-adrenomedullary (SAM) system, which produces adrenaline, and the hypothalamic-pituitary-adrenocortical (HPA) system, which produces cortisol. Increases in adrenaline help the body engage energy stores and alter blood flow. Increases in cortisol also help the body engage energy stores and also can enhance certain types of memory and activate immune responses. In a healthy stress response, the hormonal levels will return to normal after the stressful experience has passed.

Effects of Maltreatment on Brain Development

Just as positive experiences can assist with healthy brain development, children's experiences with child maltreatment or other forms of toxic stress, such as domestic violence or disasters, can negatively affect brain development. This includes changes to the structure and chemical activity of the brain (e.g., decreased size or connectivity in some parts of the brain) and in the emotional and behavioral functioning of the child (e.g., over-sensitivity to stressful situations). For example, healthy brain development includes situations in which babies' babbles, gestures, or cries bring reliable, appropriate reactions from their caregivers. These caregiver-child interactions—sometimes referred to as "serve and return"—strengthen babies' neuronal pathways regarding social interactions and how to get their needs met, both physically and emotionally. If children live in a chaotic or threatening world, one in which their caregivers respond with abuse or chronically provide no response, their brains may become hyperalert for danger or not fully develop. These neuronal pathways that are developed and strengthened under negative conditions prepare children to cope in that negative environment, and their ability to respond to nurturing and kindness may be impaired.

The specific effects of maltreatment may depend on such factors as the age of the child at the time of the maltreatment, whether the maltreatment was a one-time incident or chronic, the identity of the abuser (e.g., parent or other adult), whether the child had a dependable nurturing individual in his or her life, the type and severity of the maltreatment, the intervention, how long the maltreatment lasted, and other individual and environmental characteristics.

Effects of Maltreatment on Brain Structure and Activity Toxic stress, including child maltreatment, can have a variety of negative effects on children's brains:

- **Hippocampus**: Adults who were maltreated may have reduced volume in the hippocampus, which is central to learning and memory. Toxic stress also can reduce the hippocampus's capacity to bring cortisol levels back to normal after a stressful event has occurred.

- **Corpus callosum**: Maltreated children and adolescents tend to have decreased volume in the corpus callosum, which is the largest white matter structure in the brain and is responsible for interhemispheric communication and other processes (e.g., arousal, emotion, higher cognitive abilities).

- **Cerebellum**: Maltreated children and adolescents tend to have decreased volume in the cerebellum, which helps coordinate motor behavior and executive functioning.

- **Prefrontal cortex**: Some studies on adolescents and adults who were severely neglected as children indicate they have a smaller prefrontal cortex, which is critical to behavior, cognition, and emotion regulation, but other studies show no differences. Physically abused children also may have reduced volume in the orbitofrontal cortex, a part of the prefrontal cortex that is central to emotion and social regulation.

- **Amygdala**: Although most studies have found that amygdala volume is not affected by maltreatment, abuse and neglect can cause overactivity in that area of the brain, which helps determine whether a stimulus is threatening and trigger emotional responses.

- **Cortisol levels**: Many maltreated children, both in institutional and family settings, and especially those who experienced severe neglect, tend to have lower than normal morning cortisol levels coupled with flatter release levels throughout the day. (Typically, children have a sharp increase in cortisol in the morning followed by a steady decrease throughout the day.) On the other hand, children in foster care who experienced severe emotional maltreatment had higher than normal morning cortisol levels.

These results may be due to the body reacting differently to different stressors. Abnormal cortisol levels can have many negative effects. Lower cortisol levels can lead to decreased energy resources, which could affect learning and socialization; externalizing disorders; and increased vulnerability to autoimmune disorders. Higher cortisol levels could harm cognitive processes, subdue immune and inflammatory reactions, or heighten the risk for affective disorders.

- **Other**: Children who experienced severe neglect early in life while in institutional settings often have decreased electrical activity in their brains, decreased brain metabolism, and poorer connections between areas of the brain that are key to integrating complex information. These children also may continue to have abnormal patterns of adrenaline activity years after being adopted from institutional settings. Additionally, malnutrition, a form of neglect, can impair both brain development (e.g., slowing the growth of neurons, axons, and synapses) and function (e.g., neurotransmitter syntheses, the maintenance of brain tissue).

- We also know that some cases of physical abuse can cause immediate direct structural damage to a child's brain. For example, according to the National Center on Shaken Baby Syndrome (n.d.), shaking a child can destroy brain tissue and tear blood vessels. In the short term, this can lead to seizures, loss of consciousness, or even death. In the long-term, shaking can damage the fragile brain so that a child develops a range of sensory

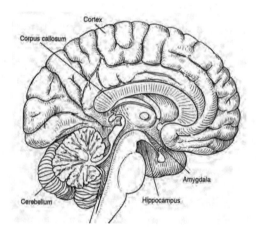

Figure 9.1. *Brain*

impairments, as well as cognitive, learning, and behavioral disabilities. Other types of head injuries caused by physical abuse can have similar effects.

Effects of Maltreatment on Behavioral, Social, and Emotional Functioning

The changes in brain structure and chemical activity caused by child maltreatment can have a wide variety of effects on children's behavioral, social, and emotional functioning.

Persistent Fear Response. Chronic stress or repeated trauma can result in a number of biological reactions, including a persistent fear state. Chronic activation of the neuronal pathways involved in the fear response can create permanent memories that shape the child's perception of and response to the environment. While this adaptation may be necessary for survival in a hostile world, it can become a way of life that is difficult to change, even if the environment improves. Children with a persistent fear response may lose their ability to differentiate between danger and safety, and they may identify a threat in a nonthreatening situation. For example, a child who has been maltreated may associate the fear caused by a specific person or place with similar people or places that pose no threat. This generalized fear response may be the foundation of future anxiety disorders, such as PTSD.

Hyperarousal. When children are exposed to chronic, traumatic stress, their brains sensitize the pathways for the fear response and create memories that automatically trigger that response without conscious thought. This is called hyperarousal. These children may be highly sensitive to nonverbal cues, such as eye contact or a touch on the arm, and they may be more likely to misinterpret them. Consumed with a need to monitor nonverbal cues for threats, their brains are less able to interpret and respond to verbal cues, even when they are in an environment typically considered nonthreatening, like a classroom. While these children are often labeled as learning disabled, the reality is that their brains have developed so that they are constantly on alert and are unable to achieve the relative calm necessary for learning.

Increased Internalizing Symptoms. Child maltreatment can lead to structural and chemical changes in the areas of the brain involved in emotion and stress regulation. For example, maltreatment can affect connectivity between the amygdala and hippocampus, which can then initiate the development of anxiety and depression by late adolescence. Additionally, early emotional abuse or severe deprivation may permanently alter the brain's ability to use serotonin, a neurotransmitter that helps produce feelings of well-being and emotional stability.

Diminished Executive Functioning. Executive functioning generally includes three components: working memory (being able to keep and use information over a short period of time), inhibitory control (filtering thoughts and impulses), and cognitive or mental flexibility (adjusting to changed demands, priorities, or perspectives). The structural and neurochemical damage caused by maltreatment can create deficits in all areas of executive functioning, even at an early age. Executive functioning skills help people achieve academic and career success, bolster social interactions, and assist in everyday activities. The brain alterations caused by a toxic stress response can result in lower academic achievement, intellectual impairment, decreased IQ, and weakened ability to maintain attention.

Delayed Developmental Milestones. Although neglect often is thought of as a failure to meet a child's physical needs for food, shelter, and safety, neglect also can be a failure to meet a child's cognitive, emotional, or social needs. For children to master developmental tasks in these areas, they need opportunities and encouragement from their caregivers. If this stimulation is lacking during children's early years, the weak neuronal pathways that developed in expectation of these experiences may wither and die, and the children may not achieve the usual developmental milestones. For example, babies need to experience face-to-face baby talk and hear countless repetitions of sounds in order to build the brain circuitry that will enable them to start making sounds and eventually say words. If babies' sounds are ignored repeatedly when they begin to babble at around 6 months, their language may be delayed. In fact, neglected children often do not show the rapid growth that normally occurs in language development at 18–24 months. These types of delays may extend to all types of normal development for neglected children, including their cognitive-behavioral, socio-emotional, and physical development.

Weakened Response to Positive Feedback. Children who have been maltreated may be less responsive to positive stimuli than non-maltreated children. A study of young adults who had been maltreated found that they rated monetary rewards less positively than their peers and demonstrated a weaker response to reward cues in the basal ganglia areas of the brain responsible for reward processing.

Complicated Social Interactions. Toxic stress can alter brain development in ways that make interaction with others more difficult. Children or youth with toxic stress may find it more challenging to navigate social situations and adapt to changing social contexts. They may perceive threats in safe situations more frequently and react accordingly, and they may have more difficulty interacting with others. For example, a maltreated child may misinterpret a peer's neutral facial expression as anger, which may cause the maltreated child to become aggressive or overly defensive toward the peer.

Implications for Practice and Policy

The knowledge we gained from research examining the effects of maltreatment on brain development can be helpful in many ways. With this information we are better able to understand what is happening within the brains of children who have been abused and neglected. In fact, much of this research is providing concrete/scientific evidence for what professionals and caregivers have long described in behavioral, emotional, and psychological terms. We also now know that children who were reared in severely stressful environments can see positive effects on brain development and functioning when their living environments improve. For example, children who lived in Romanian institutions and then moved into foster care settings had larger total volumes in cortical white matter and the posterior corpus callosum than children who remained in institutional care (though these volumes were smaller than never-institutionalized children). We can use this information to improve our systems of care and to strengthen our prevention efforts.

The Role of the Child Welfare System

While the goal of the child welfare system is to protect children, many child welfare interventions—such as investigation, appearance in court, removal from home, placement in a foster home, etc.—may actually reinforce the child's view that the world is unknown, uncontrollable, and frightening. A number of trends in child welfare may help provide a more caring view of the world to an abused or neglected child. These trends include:

- Trauma-informed care

- Family-centered practice and case planning, including parent-child interaction therapy Individualized services for children and families

- The growth of child advocacy centers, where children can be interviewed and assessed and receive services in a child-friendly environment

- The use of differential response to ensure children's safety while providing nonadversarial support to families in low-risk cases

- The promotion of evidence-based practices

Prevention. Child welfare systems that devote significant efforts to prevention may be the most successful in helping children and families and promoting healthy brain development. By the time a child who has been abused or neglected comes to the attention of professionals, some negative effects are likely. Prevention efforts should focus on supporting and strengthening children's families so that children have the best chance of remaining safely in their homes and communities while receiving proper nurturing and care. These efforts may target the general population ("primary" or "universal" prevention) by educating the public and changing policies to promote healthy brain development. Prevention efforts also may target children and families considered to be at-risk of developing problems ("secondary" or "selected" prevention).

Prevention efforts for at-risk families should focus on strengthening the family and building on the family's positive attributes. Recent prevention resource guides from the HHS Children's Bureau encourage professionals to promote six "protective factors" that can strengthen families, help prevent abuse and neglect, and promote healthy brain development:

- Nurturing and attachment
- Knowledge of parenting and of child and youth development
- Parental resilience
- Social connections
- Concrete supports for parents
- Social and emotional competence for children

Brain research underscores the importance of prevention efforts that target the youngest children. For example, early childhood home visiting programs for expectant and new mothers, who might be at-risk because of their age, income, or other circumstances, show promise for mitigating maternal stress, thus keeping adversity from becoming toxic stress. Parent education programs also serve as a prevention method that can promote protective factors and lead to positive outcomes for both parents and children. The Centers for Disease Control and Prevention (CDC) developed the Essentials for Childhood Framework to help communities prevent child maltreatment. This framework is based on establishing safe, stable, and nurturing relationships between children and caregivers.

Early Intervention. Intensive, early interventions when the brain is most plastic are much more effective than reactive services as the child ages. In recognition of this fact, Federal legislation requires States to develop referral procedures for children ages 0–36 months who are involved in a substantiated case of child abuse or neglect. Once a child is identified, States must provide intervention services through Early Intervention Plans funded under Part C of the Individuals with Disabilities Education Improvement Act. A number of States developed innovative programs to meet these requirements and to identify and help the youngest victims of abuse and neglect.

One theory about healing a damaged or altered brain is that the interventions must target those portions of the brain that have been altered. Because brain functioning is altered by repeated experiences that strengthen and sensitize neuronal pathways, interventions should not be limited to weekly therapy appointments. Interventions should address the totality of the child's life, providing frequent, consistent replacement experiences so that the child's brain can begin to incorporate a new environment—one that is safe, predictable, and nurturing.

The following are examples of models and interventions available to child welfare and related professionals to assist children and youth who have been maltreated or otherwise exposed to toxic stress:

- **The neurosequential model of therapeutics (NMT)** is based on the fact that the higher brain functions (e.g., speech, relational interactions) depend on input from lower brain functions (e.g., stress responses). Many clinical interventions, however, focus on the higher brain functions rather than the lower brain functions, which may be the source of the child's issues. NMT has three central elements: a developmental history that helps delineate the timing, nature, and severity of developmental challenges; a current assessment of functioning to help determine which neural systems and brain areas are affected and what the developmental level of the child is in various areas (e.g., speech, social skills); and specific recommendations for the interventions to be used, with a focus on the sequence of the interventions (i.e., focusing on deficits in the lower brain first and progressing to the higher brain functions).

- **The Attachment and Biobehavioral Catch-up (ABC)** for Infants and Young Children intervention is designed for the parents of young children who have experienced early adversity. ABC is implemented during 10 sessions in the parents' homes and includes both the parents and children. The sessions focus on providing clear feedback to parents about nurturance and following their child's lead, and include the review of video clips of interactions between the parents and child. A study of ABC found that children who received the intervention showed a steeper slope of cortisol production and higher wake-up cortisol values (i.e., healthier cortisol levels) than nonintervention children. These effects were still seen even at 3 years after the intervention.

- **Multidimensional Treatment Foster Care for Preschoolers (MTFC-P)**, which typically lasts 9 to 12 months, helps parents learn and practice behavior management techniques. This helps children experience a more controlled and stable environment, which, in turn, helps enhance their regulatory capabilities. Foster parents are trained prior to placement, and program staff are available 24 hours a day to provide support. A support group is available, too. Children also participate in a weekly therapeutic playgroup to practice self-regulatory skills. If children will be returning to their birth families, MTFC-P staff provide training to the birth parents as well. Similar to the ABC intervention, children receiving MTFC-P had more stable cortisol levels than those who did not receive MTFC-P. Children's recovery depends on a variety of factors, including the timing, severity, and duration of the maltreatment or other toxic stress, the intervention itself, and the individual child's response to the maltreatment.

In some cases, doctors may prescribe psychotropic medications for certain mental health conditions, such as depression or anxiety. The Children's Bureau developed a guide, *Making Healthy Choices: A Guide on Psychotropic Medications for Youth in Foster Care,* to help adolescents better understand their options.

The Role of Caregivers

Many children who suffered abuse and neglect are removed from their homes (for their safety) by the child welfare system. Extended family, foster parents, or group home staff may temporarily care for these children, and some will be adopted. In these cases, educating caregivers about the possible effects of maltreatment on brain development, and the resulting symptoms, may help them to better understand and support the children in their care. Child welfare workers may also want to explore any past abuse or trauma experienced by parents that may influence their parenting skills and behaviors.

It is important for caregivers to have realistic expectations for their children. Children who have been abused or neglected may not be functioning at their chronological age in terms of their physical, social, emotional, and cognitive skills. They may also be displaying unusual and/or difficult coping behaviors. For example, abused or neglected children may:

- Be unable to control their emotions and have frequent outbursts

- Be quiet and submissive

- Have difficulties learning in school

- Have difficulties getting along with siblings or classmates

- Have unusual eating or sleeping behaviors

- Attempt to provoke fights or solicit sexual experiences

- Be socially or emotionally inappropriate for their age

- Be unresponsive to affection

Understanding some basic information about the neurobiology underlying many challenging behaviors may help caregivers shape their responses more effectively. They also need to know as much as possible about the particular circumstances and background of the individual children in their care.

In general, children who have been abused or neglected need nurturance, stability, predictability, understanding, and support. They may need frequent, repeated experiences of these kinds to begin altering their view of the world from one that is uncaring or hostile to one that is caring and supportive. Until that view begins to take hold in a child's mind, the child may not be able to engage in a truly positive relationship, and the longer a child lives in an abusive or neglectful environment, the harder it will be to convince the child's brain that the world can change. Consistent nurturing from caregivers who receive training and support may offer the best hope for the children who need it most.

Section 9.2

Child Abuse Leaves Epigenetic Marks

This section includes text excerpted from "Child Abuse Leaves Epigenetic Marks," National Human Genome Research Institute (NHGRI), July 3, 2013.

Child abuse is a serious national and global problem that cuts across economic, racial and cultural lines. Each year, more than 1.25 million children are abused or neglected in the United States, with that number expanding to at least 40 million per year worldwide.

In addition to harming the immediate well being of the child, maltreatment and extreme stress during childhood can impair early brain development and metabolic and immune system function, leading to chronic health problems. As a consequence, abused children are at increased risk for a wide range of physical health conditions including obesity, heart disease, and cancer, as well as psychiatric conditions such as depression, suicide, drug and alcohol abuse, high-risk behaviors and violence.

They are also more susceptible to developing posttraumatic stress disorder (PTSD) a severe and debilitating stress-related psychiatric disorder-after experiencing other types of trauma later in life.

Part of the explanation is that child abuse can leave marks, not only physically and emotionally, but also in the form of epigenetic marks on a child's genes. Although these *epigenetic marks* do not cause mutations in the DNA itself, the chemical modifications-including DNA methylation-change gene expression by silencing (or activating) genes. This can alter fundamental biological processes and adversely affect health outcomes throughout life.

New research, published in the May 14, 2013, issue of the *Proceedings for the National Academy of Sciences*, shows that PTSD patients

72

who were abused as children have different patterns of DNA methylation and gene expression compared to those who were not.

Researchers from the Max Planck Institute in Germany and Emory University in the United States investigated whether the timing of trauma, specifically childhood abuse early in life, had an effect on the underlying biology of PTSD at the genome-wide level. To address this question, the authors examined a subset of 169 participants from the Grady Trauma Project-a survey of more than 5,000 individuals in Atlanta with a high lifetime exposure to multiple types of trauma, violence and abuse.

Among the 169 participants in the current study, most were African Americans in their late thirties and forties, and all had suffered from at least two types of trauma other than child abuse and seven types of trauma on average. In spite of multiple trauma exposure, the majority (108 people) did not develop PTSD. Of the 61 that did, however, 32 reported a history of childhood abuse and 29 did not.

To focus on the effect of childhood abuse in PTSD, the researchers examined genetic changes in peripheral blood cells from PTSD patients with and without previous exposure to childhood maltreatment. These were then compared to the trauma-exposed group that did not develop PTSD to rule out changes associated with trauma exposure alone.

Despite sharing a few common biological pathways, 98 percent of the changes in gene expression patterns in PTSD patients with childhood abuse did not overlap with those found in PTSD patients without childhood abuse. Interestingly, PTSD patients who experienced significant abuse as children exhibited more changes in genes associated with central nervous system development and immune system regulation, whereas those without a history of childhood abuse displayed more changes in genes associated with cell death and growth rate regulation.

Furthermore, the researchers found that epigenetic marks associated with gene expression changes were up to 12-fold higher in PTSD patients with a history of childhood abuse. This suggests that although all patients with PTSD may show similar symptoms, abused children who subsequently develop PTSD may experience a systematically and biologically different form of the disorder compared to those without childhood abuse.

What this means is that we may need to rethink our classification of PTSD and the notion of providing the same treatment for all PTSD patients, said Dr. Divya Mehta, corresponding author at the Max Planck Institute of Psychiatry.

"At the biological level, these individuals may be very distinct, as we see with the epigenetics," Dr. Mehta explained. "As we move forward with more personalized medicine, we will need to delve a bit further into the environment and history of each individual to understand the biology of their PTSD and to determine the best treatment for their disorder."

Although, it is currently unclear whether the epigenetic marks left by child abuse can be removed or the damage reversed, this discovery is important in the search for biomarkers with clinical indications that can be used to identify different forms of PTSD. This will help to direct more precise avenues for therapy and guide treatments tailored specifically to the biological process of individual patients.

By starting to distinguish subtypes of PTSD, this study highlights the multi-factorial nature of psychiatric disorders triggered by a combination of environmental and genetic factors. As the next step, Dr. Mehta and her team plan to study whether the age at which abuse occurs or the type of abuse affects the biology of PTSD.

Since even small changes in DNA methylation signatures in child abuse can have long-term implications for fundamental biological processes and health, Dr. Mehta hopes their research will also increase public awareness and strengthen efforts to protect children from the consequences of childhood abuse and neglect.

Section 9.3

Child Abuse – A National Burden

This section includes text excerpted from "Child Maltreatment: Consequences," Centers for Disease Control and Prevention (CDC), January 14, 2014.

Child Maltreatment: Consequences

Child maltreatment affects children's health now and later, and costs our country as much as other high profile public health problems. Neglect, physical abuse, custodial interference and sexual abuse are types of child maltreatment that can lead to poor physical and mental health well into adulthood. The physical, psychological, behavioral and economic consequences of child maltreatment are explained below.

Prevalence: About 14% of Children Suffer

- An estimated 681,000 children were confirmed by Child Protective Services as being victims of maltreatment in 2011.

- A cross-sectional, U.S. national telephone survey of the child maltreatment experiences of 4,503 children and youth aged 1 month to 17 years in 2011 found that 13.8% experienced child maltreatment in the last year (included neglect, physical abuse, emotional abuse, custodial interference, or sexual abuse by a known adult).

Physical

- In 2011, approximately 1,570 children died from abuse and neglect across the country—a rate of 2.10 deaths per 100,000 children.

- Maltreatment during infancy or early childhood can cause important regions of the brain to form and function improperly with long-term consequences on cognitive, language, and socioemotional development, and mental health. For example, the stress of chronic abuse may cause a "hyperarousal" response in certain areas of the brain, which may result in hyperactivity and sleep disturbances.

- Children may experience severe or fatal head trauma as a result of abuse. Nonfatal consequences of abusive head trauma include varying degrees of visual impairment (e.g., blindness), motor impairment (e.g., cerebral palsy) and cognitive impairments.

- Children who experience maltreatment are also at increased risk for adverse health effects and certain chronic diseases as adults, including heart disease, cancer, chronic lung disease, liver disease, obesity, high blood pressure, high cholesterol, and high levels of C-reactive protein.

Psychological

- In one long-term study, as many as 80 percent of young adults who had been abused met the diagnostic criteria for at least one psychiatric disorder at age 21. These young adults exhibited many problems, including depression, anxiety, eating disorders, and suicide attempts.

- In addition to physical and developmental problems, the stress of chronic abuse may result in anxiety and may make victims more vulnerable to problems such as posttraumatic stress disorder, conduct disorder, and learning, attention, and memory difficulties.

Behavioral

- Children who experience maltreatment are at increased risk for smoking, alcoholism, and drug abuse as adults, as well as engaging in high-risk sexual behaviors.

- Those with a history of child abuse and neglect are 1.5 times more likely to use illicit drugs, especially marijuana, in middle adulthood.

- Studies have found abused and neglected children to be at least 25 percent more likely to experience problems such as delinquency, teen pregnancy, and low academic achievement. Similarly, a longitudinal study found that physically abused children were at greater risk of being arrested as juveniles. This same study also found that abused youth were less likely to have graduated from high school and more likely to have been a teen parent. A National Institute of Justice study indicated that being abused or neglected as a child increased the likelihood of arrest as a juvenile by 59 percent. Abuse and neglect also increased the likelihood of adult criminal behavior by 28 percent and violent crime by 30 percent.

- Early child maltreatment can have a negative effect on the ability of both men and women to establish and maintain healthy intimate relationships in adulthood.

Economic Consequences

- The total lifetime economic burden resulting from new cases of fatal and nonfatal child maltreatment in the United States in 2008 is approximately $124 billion in 2010 dollars. This economic burden rivals the cost of other high profile public health problems, such as stroke and Type 2 diabetes.

- The estimated average lifetime cost per victim of nonfatal child maltreatment is $210,012 including:
  - childhood health care costs

- adult medical costs

- productivity losses

- child welfare costs

- criminal justice costs

- special education costs

- The estimated average lifetime cost per death is $1,272,900, including medical costs and productivity losses.

- Research suggests the benefits of effective prevention likely outweigh the costs of child maltreatment.

Most of the studies examining the consequences of child maltreatment have used a retrospective approach. This requires conducting studies to determine if any association exists between a history of childhood abuse and/or neglect and current health conditions in adults. Fewer research projects have employed a more rigorous longitudinal approach. This type of research strategy identifies children who are at risk or who have already been maltreated and follows them for a long period of time, sometimes decades, to see what conditions develop.

Part Two

Physical and Sexual Abuse of Children

Chapter 10

Physical Abuse of Children

Chapter Contents

Section 10.1

Recognizing Physical Abuse in Children

This section includes text excerpted from "What Is Child Abuse and Neglect? Recognizing the Signs and Symptoms," Child Welfare Information Gateway, U.S. Department of Health and Human Services (HHS), July 2013.

Recognizing Signs of Abuse and Neglect

In addition to working to prevent a child from experiencing abuse or neglect, it is important to recognize high-risk situations and the signs and symptoms of maltreatment. If you do suspect a child is being harmed, reporting your suspicions may protect him or her and get help for the family. Any concerned person can report suspicions of child abuse or neglect. Reporting your concerns is not making an accusation; rather, it is a request for an investigation and assessment to determine if help is needed.

Some people (typically certain types of professionals, such as teachers or physicians) are required by State law to make a report of child maltreatment under specific circumstances—these are called mandatory reporters. Some States require all adults to report suspicions of child abuse or neglect.

For information about where and how to file a report, contact your local child protective services agency or police department. Childhelp National Child Abuse Hotline (1-800-4-A-CHILD (1-800-422-4453)) and its website offer crisis intervention, information, resources, and referrals to support services and provide assistance in 170 languages.

The following signs may signal the presence of child abuse or neglect.

The Child:

- Shows sudden changes in behavior or school performance
- Has not received help for physical or medical problems brought to the parents' attention
- Has learning problems (or difficulty concentrating) that cannot be attributed to specific physical or psychological causes

- Is always watchful, as though preparing for something bad to happen
- Lacks adult supervision
- Is overly compliant, passive, or withdrawn
- Comes to school or other activities early, stays late, and does not want to go home
- Is reluctant to be around a particular person
- Discloses maltreatment

The Parent:

- Denies the existence of—or blames the child for—the child's problems in school or at home Asks teachers or other caregivers to use harsh physical discipline if the child misbehaves
- Sees the child as entirely bad, worthless, or burdensome
- Demands a level of physical or academic performance the child cannot achieve
- Looks primarily to the child for care, attention, and satisfaction of the parent's emotional needs Shows little concern for the child

The Parent and Child:

- Rarely touch or look at each other
- Consider their relationship entirely negative
- State that they do not like each other

The above list may not be all the signs of abuse or neglect. It is important to pay attention to other behaviors that may seem unusual or concerning.

Signs of Physical Abuse

Consider the possibility of physical abuse when the **child:**

- Has unexplained burns, bites, bruises, broken bones, or black eyes
- Has fading bruises or other marks noticeable after an absence from school
- Seems frightened of the parents and protests or cries when it is time to go home

- Shrinks at the approach of adults
- Reports injury by a parent or another adult caregiver
- Abuses animals or pets

Consider the possibility of physical abuse when the **parent or other adult caregiver:**

- Offers conflicting, unconvincing, or no explanation for the child's injury, or provides an explanation that is not consistent with the injury
- Describes the child as "evil" or in some other very negative way
- Uses harsh physical discipline with the child
- Has a history of abuse as a child
- Has a history of abusing animals or pets

Signs of Neglect

Consider the possibility of neglect when the **child:**

- Is frequently absent from school
- Begs or steals food or money
- Lacks needed medical or dental care, immunizations, or glasses
- Is consistently dirty and has severe body odor
- Lacks sufficient clothing for the weather
- Abuses alcohol or other drugs
- States that there is no one at home to provide care

Consider the possibility of neglect when the **parent or other adult caregiver:**

- Appears to be indifferent to the child
- Seems apathetic or depressed
- Behaves irrationally or in a bizarre manner
- Is abusing alcohol or other drugs

Signs of Sexual Abuse

Consider the possibility of sexual abuse when the **child:**

- Has difficulty walking or sitting
- Suddenly refuses to change for gym or to participate in physical activities
- Reports nightmares or bedwetting
- Experiences a sudden change in appetite
- Demonstrates bizarre, sophisticated, or unusual sexual knowledge or behavior
- Becomes pregnant or contracts a venereal disease, particularly if under age 14
- Runs away
- Reports sexual abuse by a parent or another adult caregiver
- Attaches very quickly to strangers or new adults in their environment

Consider the possibility of sexual abuse when the **parent or other adult caregiver:**

- Is unduly protective of the child or severely limits the child's contact with other children, especially of the opposite sex
- Is secretive and isolated
- Is jealous or controlling with family members

Signs of Emotional Maltreatment

Consider the possibility of emotional maltreatment when the **child:**

- Shows extremes in behavior, such as overly compliant or demanding behavior, extreme passivity, or aggression
- Is either inappropriately adult (parenting other children, for example) or inappropriately infantile (frequently rocking or head-banging, for example)
- Is delayed in physical or emotional development
- Has attempted suicide
- Reports a lack of attachment to the parent

Consider the possibility of emotional maltreatment when the **parent or other adult caregiver:**

- Constantly blames, belittles, or berates the child

- Is unconcerned about the child and refuses to consider offers of help for the child's problems

- Overtly rejects the child

Section 10.2

Helping First Responders Identify Child Abuse

This section includes text excerpted from "The Role of First Responders in Child Maltreatment Cases: Disaster and Nondisaster Situations," Child Welfare Information Gateway, U.S. Department of Health and Human Services (HHS), 2010. Reviewed May 2016.

First responders have various levels of experience and training regarding the detection of possible child abuse and neglect. While some effects of child maltreatment are easily observable, many require a more in depth assessment by first responders. The physical, emotional, and behavioral effects of child abuse or neglect are wide-ranging, but many of these also may be caused by something other than maltreatment. First responders should be able to recognize and to assess any possible maltreatment within the context of other problematic situations that may occur in the home, such as domestic violence or substance abuse.

Federal Child Welfare Laws

State laws, sound professional standards for practice, and strong philosophical underpinnings should guide any intervention into family life on behalf of children. The key principles guiding State child protection laws are based largely on Federal statutes, primarily the Child Abuse Prevention and Treatment Act (CAPTA), as amended by the Keeping Children and Families Safe Act of 2003, and the Adoption and Safe Families Act (ASFA) of 1997. CAPTA provides definitions and guidelines regarding child maltreatment issues, and ASFA promotes three national goals for child protection:

1. **Safety**–All children have the right to live in an environment free from abuse and neglect. The safety of children is the paramount concern that must guide child protection efforts.

2. **Permanency**–Children need a family and a permanent place to call home. A sense of continuity and connectedness is central to children's healthy development.

3. **Well-being**–Children deserve nurturing families and environments in which their physical, emotional, educational, and social needs are met. Child protection practices must take into account each child's needs and should promote the healthy development of family relationships.

Types of Child Maltreatment

There are four commonly recognized forms of child maltreatment—physical abuse, neglect, psychological abuse, and sexual abuse. The definitions of these types of child maltreatment may vary depending on the State or the locality in which the first responder works. First responders should become familiar with the definitions that apply in their jurisdictions. Actual child maltreatment, as well as the perpetrator's identity, can be determined only after a thorough response and investigation.

Physical Abuse

The physical abuse of children includes any nonaccidental physical injury caused by the child's caretaker. Physical abuse can vary greatly in frequency and severity. It may include injuries sustained from burning, beating, kicking, or punching. Although the injury is not an accident, neither is it necessarily the intent of the child's caretaker to injure the child. Physical abuse may result from punishment that is inappropriate to the child's age, developmental level, or condition. Additionally, it may be caused by a parent's recurrent lapses in self-control that are brought on by immaturity, stress, or the use of alcohol or illicit drugs. Caretakers may physically abuse children during discipline or as a way to "teach the child a lesson."

Signs of Possible Physical Abuse

Signs of possible physical abuse include:

- Fractures unexpectedly discovered in the course of an otherwise routine medical examination (e.g., discovering a broken rib while listening to the child's heartbeat)

- Injuries that are inconsistent with, or out of proportion to, the history provided by the caretaker or with the child's age or developmental stage (e.g., a 3-month old burning herself by crawling on top of the stove)

- Multiple fractures, often symmetrical (e.g., in both arms or legs), or fractures at different stages of healing

- Fractures in children who are not able to walk

- Skeletal trauma (e.g., fractures) combined with other types of injuries, such as burns

- Subdural hematomas, which are hemorrhages between the brain and its outer lining that are caused by ruptured blood vessels

- Burns on the buttocks, around the anogenital region, on the backs of the hands, or on both hands, as well as those that are severe.

Some injuries that may have been caused by physical abuse have distinct marks. Some injuries, however, may not be visible without a complete medical examination. For instance, injuries caused by abuse directed to the abdomen or to the head often are undetected because many of the injuries are internal.

The first response in child physical abuse cases is handled predominately by social service agencies, such as child protective services (CPS). Many jurisdictions across the country have interagency agreements and protocols that define when a joint investigation by law enforcement and CPS will be conducted. Some have put guidelines in place for law enforcement to respond to all physical abuse cases involving young children, as well as to all cases of serious physical abuse. Serious physical abuse cases generally are defined as those requiring medical treatment or hospitalization. A response by law enforcement is also often required in cases involving any blows to the face or the head or the use of a particular instrument (e.g., clubs, bats, sticks, chains), which can indicate an attempt to do serious harm.

Neglect

Neglect involves a caregiver's failure to meet the basic needs of a child, such as food, clothing, shelter, medical care, or supervision. Types of neglect include physical, environmental, emotional, and educational neglect, as well as inadequate supervision. Neglect follows a continuum from mild to severe and often is very difficult to define. Most laws today include some mention of "failure or inability to provide" in their definitions. There is still a lack of consensus, however, as to what constitutes failure to provide adequate food, shelter, protection, or clothing. Some State definitions include "failure or inability to protect," which refers to a situation in which a child is exposed to someone who may harm him, such as being left with a parent's drug dealer or a known child molester. In addition, parents might be accused of failing to provide a safe environment by not protecting a child from unsanitary or hazardous living conditions.

Caregivers may not provide proper care for a variety of reasons, including a lack of knowledge or understanding about meeting the child's needs, inadequate bonding with the child, or impairment due to substance abuse or to mental illness. Although there are cases of co-occurring maltreatment and poverty, living in poverty, in and of itself, does not mean that a child is being neglected.

Signs of Possible Neglect

Children who possibly are neglected may:

- Seem inadequately dressed for the weather (e.g., wearing shorts and sandals in freezing weather)

- Appear excessively listless and tired (due to no routine or structure around bedtimes)

- Report caring for younger siblings (when they themselves are underage or are developmentally not ready to do so)

- Demonstrate poor hygiene or smell of urine or feces

- Seem unusually small or thin or have a distended stomach (indicative of malnutrition)

- Have unattended medical or dental problems, such as infected sores or badly decayed or abscessed teeth

- Appear withdrawn

- Crave unusual amounts of attention, even eliciting negative responses in order to obtain it

- Be chronically truant.

Additionally, the first responder should check the home environment for signs of neglect, such as health or safety hazards, no heat, or unsanitary conditions.

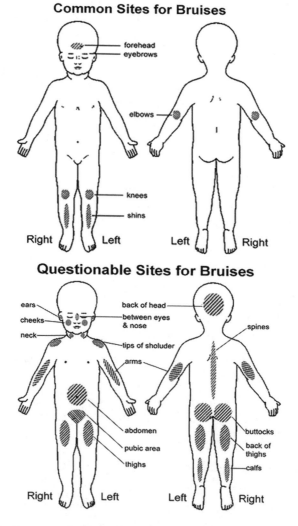

Figure 10.1. *Common Sites for Bruises*

Distinguishing Physical Abuse from Nonintentional Injury

Children may receive bruises during the course of play or while being active. The areas that are bruised most commonly during normal play include the leading or bony edges of the body, such as knees, elbows, forearms, or eyebrows. The soft tissue areas, such as cheeks, buttocks, and thighs, are not normally injured during play. Additionally, bruises received during the normal course of childhood activity rarely are in distinct shapes, such as a hand, a belt buckle, or adult teeth marks. Bruises in soft tissue areas or in distinct shapes may be indicative of physical abuse.

Chapter 11

Abusive Head Trauma

What Is Abusive Head Trauma

Abusive head trauma, also called shaken baby syndrome (or SBS), goes by many other names, including inflicted traumatic brain injury and shaken impact syndrome. All of these names mean the same thing: an injury to a child's brain as a result of child abuse.

Abusive head trauma (AHT) can be caused by direct blows to the head, dropping or throwing a child, or shaking a child. Head trauma is the leading cause of death in child abuse cases in the United States. Because the anatomy of infants puts them at particular risk for injury from this kind of action, the majority of victims are infants younger than 1 year old.

AHT can happen in children up to 5 years old, and the average age of victims is between 3 and 8 months. However, the highest rate of cases occur among infants just 6 to 8 weeks old, which is when babies tend to cry the most.

How These Injuries Happen

Abusive head trauma results from injuries caused by someone (most often a parent or other caregiver) vigorously shaking a child or striking

This chapter includes text excerpted from "Abusive Head Trauma (Shaken Baby Syndrome)," © 1995–2016. The Nemours Foundation/KidsHealth®. Reprinted with permission.

the child's head against a surface. In many cases, the caregiver cannot get the baby to stop crying and, out of frustration or anger, will shake the baby. Unfortunately, the shaking may have the desired effect: Although at first the baby cries more, he or she may stop crying as the brain is damaged.

Children with special needs, multiple siblings, or conditions like colic or GERD have an increased risk of AHT. Boys are more likely to be victims of AHT than girls, and children of families who live at or below the poverty level are at an increased risk for these injuries and other types of child abuse.

The perpetrators in about 70% of cases are males—usually either the baby's father or the mother's boyfriend, often someone in his early twenties. But anyone has the potential to shake a baby if he or she isn't able to handle stressful situations well, has poor impulse control, or has a tendency toward aggressive behavior. Substance abuse often plays a role in AHT.

When someone forcefully shakes a baby, the child's head rotates uncontrollably. This is because infants' neck muscles aren't well developed and provide little support for their heads. This violent movement pitches the infant's brain back and forth within the skull, sometimes rupturing blood vessels and nerves throughout the brain and tearing the brain tissue. The brain may strike the inside of the skull, causing bruising and bleeding to the brain.

The damage can be even greater when a shaking episode ends with an impact (hitting a wall or a crib mattress, for example), because the forces of acceleration and deceleration associated with an impact are so strong. After the shaking, swelling in the brain can cause enormous pressure within the skull, compressing blood vessels and increasing overall injury to the brain's delicate structure.

Normal interaction with a child, like bouncing the baby on a knee or tossing the baby up in the air, will **not** cause these injuries. But it's important to **never** shake a baby under **any** circumstances.

What Are the Effects?

AHT often causes irreversible damage, and about 1 out of every 4 cases results in the child's death.

Children who survive may have:

- partial or total blindness

- hearing loss

- seizures

- developmental delays
- impaired intellect
- speech and learning difficulties
- problems with memory and attention
- severe mental retardation
- cerebral palsy

Even in milder cases, in which babies look normal immediately after the shaking, they may eventually develop one or more of these problems. Sometimes the first sign of a problem isn't noticed until the child enters the school system and exhibits behavioral problems or learning difficulties. But by that time, it's more difficult to link these problems to a shaking incident from several years before.

Signs and Symptoms

In any abusive head trauma case, the duration and force of the shaking, the number of episodes, and whether impact is involved all affect the severity of the child's injuries. In the most violent cases, children may arrive at the emergency room unconscious, suffering seizures, or in shock. But in many cases, infants may never be brought to medical attention if they don't exhibit such severe symptoms.

In less severe cases, a child who has been shaken may experience:

- lethargy
- irritability
- vomiting
- poor sucking or swallowing
- decreased appetite
- lack of smiling or vocalizing
- rigidity
- seizures
- difficulty breathing
- blue color due to lack of oxygen
- altered consciousness
- unequal pupil size

- an inability to lift the head

- an inability to focus the eyes or track movement

Diagnosis

Many cases of AHT are brought in for medical care as "silent injuries." In other words, parents or caregivers don't often provide a history that the child has had abusive head trauma or a shaking injury, so doctors don't know to look for subtle or physical signs. This can sometimes result in children having injuries that aren't identified in the medical system.

In many cases, babies who don't have severe symptoms may never be brought to a doctor. Many of the less severe symptoms such as vomiting or irritability may resolve and can have many non-abuse-related causes.

Unfortunately, unless a doctor has reason to suspect child abuse, mild cases (in which the infant seems lethargic, fussy, or perhaps isn't feeding well) are often misdiagnosed as a viral illness or colic. Without a suspicion of child abuse and any resulting intervention with the parents or caregivers, these children may be shaken again, worsening any brain injury or damage.

If shaken baby syndrome is suspected, doctors may look for:

- hemorrhages in the retinas of the eyes

- skull fractures

- swelling of the brain

- subdural hematomas (blood collections pressing on the surface of the brain)

- rib and long bone (bones in the arms and legs) fractures

- bruises around the head, neck, or chest

The Child's Development and Education

What makes AHT so devastating is that it often involves a total brain injury. For example, a child whose vision is severely impaired won't be able to learn through observation, which decreases the child's overall ability to learn.

The development of language, vision, balance, and motor coordination, all of which occur to varying degrees after birth, are particularly likely to be affected in any child who has AHT. Such impairment can require intensive physical and occupational therapy to help the child acquire skills that would have developed normally had the brain injury not occurred.

Before age 3, a child can receive free speech or physical therapy through state-run early intervention programs. Federal law requires that each state provide these services for children who have developmental disabilities as a result of being abused. After a child turns 3, it's the school district's responsibility to provide any needed additional special educational services.

As kids get older, they may require special education and continued therapy to help with language development and daily living skills, like dressing.

Preventing AHT

Abusive head trauma is *100% preventable*. A key aspect of prevention is increasing awareness of the potential dangers of shaking.

Finding ways to alleviate the parent or caregiver's stress at the critical moments when a baby is crying can significantly reduce the risk to a child. Some hospital-based programs have helped new parents identify and prevent shaking injuries and understand how to respond when infants cry.

All Babies Cry is a national program that promotes healthy parenting behavior through practical demonstrations of infant soothing and ways to manage the stress of parenting. The program is divided into four parts:

1. What's normal about crying?

2. Comforting your baby.

3. Self-care tips for parents.

4. Colic and how to cope.

The National Center on Shaken Baby Syndrome offers a prevention program, **the Period of Purple Crying**, which can help parents and other caregivers understand crying in healthy infants and how to handle it.

Another method that can help is the **"five S's" approach**, which stands for:

1. Shushing (by using "white noise" or rhythmic sounds that mimic the constant whir of noise in the womb. Vacuum cleaners, hair dryers, clothes dryers, a running tub, or a white noise machine can all create this effect.)

2. Side/stomach positioning (placing the baby on the left side—to help with digestion—or on the belly while holding him or her. Babies should always be placed on their backs to sleep.)

3. Sucking (letting the baby breastfeed or bottle-feed, or giving the baby a pacifier or finger to suck on).

4. Swaddling (wrapping the baby in a blanket like a "burrrito" to help him or her feel more secure. Hips and knees should be slightly bent and turned out).

5. Swinging gently (rocking in a chair, using an infant swing, or taking a car ride to help duplicate the constant motion the baby felt in the womb).

If a baby in your care won't stop crying, you can also try the following:

*   Make sure the baby's basic needs are met (for example, he or she isn't hungry and doesn't need to be changed).

*   Check for signs of illness, like fever or swollen gums.

*   Rock or walk with the baby.

*   Sing or talk to the baby.

*   Offer the baby a pacifier or a noisy toy.

*   Take the baby for a ride in a stroller or strapped into a child safety seat in the car.

*   Hold the baby close against your body and breathe calmly and slowly.

*   Give the baby a warm bath.

*   Pat or rub the baby's back.

*   Call a friend or relative for support or to take care of the baby while you take a break.

*   If nothing else works, put the baby on his or her back in the crib, close the door, and check on the baby in 10 minutes.

*   Call your doctor if nothing seems to be helping your infant, in case there is a medical reason for the fussiness.

To prevent potential AHT, parents and caregivers of infants need to learn how to respond to their own stress. It's important to tell *anyone* caring for a baby to never shake him or her. Talk about the dangers of shaking and how it can be prevented.

Chapter 12

Munchausen by Proxy Syndrome

What Is Munchausen by Proxy Syndrome?

Munchausen by proxy syndrome (MBPS) is a relatively rare form of child abuse that involves the exaggeration or fabrication of illnesses or symptoms by a primary caretaker.

Also known as "medical child abuse," MBPS was named after Baron von Munchausen, an 18th-century German dignitary known for making up stories about his travels and experiences in order to get attention. "By proxy" indicates that a parent or other adult is making up or exaggerating symptoms in a child, not in himself or herself.

Munchausen by proxy syndrome is a mental illness and requires treatment.

About MBPS

In MBPS, an individual—usually a parent or caregiver—causes or fabricates symptoms in a child. The adult deliberately misleads others (particularly medical professionals), and may go as far as to actually cause symptoms in the child through poisoning, medication, or even suffocation. In most cases (85%), the mother is responsible for causing the illness or symptoms.

This chapter includes text excerpted from "Munchausen by Proxy Syndrome," © 1995–2016. The Nemours Foundation/KidsHealth®. Reprinted with permission.

99

Usually, the cause of MBPS is a need for attention and sympathy from doctors, nurses, and other professionals. Some experts believe that it isn't just the attention that's gained from the "illness" of the child that drives this behavior, but also the satisfaction in deceiving individuals whom they consider to be more important and powerful than themselves.

Because the parent or caregiver appears to be so caring and attentive, often no one suspects any wrongdoing. Diagnosis is made extremely difficult due to the ability of the parent or caregiver to manipulate doctors and induce symptoms in the child.

Often, the perpetrator is familiar with the medical profession and knowledgeable about how to bring on illness or impairment in the child. Medical personnel often overlook the possibility of MBPS because it goes against the belief that parents and caregivers would never deliberately hurt their child.

Most victims of MBPS are preschoolers (although there have been cases in kids up to 16 years old), and there are equal numbers of boys and girls.

Diagnosing MBPS

Diagnosis is very difficult, but could involve some of the following:

- a child who has multiple medical problems that don't respond to treatment or that follow a persistent and puzzling course

- physical or laboratory findings that are highly unusual, don't correspond with the child's medical history, or are physically or clinically impossible

- short-term symptoms that tend to stop or improve when the victim is not with the perpetrator (for example, when the child is hospitalized)

- a parent or caregiver who isn't reassured by "good news" when test results find no medical problems, but continues to insist that the child is ill and may "doctor shop" to find a professional who believes that

- a parent or caregiver who appears to be medically knowledgeable or fascinated with medical details or seems to enjoy the hospital environment and attention the sick child receives

- a parent or caregiver who's overly supportive and encouraging of the doctor, or one who is angry and demands further intervention, more procedures, second opinions, or transfers to more sophisticated facilities

If you have any concerns about a child you know, it is important to speak to someone at your local child protective services agency—even if you prefer to call in anonymously.

Causes of MBPS

MBPS is a psychiatric condition. In some cases, the perpetrators were themselves abused, physically and/or and sexually, as children. They may have come from families in which being sick was a way to get love.

The parent's or caregiver's own personal needs overcome his or her ability to see the child as a person with feelings and rights, possibly because the parent or caregiver may have grown up being treated like he or she wasn't a person with rights or feelings.

In rare cases, MBPS is not caused by a parent or family member, but by a medical professional (such as a nurse or doctor), who induces illness in a child who is hospitalized for other reasons.

What Happens to the Child?

In the most severe instances, parents or caregivers with MBPS may go to great lengths to make their children sick. When cameras were placed in some children's hospital rooms, some perpetrators were filmed switching medicines, injecting kids with urine to cause an infection, or placing drops of blood in urine specimens.

In most cases, victims of MBPS need hospitalization. And because they may be deemed a "medical mystery," hospital stays tend to be longer than usual. Whatever the cause, the child's symptoms—whether created or fabricated—ease or completely disappear when the perpetrator isn't present.

According to experts, common conditions and symptoms that are created or fabricated by parents or caregivers with MBPS can include: failure to thrive, allergies, asthma, vomiting, diarrhea, seizures, and infections.

The long-term prognosis for these children depends on the degree of damage done by the illness or impairment and the amount of time it takes to recognize and diagnose MBPS. Some extreme cases have been reported in which children developed destructive skeletal changes, limps, mental retardation, brain damage, and blindness from symptoms caused by the parent or caregiver. Often, these children need multiple surgeries, each with the risk for future medical problems.

For a child who is old enough to understand what's happening, the psychological damage can be significant. The child may come to feel that he or she will only be loved when ill and may, therefore, help the parent try to deceive doctors, using self-abuse to avoid being abandoned. And so, some victims of MBPS are at risk of repeating the cycle of abuse.

Getting Help for the Child

If MBPS is suspected, health care providers are required by law to report their concerns. However, after a parent or caregiver is charged, the child's symptoms may increase as the person who is accused attempts to prove the presence of the illness. If the parent or caregiver repeatedly denies the charges, the child would likely be removed from the home and legal action would be taken on the child's behalf.

In some cases, the parent or caregiver may deny the charges and move to another location, only to continue the behavior. If the child is returned to the perpetrator's custody while protective services are involved, the child may continue to be a victim of abuse while the perpetrator avoids treatment and interventions.

Getting Help for the Parent or Caregiver

To get help, the parent or caregiver must admit to the abuse and seek psychological treatment.

But if the perpetrator doesn't admit to the wrongdoing, psychological treatment has little chance of helping the situation. Recognizing MBPS as an illness that has the potential for treatment is one way to give hope to the family in these rare situations.

Chapter 13

Sexual Abuse of Children

What Is Child Sexual Abuse?

Child sexual abuse includes a wide range of sexual behaviors that take place between a child and an older person. These behaviors are meant to arouse the older person in a sexual way. In general, no thought is given to what effect the behavior may have on the child. For the most part, the abuser does not care about the reactions or choices of the child.

Child sexual abuse often involves body contact. This could include sexual kissing, touching, and oral, anal, or vaginal sex. Not all sexual abuse involves body contact, though. Showing private parts ("flashing"), forcing children to watch pornography, verbal pressure for sex, and exploiting children as prostitutes or for pornography can be sexual abuse as well. Researchers estimate that in our country about one out of six boys and one out of four girls are sexually abused.

Under the child sexual abuse laws, the abuser must be older than the victim in most cases. Some states require the abuser to be at least five years older.

Who Commits Child Sexual Abuse?

- Most often, sexual abusers know the child they abuse, but are not family. For example, the abuser might be a friend of the

This chapter includes text excerpted from "Child Sexual Abuse," U.S. Department of Veterans Affairs (VA), September 2, 2015.

family, babysitter, or neighbor. About 6 out of 10 abusers fall into that group.

- About 3 out of 10 of those who sexually abuse children are family members of the child. This includes fathers, uncles, or cousins.

- The abuser is a stranger in only about 1 out of 10 child sexual abuse cases.

- Abusers are men in most cases, whether the victim is a boy or a girl.

- Women are the abusers in about 14% of cases reported against boys and about 6% of cases reported against girls.

- Child pornographers and other abusers who are strangers may make contact with children using the Internet.

What Are the Effects of Childhood Sexual Abuse?

It is not always easy to tell whether a child has been sexually abused. Sexual abuse often occurs in secret, and there is not always physical proof of the abuse. For these reasons, child sexual abuse can be hard to detect.

Some child sexual abuse survivors may show symptoms of PTSD. They may behave in a nervous, upset way. Survivors may have bad dreams. They may act out aspects of the abuse in their play. They might show other fears and worries. Young children may lose skills they once learned and act younger than they are. For example, an abused child might start wetting the bed or sucking his or her thumb. Some sexual abuse survivors show out-of-place sexual behaviors that are not expected in a child. They may act seductive or they may not maintain safe limits with others. Children, especially boys, might "act out" with behavior problems. This could include being cruel to others and running away. Other children "act in" by becoming depressed. They may withdraw from friends or family. Older children or teens might try to hurt or even kill themselves.

Sexual abuse can be very confusing for children. For a child, it often involves being used or hurt by a trusted adult. The child might learn that the only way to get attention or love is to give something sexual or give up their self-respect. Some children believe the abuse is their fault somehow. They may think the abuser chose them because they must have wanted it or because there is something wrong with them. If the abuser was of the same sex, children (and parents) might wonder if that means they are "gay."

Almost every child sexual abuse victim describes the abuse as negative. Most children know it is wrong. They usually have feelings of fear, shock, anger, and disgust. A small number of abused children might not realize it is wrong, though. These children tend to be very young or have mental delays. Also some victims might enjoy the attention, closeness, or physical contact with the abuser. This is more likely if these basic needs are not met by a caregiver. All told, these reactions make the abuse very hard and confusing for children.

If childhood sexual abuse is not treated, long-term symptoms can go on through adulthood. These may include:

- PTSD and anxiety.

- Depression and thoughts of suicide.

- Sexual anxiety and disorders, including having too many or unsafe sexual partners.

- Difficulty setting safe limits with others (e.g., saying no to people) and relationship problems.

- Poor body image and low self-esteem.

- Unhealthy behaviors, such as alcohol, drugs, self-harm, or eating problems. These behaviors are often used to try to hide painful emotions related to the abuse.

- If you were sexually abused as a child and have some of these symptoms, it is important for you to get help.

What Can Caregivers Do to Help Keep Children Safe?

Although caregivers cannot protect their children 100% of the time, it is important to get to know the people that come around your child. You can find out whether someone has been charged with sexual abuse and find out where sexual abusers live in your area by going to the website FamilyWatchdog.com

Most importantly, provide a safe, caring setting so children feel able to talk to you about sexual abuse.

Other tips to keep your children safe include:

- Talk to others who know the people with whom your child comes in contact.

- Talk to your children about the difference between safe touching and unsafe touching.

- Tell the child that if someone tries to touch his or her body in their private areas or do things that make the child feel unsafe, he should say NO to the person. He needs to tell you or a trusted adult about it right away.

- Let children know that their bodies are private and that they have the right not to allow others to touch their bodies in an unsafe way.

- Let them know that they do not have to do EVERYTHING the babysitter, family member, or group leader tells them to do.

- Alert your children that abusers may use the Internet. Watch over your child on the Internet.

What Should You Do If You Think Your Child Has Been Sexually Abused?

If a child says she or he has been abused, try to stay calm. Reassure the child that what happened is not her fault, that you believe her, that you are proud of her for telling you (or another person), and that you are there to keep her safe. Take your child to a mental health and medical professional right away. Many cities have child advocacy centers where a child and her family can get help. These centers interview children and family members in a sensitive, warm place. They can help you report the abuse to legal authorities. They can help you find a medical examiner and therapist skilled in child sexual abuse.

Children can recover from sexual abuse and go on to live good lives. The best predictor of recovery is support and love from their main caregiver. As a caregiver, you might also consider getting help for yourself. It is often very hard to accept that a child has been sexually abused. You will not be supporting your child, though, if you respond in certain unhelpful ways. For example, you will not be able to provide support if you are overwhelmed with your own emotions. Don't downplay the abuse ("it wasn't that bad"), but also try not to have extreme fears related to the abuse ("my child will never be safe again"). It will not help children if you force them to talk, or if you blame the child. Getting therapy for yourself can help you deal with your own feelings about the abuse. Then you might be better able to provide support to your child.

Chapter 14

Incest

One of the least discussed issues related to child abuse is incest. The victims of incest often don't want to talk about it, because of the powerful societal taboo attached to the act. According to U.S. Bureau of Justice statistics, about 44 percent of sexual-assault victims are under the age of 18. The data also show that many perpetrators are known to the victims, and one-third are members of the victims' own families. And although it is commonly believed that only men initiate incest, in fact women can be the perpetrators of such abuse. But since this takes place at a much lower rate than incest by men, and since so many of such cases are not reported, it often goes unnoticed.

Considering the gravity of the issue, it is vital to understand what incest is and what can be done about it. This chapter aims to define incest, identify the causes of incest, elucidate the reasons behind the difficulty in sharing information about sexual abuse by a family member, and suggest ways to find help and support for the victim.

Defining Incest

Incest is defined as sexual contact, including intercourse, between close relatives. In most cultures incest is considered immoral, and in virtually all parts of the United States and many other countries it is also illegal. An adult engaging in incest with a child, however, is

"Incest," © 2016 Omnigraphics, Inc. Reviewed May 2016.

considered child abuse under the law, and while the laws legislation pertaining to sexual assaults varies incest with a minor is illegal in all U.S. jurisdictions. The trauma experienced by a young victim of incest has to undergo can be severe, and the incident can have a serious impact upon the life of the survivor.

Although incest can take place between consenting adults, when it occurs between adults and children some common forms include:

- Incest between a parent and a child

- Incest between an older and younger sibling

- Incest between another older relative (for example, an uncle or aunt) and a child

Signs and Symptoms of Abuse

To identify whether a child has been a victim of incest, both physical and psychological symptoms must be considered. The physical symptoms include vaginal or rectal pain, vaginal discharge, bleeding, painful urination, bed-wetting, and constipation. The psychological signs include self-harm, nightmares, eating disorders, sleep disorders, aggressive behavior, withdrawal from social interactions, post-traumatic stress disorder (PTSD), lack of concentration, poor performance at school, depression, phobias, and precocious sexual behavior.

Characteristics of Incest Offenders

Learning to identify offenders is very important in order to protect children from becoming victims of incest. There are certain characteristics, conditions, are often evident in abusive incest situations. Some examples:

- Adolescent perpetrators often seek victims who are quite young. They tend to abuse the victims for long period of time, and they may behave more violently than adult perpetrators.

- The absence or unavailability of parents may present the opportunity for incest by siblings or other relatives.

- Dominant or abusive siblings often tend to use incest as a way of expressing their power over the other(s).

- Incest is not always between an adult and a child. Studies have revealed that sibling incest is the most prevalent form of incest.

The Difficulty in Sharing Information on Sexual Abuse with a Family Member

The very thought of sexual abuse can be disturbing, and talking about it can often be very traumatic. It can become even more difficult to share such incidents if the survivor and the perpetrator are part of the same family.

Some struggles that a victim might face while sharing such information with another family member include:

- Concern about the abuser's future.

- Response or reaction by the family towards the incident, perpetrator, and also the survivor.

- Negligence or downplaying the issue by the family.

- Being told that such things are normal in most families.

- Inability of the family to recognize the incest as a type of abuse.

- The victim being unaware of available help or difficulty in finding a trustworthy person.

- Fear of being harassed by the perpetrator.

Helping the Victims of Incest

Victims of incest may feel hopeless and can thus be hesitant to seek help. If you observe any symptoms of this type of abuse, some ways to help include:

- **Have a Talk.** By talking to a child who has experienced abuse, you can provide them with comfort and try to ease their pain.

- **Show Faith.** When a victim of abuse reveals their traumatic experience, lend a patient ear. Assure them that you are absolutely serious about what they are saying, and let them know that you are on their side. If you are not sure, then seek the assistance of Child Protective Services.

- **Child Protective Services.** Reporting to Child Protective Services is an option whether the victim happens to be a minor or a vulnerable adult (that is, one who is susceptible to harm due to mental illness, age, or other factors). Contacting the Department of Human Services or the police are other options available to help get assistance for the victim.

References

1. "Incest." Rape, Abuse and Incest National Network, July 2, 2015.

2. U.S. Marshals Service, U.S. Department of Justice, October 5, 2012.

3. Willacy, Hayley, Dr. "Incest." Patient, February 21, 2013.

Chapter 15

Teen Dating Abuse

Chapter Contents

Section 15.1

Dating Violence

This section includes text excerpted from "Understanding Teen Dating Violence," Centers for Disease Control and Prevention (CDC), March 4, 2016.

What Is Dating Violence?

Dating violence is a type of intimate partner violence. It occurs between two people in a close relationship. The nature of dating violence can be physical, emotional, or sexual.

- **Physical.** This occurs when a partner is pinched, hit, shoved, slapped, punched, or kicked.

- **Psychological/Emotional.** This means threatening a partner or harming his or her sense of self-worth. Examples include name calling, shaming, bullying, embarrassing on purpose, or keeping him/her away from friends and family.

- **Sexual.** This is forcing a partner to engage in a sex act when he or she does not or cannot consent. This can be physical or non-physical, like threatening to spread rumors if a partner refuses to have sex.

- **Stalking.** This refers to a pattern of harassing or threatening tactics that are unwanted and cause fear in the victim. Dating violence can take place in person or electronically, such as repeated texting or posting sexual pictures of a partner online. Unhealthy relationships can start early and last a lifetime. Teens often think some behaviors, like teasing and name calling, are a "normal" part of a relationship. However, these behaviors can become abusive and develop into more serious forms of violence.

Why Is Dating Violence a Public Health Problem?

Dating violence is a widespread issue that has serious long-term and short-term effects. Many teens do not report it because they are afraid to tell friends and family.

- Among high school students who dated, 21% of females and 10% of males experienced physical and/or sexual dating violence.

- Among adult victims of rape, physical violence, and/ or stalking by an intimate partner, 22% of women and 15% of men first experienced some form of partner violence between 11 and 17 years of age.

How Does Dating Violence Affect Health?

Dating violence can have a negative effect on health throughout life. Youth who are victims are more likely to experience symptoms of depression and anxiety, engage in unhealthy behaviors, like using tobacco, drugs, and alcohol, or exhibit antisocial behaviors and think about suicide. Youth who are victims of dating violence in high school are at higher risk for victimization during college.

Who Is at Risk for Dating Violence?

Factors that increase risk for harming a dating partner include the following:

- Belief that dating violence is acceptable
- Depression, anxiety, and other trauma symptoms
- Aggression towards peers and other aggressive behavior
- Substance use
- Early sexual activity and having multiple sexual partners
- Having a friend involved in dating violence
- Conflict with partner
- Witnessing or experiencing violence in the home

How Can We Prevent Dating Violence?

The ultimate goal is to stop dating violence before it starts. Strategies that promote healthy relationships are vital. During the preteen and teen years, young people are learning skills they need to form positive relationships with others. This is an ideal time to promote healthy relationships and prevent patterns of dating violence that can last into adulthood.

Many prevention strategies are proven to prevent or reduce dating violence. Some effective school-based programs change norms, improve problem-solving, and address dating violence in addition to other youth risk behaviors, such as substance use and sexual risk behaviors. Other programs prevent dating violence through changes to the school environment or training influential adults, like parents/caregivers and coaches, to work with youth to prevent dating violence.

Section 15.2

Dating Violence and the Role of Peers

This section includes text excerpted from "Teen Dating Violence,"
U.S. Department of Justice (DOJ), November 24, 2014.

Peer Roles in Teen Dating Violence

Peer roles are best understood within a multisystemic framework. That is, when teens begin dating, each partner enters into the relationship with his or her own set of perceptions, attitudes and behaviors shaped, in part, by the broader social "contexts," or environments, in which they live. Teens interact with peers in many different social contexts, for example, schools, social clubs, sports teams, neighborhood parks or community centers. Each social context can promote attitudes and behaviors that encourage or discourage dating violence. For example, teens' and their peers' perceptions of whether violence is acceptable within romantic relationships might depend on the level of violence they witness at school or in their neighborhood.

Thus, when considering how peers might shape dating experiences, it is important to consider not only the context of teens' close peer group but also the larger school and community contexts in which teens and their peers interact.

Teens' peers have the potential to considerably shape their dating experiences. Teens spend most of their days in school with peers and, in their free time, spend proportionally more time with peers than with parents or any other adults. The desire to fit in and be liked by peers heightens in adolescence, and teens begin to rely on peers as a primary source of support and guidance. In addition, peer groups often set norms and offer social rewards for dating; for example, youth who date are often perceived as more socially accepted or popular than youth who do not date. As such, peers are likely to have a significant impact on teens' decisions about whether to date, whom to date, and when to break up with romantic partners. Furthermore, the experiences that teens witness or perceive their peers to have within romantic relationships might shape teens' perceptions of what is normal or acceptable in their own romantic relationships.

It is critical to consider the very public nature of teens' romantic relationships. Teen couples often interact in the presence of peers at school or in other social settings where other teens and adults are present, such as a mall, a movie theatre, or at home. Because of this, interactions that occur in public, or that happen in private but are shared with peers, might quickly become public knowledge to the larger peer network. This is particularly true in today's digital world. Even when teens are not physically together, they are often still interacting by cell phone, text messages, social media sites, online video games and other electronic outlets that allow them to disseminate information quickly and widely.

As a result, when relationships become violent or unhealthy in other ways, teens are at risk for experiencing embarrassment, being publicly ridiculed, or developing negative reputations among their peers. These concerns are very real to teens; they have to contend with their image among close friends and the larger peer network on a daily basis. Of particular interest to service providers is that the presence of peers might instigate, elevate or reduce the likelihood of teen dating violence, depending on the situation. For example, if a girl hits a boy in front of his friends, the boy might feel pressure to "save face" and hit her in return. On the other hand, if peers are present when a couple is arguing, the peers might help defuse the situation and prevent the argument from escalating to violence—or peers who witness or hear about violence occurring also might seek help from an adult.

Clearly, teens' orientation toward peers and the significant amount of time spent with them affords numerous opportunities for peers to impact teens' behaviors and decisions within romantic relationships. Findings emerging from NIJ-funded research on peer roles in teen dating violence can be viewed in terms of three overarching questions:

1. Do risky peer contexts increase the likelihood that teens will experience dating violence?

2. What roles do peers play in seeking help after teens experience violence?

3. Can group interventions or those focused on social contexts reduce the risk for teen dating violence?

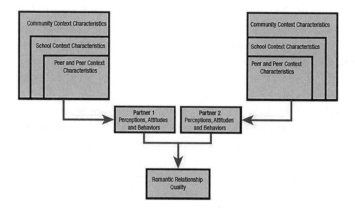

Figure 15.1. *Peer Roles in Teen Dating Violence: A Multisystemic Framework*

This figure illustrates the theoretical framework guiding our review of research on peers, peer contexts and teen dating violence. It is not intended to depict all potential influences on the quality of the romantic relationships among teens; there are a number of individual- and family-level factors, for example, that are not depicted in this figure.

Do Risky Peer Contexts Increase the Likelihood That Teens Will Experience Dating Violence?

Research consistently shows the tendency for dating violence to overlap with peer victimization, suggesting that youth who are victims or perpetrators of peer violence tend to be the same youth at risk for experiencing violence within romantic relationships. As such, researchers have begun to identify risky or antisocial characteristics of teens' broader peer social environments that increase the risk for dating violence.

Peer Violence and Dating Violence Tend to Co-Occur

Two studies using community-based samples directly examined the links between dating violence and peer violence, including the associations between bullying among peers and dating violence. One study of 1,162 teens attending high school in Illinois revealed concurrent links between youth who bully and youth who perpetrate teen dating violence, suggesting an overlap in teens who victimize peers and those who victimize dating partners. Specifically, female teens who bullied others were also likely to perpetrate sexual harassment and sexual, verbal and physical dating violence. Similarly, male teens who bullied others were also likely to perpetrate sexual harassment, physical dating violence and verbal dating violence.

A survey of 5,647 teens across three northeastern states focused more specifically on the co-occurrence of cyberbullying and teen dating violence. Results revealed significant overlaps in who perpetrated cyberbullying and cyberdating violence—26 percent of teens who perpetrated cyberbullying also perpetrated cyberdating violence, compared with only 7 percent of teens who did not perpetrate cyberbullying. Overlap also existed in victimization experiences. Teens who experienced cyberbullying by peers were more than three times as likely to experience cyberdating violence, compared with those who did not experience cyberbullying (38 percent versus 13 percent, respectively).

Furthermore, a national study of 1,525 Latino teens revealed links between victimization by dating partners and a wide range of other forms of victimization. About 71 percent of dating violence victims experienced peer/sibling violence, sexual victimization, stalking, conventional crime or another form of victimization in the prior year. Dating violence and peer/sibling violence were the two most common forms of victimization to co-occur. About 57 percent of teen victims of dating violence were also victims of peer/sibling violence.

The consistency with which peer violence and teen dating violence have been found to co-occur illustrates that teens who struggle with establishing healthy peer relationships also have difficulties in romantic relationships. Although we know little about the details of how this occurs, these findings are in line with theories that suggest that outcomes in one relationship tend to be shaped by experiences, beliefs and attitudes learned in other relationships.

Youth in Risky, Antisocial Environments Are at Significant Risk for Teen Dating Violence

Practitioners often must provide services to teens who have multiple risk factors for dating violence and thus would benefit by knowing which risk factors are most important to address in situations where time and resources might be limited. One study simultaneously examined multiple risk factors, including social context, within a sample of low-income teens who were receiving community-based services allocated to at-risk populations. Among the 223 youth in that study, there were 11 known risk factors for dating violence, divided into four categories: risky social environment, risky sexual history, risky family background and poor ability to self-regulate. Risky social environment represented a combination of teens' ratings of peer delinquency, exposure to peer dating abuse, negative neighborhood quality and attitudes toward relationship abuse.

When the four categories of risk factors were examined simultaneously, risky social environment was the strongest correlate of physical and emotional dating violence victimization and perpetration within a romantic relationship. Teens from risky family backgrounds were also more likely to experience and perpetrate emotional and physical dating violence. However, this finding was partly explained by the fact that the more high-risk the teens' family backgrounds were, the more likely they were to become involved in risky social contexts, such as having delinquent peers or witnessing dating violence among their peers.

Studies consistently show that teens who engage in delinquent behaviors are at risk for experiencing and perpetrating dating violence. Indeed, teens' own participation in delinquent behaviors is a likely indicator that they are embedded within a risky social environment. The vast majority of adolescent delinquency is committed in groups of peers, and teens' and their peers' levels of delinquency tend to be similarly aligned. Moreover, teens who engage in delinquency are also likely to choose delinquent romantic partners, creating risky romantic relationship contexts that are, in turn, associated with higher levels of dating violence and other health-risk behaviors.

Findings from NIJ-funded studies contribute to a growing body of literature suggesting that a diverse set of peer attributes are linked to whether teens experience or perpetrate dating violence, including close peers' and the broader peer group's behaviors, attitudes and guidance; teens' social standing among the broader peer group; and the quality of relationships with close peers. Moreover, peer risk factors tend to be more strongly associated with dating violence perpetration and victimization in adolescence than with family risk factors.

What Roles Do Peers Play in Help-Seeking after Teens Experience Violence?

Teen dating violence has been associated with negative psychosocial health outcomes, including delinquency, hostility and depression. Once teens experience violence in one relationship, they are at significant risk for experiencing violence in another relationship. Thus, it is important that teens who experience dating violence seek help soon after, so they can receive services to protect against the potential psychosocial impacts of violence and reduce the likelihood of future violence.

Peers also can have a significant impact on how teens respond to dating violence. Studies have identified two ways in which peers play a role in the aftermath of dating violence:

1. Peers often serve as first responders to dating violence, and

2. Peers can hinder or encourage legal help-seeking in the form of a protection order.

Peers as First Responders to Dating Violence

It is difficult to determine how many teens seek help after violence occurs because researchers often ask different questions about help-seeking and dating abuse. For example, some researchers examine the percentage of teens who sought help after experiencing certain forms of serious physical or sexual abuse, whereas others examine help-seeking among teens who experienced any form of dating violence. Regardless, one clear message has emerged: *Many teens do not seek help from anyone after violence has occurred, and those who do seek help most frequently turn to a friend.*

In a study of 2,173 teens who reported being the victim of cyber, physical, psychological or sexual dating abuse, only 8.6 percent reported seeking help from at least one person; more females (11 percent) sought help than males (5.7 percent). Very few teens—only 4.1 percent of females and 2 percent of males—sought help after they experienced dating abuse for the first time. Among the teens who did seek help, more than three-quarters (77.2 percent) turned to a friend for help and 48.5 percent turned to parents. Less than 10 percent sought help from other service providers, such as a teacher or police officer. For those who did seek help, both males (69.2 percent) and females (82 percent) were most likely to seek help from friends.

Somewhat higher rates were reported in another study that asked only about help-seeking after experiencing physical, sexual or stalking dating violence in the past year. Of the roughly 90 Latino teens who had experienced such violence, about 63 percent sought help afterward (60 percent of males and 69 percent of females). Compared with psychological or cyber forms of abuse, it is possible that teens are more likely to recognize physical, sexual and stalking dating violence as abuse and thus seek help. Nonetheless, few teens (15.6 percent) sought help from formal sources such as school, social services or legal professionals. Instead, male and female teens were most likely to turn

119

to friends for help (43.6 percent and 41.4 percent, respectively). These findings add to the growing evidence that peers tend to be the most frequent first responders to teen dating violence among male and female teens, teens of varying racial and ethnic backgrounds, and teens who experience different forms of dating violence.

Peers Play a Role in Teens' Help-Seeking

A recent exploratory study examined teens' use of protection orders, also called civil orders of protection or restraining orders. In July 2008, New York state law was modified to give teens access to protection orders without parental consent and without having a child in common with their partner. The study examined all petitions filed by dating violence victims age 18 and younger throughout 2009 and 2010—a 2-year period shortly after the law took effect. The study found that the orders were not being used widely; victims filed only 1,200 petitions during the 2-year period. To better understand potential barriers to obtaining protection orders, the researchers conducted focus groups and interviewed teens who were potentially at risk for dating violence or had begun the process of filing for a protection order.

These conversations revealed that many youth were hesitant to obtain protection orders because they were afraid of escalating violence, were reluctant to end the relationship, or felt overwhelmed with other responsibilities. Another common barrier to seeking a protection order was how family and friends would feel about it. For example, teens were concerned about being viewed as a "snitch" or as responsible for the violence. Some teens felt ashamed to admit their victimization to others, as shown in the following examples:

"I feel like you'd get talked about at school. 'Cause, like, I feel like we live in a small town, so everyone would know and figure out, and they'd talk about you." "Your friends whatever, like, might look at you a different way ... they see it as you went to the police and you couldn't handle it—that's really not for guys."

Teens also were concerned that protection orders place victims at risk for retaliation by the abusive partners' peer network and might lead to social isolation resulting from losing mutual friends after the breakup. For example, one teen's decision to end the relationship and seek a protective order led to the dissolution of nearly her entire peer network: "It's like I don't have anybody." Another teen stated,

"[His] friends target you. When I was with him he got some other girls, and they were all, like, gang members ... and now there's, like, a whole group of girls after me and, like, I don't feel safe at all."

On the other hand, teens' social networks can also be a source of motivation to seek legal protection. Teens reported that moral support from their friends and family is what helped them make it through the process of obtaining a protection order. Teens who had obtained a protection order recommended making peer support networks available for those who are considering taking legal action against an abusive partner.

Although research on protection orders in abusive teen relationships is nascent, preliminary work illustrates that teens' decisions to bring legal action against an abusive partner are shaped by more than the abusiveness of the relationship and guidance from caring adults. Teens also weigh the potential benefits of the protection order against the potential negative consequences such legal action might have on their image and social well-being among peers.

Chapter 16

Statutory Rape

Statutory Rape—Criminal Offenses

Few states use the term statutory rape in their codes. Instead, criminal codes specify the legality of specific sexual acts. The applicable laws are often embedded in the section of the code dealing with other sexual offenses (e.g., sexual assault, forcible rape).

Sexual Intercourse with Minors

States' statutory rape offenses detail the age at which an individual can legally consent to sexual activity. This section focuses on laws addressing sexual intercourse. *Table 16.1* summarizes, where applicable, each state's:

- *Age of consent.* This is the age at which an individual can legally consent to sexual intercourse under any circumstances;

- *Minimum age of victim.* This is the age below which an individual cannot consent to sexual intercourse under any circumstances;

- *Age differential.* If the victim is above the minimum age and below the age of consent, the age differential is the maximum

---

This chapter includes text excerpted from "Statutory Rape: A Guide to State Laws and Reporting Requirements," Office of the Assistant Secretary for Planning and Evaluation (ASPE), U.S. Department of Health and Human Services (HHS), December 15, 2004. Reviewed May 2016.

difference in age between the victim and the defendant where an individual can legally consent to sexual intercourse; and

- *Minimum age of defendant in order to prosecute.* This is the age below which an individual cannot be prosecuted for engaging in sexual activities with minors. The table notes those states in which this law only applies when the victim is above a certain age.

As the first column in Table 15.1 shows, the age of consent varies by state. In the majority of states (34), it is 16 years of age. In the remaining states, the age of consent is either 17 or 18 years old (6 and 11 states, respectively).

Table 16.1. State Age Requirements

State	Age of consent	Minimum age of victim	Age differential between the victim and defendant (if victim is above minimum age)	Minimum age of defendant in order to prosecute
Alabama	16	12	2	16
Alaska	16	N/A	3	N/A
Arizona	18	15	2 (defendant must be in high school and < 19)	N/A
Arkansas	16	N/A	3 (if victim is < 14)	20 (if victim is > 14)
California	18	18	N/A	N/A
Colorado	17	N/A	4 (if victim is < 15), 10 (if victim is < 17)	N/A
Connecticut	16	N/A	2	N/A
Delaware	18	16	N/A	N/A
District of Columbia	16	0	4	N/A
Florida	18	16	N/A	24 (if victim is > 16)
Georgia	16	16	N/A	N/A
Hawaii	16	14	5	N/A
Idaho	18	18	N/A	N/A
Illinois	17	17	N/A	N/A
Indiana	16	14	N/A	18 (if victim is > 14)

Table 16.1. Continued

State	Age of consent	Minimum age of victim	Age differential between the victim and defendant (if victim is above minimum age)	Minimum age of defendant in order to prosecute
Iowa	16	14	4	N/A
Kansas	16	16	N/A	N/A
Kentucky	16	16	N/A	N/A
Louisiana	17	13	3 (if victim is < 15), 2 (if victim is < 17)	N/A
Maine	16	14	5	N/A
Maryland	16	N/A	4	N/A
Massachusetts	16	16	N/A	N/A
Michigan	16	16	N/A	N/A
Minnesota	16	N/A	3 (if victim is < 13), 2 (if victim is < 16)	N/A
Mississippi	16	N/A	2 (if victim is < 14), 3 (if victim is < 16)	N/A
Missouri	17	14	N/A	21 (if victim is ≥ 14)
Montana	16	16	N/A	N/A
Nebraska	16	16	N/A	19
Nevada	16	16	N/A	18
New Hampshire	16	16	N/A	N/A
New Jersey	16	13	4	N/A
New Mexico	16	13	4	18 (if victim is ≥ 13)
New York	17	17	N/A	N/A
North Carolina	16	N/A	4	12
North Dakota	18	15	N/A	18 (if victim is ≥ 15)
Ohio	16	13	N/A	18 (if victim is ≥ 13)
Oklahoma	16	14	N/A	18 (if victim is > 14)
Oregon	18	15	3	N/A
Pennsylvania	16	13	4	N/A

Table 16.1. Continued

State	Age of consent	Minimum age of victim	Age differential between the victim and defendant (if victim is above minimum age)	Minimum age of defendant in order to prosecute
Rhode Island	16	14	N/A	18 (if victim is ≥ 14)
South Carolina	16	14	Illegal if victim is 14 to 16 and defendant is older than victim	N/A
South Dakota	16	10	3	N/A
Tennessee	18	13	4	N/A
Texas	17	14	3	N/A
Utah	18	16	10	N/A
Vermont	16	16	N/A	16
Virginia	18	15	N/A	18 (if victim is ≥ 15
Washington	16	N/A	2 (if victim is < 12), 3 (if victim is < 14), 4 (if victim is < 16)	N/A
West Virginia	16	N/A	4 (if victim is ≥ 11)	16, 14 (if victim is < 11)
Wisconsin	18	18	N/A	N/A
Wyoming	16	N/A	4	N/A

Note: Some states have marital exemptions. This Table assumes the two parties are not married to one another.

A common misperception about statutory rape is that state codes define a single age at which an individual can legally consent to sex. Only 12 states have a *single age of consent,* below which an individual cannot consent to sexual intercourse under any circumstances, and above which it is legal to engage in sexual intercourse with another person above the age of consent. For example, in Massachusetts, the age of consent is 16.

In the remaining 39 states, other factors come into play: age differentials, minimum age of the victim, and minimum age of the defendant. Each is described below.

Minimum age requirement. In 27 states that do not have a single age of consent, statutes specify the age below which an individual cannot legally engage in sexual intercourse regardless of the age of the defendant (see the second column in *Table 16.1*). The minimum age requirements in these states range from 10 to 16 years of age. The legality of sexual intercourse with an individual who is above the minimum age requirement and below the age of consent is dependent on the difference in ages between the two parties and/or the age of the defendant.

- In New Jersey, the age of consent is 16, but individuals who are at least 13 years of age can legally engage in sexual activities if the defendant is less than 4 years older than the victim.

Age differential. In 27 states, the legality of engaging in sexual intercourse with minors is, at least in some circumstances, based on the difference in age between the two parties (see the third column in *Table 16.1*). In 12 of these states, the legality is based solely on the difference between the ages of the two parties. For example:

- In the District of Columbia it is illegal to engage in sexual intercourse with someone who is under the age of consent (16) if the defendant is 4 or more years older than the victim.

Although it is less common, the age differentials in some states vary depending on the age of the victim.

- In Washington, sexual intercourse with someone who is at least 14 years of age and less than 16 years of age is illegal if the defendant is 4 or more years older than the victim. The age differential decreases in cases where the victim is less than 14 years of age (3 years), further decreasing if the victim is less than 12 years of age (2 years).

Minimum age of defendant in order to prosecute. Sixteen states set age thresholds for defendants, below which individuals cannot be prosecuted for engaging in sexual intercourse with minors (see the last column in *Table 15.1*).

- In Nevada, the age of consent is 16; however, sexual intercourse with someone who is under 16 years of age is illegal only if the defendant is at least 18 years of age (the age at which the defendant can be prosecuted).

States that set a minimum age of the defendant also tend to have minimum age requirements for the victim. Often, the age of the defendant is only relevant if the victim is above the minimum age requirement.

- In Ohio, sexual intercourse with someone under 13 years of age is illegal regardless of the age of the defendant. However, if the victim is above this minimum age requirement (13) and below the age of consent (16), it is only illegal to engage in sexual intercourse with that individual if the defendant is at least 18 years of age.

Some states define minimum age thresholds for defendants *and* age differentials.

- In North Carolina, the age of consent is 16. Sexual intercourse with someone who is under the age of consent is only illegal if the defendant is: (1) at least 4 years older than the victim *and* (2) at least 12 years of age (the age at which the defendant can be prosecuted).

Definition of Offenses

States' laws addressing sexual activity involving minors are usually included in the section of the criminal code devoted to sexual offenses.

As noted above, most states do not have laws that specifically use the term "statutory rape;" only five include the offense of statutory rape. More often, state statutes include a variety of offenses addressing voluntary sexual activity involving minors. In New Jersey, for example, sexual activities involving minors is addressed in three offenses: criminal sexual contact, sexual assault, and aggravated sexual assault. The ages of the victim and the defendant as well as the nature of the sexual activity dictate under which offense the conduct falls.

In some cases, provisions addressing statutory rape are embedded in rape or sexual assault laws that typically apply to violent offenses. For example, New Hampshire defines "felonious sexual assault" as voluntary sexual penetration with someone who is at least 13 years of age and under 16 years of age, as well as acts involving the use of physical force irrespective of the age of either party. Other states have separate offenses specifically concerned with sexual crimes involving a minor. For example, Alaska's statute includes four offenses that deal specifically with the sexual abuse of a minor.

State statutes also use a variety of terms when referring to sexual acts (for example, sexual intercourse, sexual penetration, sexual contact, indecent contact), and the definitions of these terms are not always consistent across states.

Understanding the different terms used in a state statute is especially important in those states where an individual may be able to legally consent to one type of sexual activity but not another. For example, Alabama's laws regarding the legality of sexual activities with individuals who are under 16 years of age and more than 12 years of age differ depending on the nature of the activities. In cases involving *sexual intercourse,* defendants over 16 years of age who are at least two years older than the victim are guilty of rape in the second degree. However, *sexual contact* is only illegal in cases where the defendant is at least 19 years of age.

More often though, all of the acts will be illegal (with the same age requirements), but the severity of the punishment will differ based on the type of sexual activity. In Kentucky for example, sexual activities with children under 12 years of age are illegal regardless of the age of the defendant. If the activities amount to sexual contact, the defendant is guilty of first degree *sexual abuse* (a Class D felony); if they amount to *sexual intercourse,* the defendant is guilty of first degree rape (a Class A felony).

Depending on the state, defendants may be exempt from prosecution if they are married to the victim. In some states, marriage is a defense to all of the crimes listed (for example, Alaska, District of Columbia, West Virginia); other states exclude some of the more aggravated offenses from this exemption (for example, Arkansas, Louisiana, Mississippi). In a few states, the criminal statutes identify age limits for the marriage exemptions.

Child Abuse Reporting Requirements

Statutory rape reporting requirements are generally found in the sections of states' codes that deal with juveniles, children and families, domestic relationships, or social services, whereas the criminal or penal codes address the legality of specific offenses. This section of the report summarizes states' child abuse reporting requirements and the extent to which they address the issue of statutory rape. It is divided into four subsections.

- *Subsection 1* examines differences in how state statutes define child abuse and whether these definitions include statutory rape.

- *Subsection 2* discusses which individuals states designate as mandated reporters.

- *Subsection 3* details the actions mandated reporters must take upon encountering cases of child abuse.

- *Subsection 4* deals with agencies' responsibilities upon receiving reports.

Inclusion of Statutory Rape in Reporting Requirements

State statutes vary in the extent to which statutory rape is included in the reporting requirements. In approximately one-third of the states, mandated reporting is limited to those situations where the abuse was perpetrated or allowed by a person responsible for the care of the child. Consider the example of Virginia. Child abuse, a reportable offense, is defined to include any sexual act that is in violation of the state's criminal law, but it is limited to those acts perpetrated by the victim's parent or other person responsible for the child's care.

In two-thirds of the states, the statutes specify circumstances under which child abuse is a reportable offense irrespective of the defendant's relationship to the victim. In some states, the definition of child abuse includes all of the statutory rape offenses detailed in the criminal code (e.g., North Dakota, Ohio, and Wyoming). In such cases, mandated reporters are required to notify the proper authorities if they suspect that a child has been a victim of any of these offenses. More often, states vary in terms of the applicability of the reporting requirements. The following examples illustrate the variation among these states.

In some states, there are only a few specific circumstances under which offenses not involving a person responsible for a child are considered reportable offenses. In Minnesota, for example, such a case is only a reportable offense if the reporter suspects that a defendant has sexually abused two or more children not related to the defendant in the past 10 years. Rhode Island law only requires reports of non-familial cases in two situations: (1) if the defendant is less than 18 years of age; or (2) if the mandated reporter is a physician or nurse practitioner who treats a child who is less than 12 years of age and has been infected with a sexually transmitted disease.

In Iowa, the reporting requirements only pertain to cases involving someone responsible for the care of the child in question. However, a separate provision requires mandated reporters to notify the proper authorities of all cases of sexual abuse involving a victim under 12 years of age regardless of the defendant's relationship to the victim.

In other states there are fewer limits on the applicability of reporting requirements to statutory rape. Often, such limitations are based on the age of the victim and/or the defendant. For example, in California all sexual activity involving minors is illegal. However, the reporting requirements only apply to the violations of certain criminal offenses—namely, those addressing situations involving victims under 16 years of age where there is an especially large difference in the age of the two parties.

In those states where the definition of child abuse does not explicitly refer to statutory rape, discrepancies between the legality of certain sexual activities and whether they are reportable offenses are more common. Take the following examples:

- *Georgia.* The reporting requirements in Georgia are less strict than the state's statutory rape laws. Even though all sexual activities involving someone who is less 16 years of age are illegal (per the criminal code), such acts only constitute a reportable offense if the defendant is more than five years older than the victim.

- *Utah.* In contrast, Utah's reporting requirements define as reportable offenses some activities that are legal according to the state's criminal code. For example, *sexual conduct* with someone who is at least 16 years of age and less than 18 years of age is only illegal if the defendant is 10 or more years older than the victim. However, *sexual abuse*, a reportable offense, is defined to include all acts of sexual intercourse, molestation, or sodomy directed towards someone under 18 years of age regardless of the age of the defendant.

- *Connecticut.* Due to some confusion on the part of providers in the state, the Attorney General's office issued an opinion addressing this issue. Specifically, the Commissioner of the Department of Children and Families sought clarification with respect to the reporting laws as they relate to cases involving defendants under 21 years of age who engage in sexual activities with teenagers under the age of consent. The Attorney General concluded that, although such relationships are illegal if the defendant is more than 2 years older than the victim, mandated reporters are not required to make a report if no other evidence of abuse exists. In justifying the opinion, the Attorney General cited the statute related to the treatment of minors for sexually transmitted diseases, which only requires providers to report cases where the minor seeking treatment is less than 13 years of age.

Mandatory Reporters

Each state's reporting requirements identify certain individuals who are required to notify the authorities of suspected abuse. Although it varies by state, *mandated reporters are typically individuals who*

131

encounter children through their professional capacity. In Pennsylvania, the statute requires *all* individuals who encounter a case of abuse through their professional capacity to make a report. More often, a state's statute will refer to a number of specific professions. Common professions include: physical and mental health providers, teachers, child care workers, legal professionals (e.g., judges, magistrates, attorneys, law enforcement officers), clergy members, and employees of state agencies that deal with children and families. In addition, some states designate any individual who provides care or treatment to children as a mandatory reporter (e.g., Alabama, Missouri, Montana). In 18 states, any individual who suspects that a child has been the victim of abuse is required to notify the proper authorities.

In terms of physical and/or mental health providers (e.g., physicians, nurses, psychologists, psychiatrists, dentists, surgeons, osteopaths), statutes often make specific reference to providers who treat adolescents who are pregnant or infected with sexually transmitted diseases. For example, in Texas any individual who suspects child abuse is required to notify the proper authorities. However, the law also includes more specific reporting requirements for individuals who work with children in a professional capacity, including employees of a clinic or health care facility that provides reproductive services.

In some states, a child who is pregnant or infected with a sexually transmitted disease is sufficient to cause reasonable suspicion of abuse, thereby necessitating a report. In Rhode Island, as noted above, the law requires reports of non-familial cases in two situations, one of which is if the mandated reporter is a physician or nurse practitioner who treats a child less than 12 years of age who is infected with a sexually transmitted disease. Michigan also requires medical providers to report all cases where a child under 12 years of age is pregnant or has a sexually transmitted disease. In contrast, California law states that "the pregnancy of a minor does not, in and of itself, constitute a basis for a reasonable suspicion of sexual abuse." The California Court of Appeals has similarly found that mandated reporters are not required to report cases in which a minor is found to have a sexually transmitted disease.

Few states allow mandated reporters to exercise discretion in deciding which cases to report.

Consider the following three exceptions:

- *Florida.* The criminal code includes a law stating that anyone 21 years of age or older who impregnates a child under 16 years of age is guilty of contributing to the delinquency or dependency of a minor. However, the reporting requirements state that health care professionals and other individuals who provide medical or counseling services to pregnant children are not required to report abuse when the only violation is impregnation of a child under the circumstances described above if such reporting would interfere with the provision of medical services.

- *Tennessee.* A 1996 law addressing statutory rape added a number of provisions to the state statutes with respect to reporting requirements. One such provision addresses cases in which a physician or other person treating pregnant minors learns that the alleged father of the patient's child is at least 4 years older than the patient and not her spouse. The provision *encourages* the provider to notify the appropriate legal authorities. However, such a report can only be made with the consent of the patient or the patient's parent, legal guardian, or custodian.

- *Wisconsin.* Health care practitioners who provide family planning services, pregnancy testing, obstetrical health care or screening, or diagnosis and treatment for sexually transmitted diseases to minors are exempted from the reporting requirements with the following exception: If providers judge that their clients are in a dangerous situation. For example, providers are required to report cases where they believe that: the victim, because of his or her age or immaturity, is incapable of understanding the nature or consequences of sexual activities; the other participant in the sexual acts is exploiting the child; or the child's participation in the sexual acts is not voluntary.

Who to Report To

To varying degrees of specificity, all state statutes provide mandated reporters with instructions for the reporting process. States generally require that mandated reporters notify the appropriate authorities within one to three days of encountering a case of suspected abuse. Mandated reporters can usually make an initial report orally, via telephone. Approximately two-thirds of states require mandated reporters to follow their initial report with a more detailed written report.

The reporting laws usually specify one or more agencies to which reports should be made. Mandated reporters in the majority of states may notify the state or county agency (or its designee) responsible for social or human services, children and families, or child protection.

In roughly two-thirds of states, mandated reporters have the option of notifying law enforcement agencies or prosecutors' offices instead of the child protection agency.

States differ with respect to whether mandated reporters must notify an agency's state office or one of its local offices—typically the one in the local jurisdiction in which the offense took place or the victim resides.

The only states in which the child protection agency is not designated to receive reports are those with separate reporting procedures for cases not involving abuse perpetrated by a person responsible for the victim. Take the example of Louisiana. Mandated reporters must notify the local child protection unit of the Department of Social Services if they suspect abuse perpetrated by: the victim's parent or caretaker; a person who maintains an interpersonal dating or engagement relationship with the parent or caretaker; or a person living in the same residence with the parent or caretaker as a spouse whether married or not. In all other cases, the report must be made to a local or state law enforcement agency.

West Virginia is another example of a state where the reporting requirements depend on the nature of the offense. Local child protective services agencies are responsible for receiving reports of child abuse. If the report alleges sexual abuse, the mandated reporter must also notify the Division of Public Safety and the law enforcement agency with investigative jurisdiction.

State Response

Each state summary highlights the required response of the state and local agencies that receive reports of suspected child abuse. State statutes vary in the level of detail they provide. Generally they include requirements addressing which entities, if any, the agency receiving the initial report must notify, the timeframe for this notification, and the requirements for investigating reported abuse.

States have two primary objectives when responding to allegations of child abuse: (1) ensuring the health, safety, and well-being of the child in question, taking the necessary steps to prevent further harm and (2) conducting an investigation to determine if the reported abuse constitutes a criminal act and, when appropriate, prosecuting offenders.

In most states, the responsibility for the initial investigation of reported child abuse falls to law enforcement, the state agency responsible for child protective services, or some combination of the two.

- Approximately one-half of all states require child protective services or some other human services agency to conduct the initial investigation.

- Local law enforcement agencies are responsible for conducting the initial investigation in approximately one-fifth of states.

- Although rare, in some states either law enforcement or child protective services may conduct initial investigations.

- In the remaining states, the investigation is a cooperative effort among multiple agencies.

In some states, the responsibility for the initial investigation depends on the relationship between the victim and the defendant. In North Carolina, the county Department of Social Services is generally responsible for the initial investigation of reported abuse. However, cases alleging abuse by a person not responsible for the care of the victim must be immediately forwarded to law enforcement and the district attorney's office. Such provisions are common in states where the definition of child abuse does not include statutory rape. Consider Iowa, where statutory rape is only included in the definition of child abuse—thereby making it a reportable offense—if the victim is under 12 years of age. The agency responsible for receiving and investigating reports of child abuse (the Department of Human Services) must refer to the appropriate law enforcement agency all cases that would constitute child abuse if not for the fact that the act was perpetrated by someone not responsible for the care of the child.

Generally, law enforcement is responsible for conducting investigations into criminal acts, whereas child protective services and human services agencies are primarily concerned with the well-being of the victim. For example, in Rhode Island, the Department of Children, Youth, and Families investigates all reported abuse. If the Department's investigation indicates that the child in question has been the victim of criminal abuse, the Department transfers the case to law enforcement so that it may initiate a criminal investigation.

Increasingly, states are emphasizing interagency collaboration in child abuse investigations. Almost one-half of states statutes require the involvement of multiple agencies in investigations. There is wide variation among states in the level of cooperation mandated by their statutes. Often law enforcement and child protective services maintain their traditional roles, and the laws focus on information sharing and maximizing the relative strengths of each agency. Nevada law states that if the initial evaluation of the report, conducted by the child welfare services agency, indicates that if an investigation is warranted, the agency and law enforcement must cooperate with one another and coordinate their investigation. Similarly, Hawaii statutes require the Department of Human Services to provide police and prosecutors with any relevant information that would aid in the investigation or prosecution of child abuse cases.

States can formalize such cooperation by requiring relevant agencies to develop a memorandum of understanding (MOU) for responding to reported abuse. In Ohio, the county public children services agency (usually the Department of Job and Family Services) is responsible for preparing the MOU. The MOU must delineate the roles and responsibilities of each partner and establish processes for coordinating investigations. The agency must ensure that the following officials sign the MOU: a juvenile judge in the county; the county peace officer, chief municipal peace officers, and local other law enforcement officers that handle abuse cases; the prosecuting attorney of the county; and the county humane officer. The primary goal of Ohio's MOU is to eliminate unnecessary and redundant interviews with victims.

Other states require that multi-disciplinary teams assume responsibility for the investigative process. The District of Columbia Code mandates that all child sexual abuse investigations be conducted by a multi-disciplinary team that must include at least one representative from: law enforcement, social services, child advocacy centers, and the city and federal prosecutors' offices. Additional individuals eligible for inclusion in multi-disciplinary teams include: representatives from the public schools, mental and physical health practitioners, child development specialists, and victim counselors. Teams' efforts are to be governed by a written protocol outlining investigative responsibilities, prosecutorial procedures, and treatment options and services for both victims and defendants.

Chapter 17

When Your Child Is Sexually Abused

If Your Child Is Raped

Rape—forced, unwanted sexual intercourse—can happen to males and females of any age. Rape is a sexual assault. It's not about love or sex. It's about power. A rapist uses actual or threatened force or violence to exert control over another person. Some rapists use drugs or alcohol to take away a person's ability to fight back.

Rape is a crime, no matter if the person committing the rape is a stranger, acquaintance, date, friend, or family member.

Someone who has been raped needs medical care, comfort, understanding, and support. Here's what to do if your daughter or son is the victim of a rape.

How to Tell

If your child is sexually assaulted, he or she might choose not to tell you. Preteens and teenagers often confide only in friends about deeply personal issues—and, unfortunately, something as serious as rape is no exception.

Also, laws in some states don't require parents to be notified if a teenager under age 18 has called a rape crisis center or visited a clinic for evaluation.

This chapter includes text excerpted from "If Your Child Is Raped," © 1995–2016. The Nemours Foundation/KidsHealth®. Reprinted with permission.

But even if your child doesn't confide in you, some signs can indicate that he or she is struggling emotionally—whether due to rape or something else—and needs your help. For example, your child might:

- act unusually irritable, moody, or cranky

- seem angry, frightened, or confused

- feel depressed, anxious, or nervous, especially about being alone

- withdraw from friends and family

- have trouble sleeping

- have changes in appetite

- be unable to concentrate in school or to participate in everyday activities

These may be signs of post-traumatic stress disorder (PTSD) or what's sometimes called rape trauma syndrome. If you see symptoms like these, reach out and let your daughter or son know that you're always available to listen, no matter what.

If your child still won't open up and you continue to suspect some kind of trauma or distress, seek a therapist's help to get to the root of the problem.

Seeking Medical Care

If you find out that your child is the victim of rape, it's important to seek help as soon as possible. Rapes fall into two categories: **Acute rapes** (happening within the last 72 hours) and **non-acute rapes** (happening more than 72 hours ago).

Acute rapes. If the rape happened within the last 72 hours (3 days), take your child to an emergency room immediately, call the police, or call a rape crisis hotline. Hotlines can offer guidance on what to do, including finding a hospital nearby that has a program set up specially to care for rape victims. The national sexual assault hotline at 1-800-656-HOPE (1-800-656-4673) is one you can call. (You also can call the police to report the assault before going to the hospital, but know that doctors and nurses usually report sexual assaults to the authorities.)

At the hospital, your child will be checked for sexually transmitted diseases (STDs) (also called sexually transmitted infections, or STIs) and internal injuries. Many medical facilities have people who are trained to care for someone whose been raped, such as a forensic nurse examiner (FNE) or sexual assault nurse examiner (SANE).

If possible, seek medical care before your child has changed clothes, showered, or douched. It can be hard not to clean up, of course—it's a natural human instinct to wash away all traces of a sexual assault. But being examined right away is the best way to ensure timely medical treatment and help with the collection of evidence.

In most states or cities, the window of time for gathering medical evidence for an acute rape is usually within the first 72 hours. But some jurisdictions have a longer threshold of time, such as up to 96 hours or even 2 weeks.

After getting appropriate medical care, notify the police if you haven't already. The police will take a report and document the incident, as well as collect any evidence.

Non-acute rapes. If the rape happened more than 72 hours (3 days) ago, call the police. You can also call a rape crisis hotline for counseling on next steps, including talking to the police and getting a medical evaluation. The police will want to take a report and document the incident, as well as collect any evidence. After that, your child should get a medical evaluation.

What to Expect during the Exam

Before the exam, a trained doctor, nurse, counselor, or social worker will listen to your daughter or son talk about what happened. This conversation will direct medical treatment and may help with the investigation of the crime. Talking to a trained listener also helps your child release some of the emotions associated with the experience, and can help her or him begin feeling calm and safe again.

The medical professional also might talk about the exam, what it involves, and ask for parental consent. Each state or jurisdiction may have different requirements, but most medical exams (for both acute and non-acute rape cases) are likely to include these steps:

If your child has gone through puberty:

- A medical professional may test for STDs/STIs, including HIV/AIDS. These tests may involve taking blood or saliva samples. Although the thought of having an STD after a rape is extremely scary, the quicker one is diagnosed, the more effectively it can be treated. Doctors can start your child on immediate treatment courses for STDs, including HIV/AIDS, which can help protect against developing these diseases.

- If your daughter is raped, a medical professional may treat her for unwanted pregnancy, if she chooses.

- A medical professional will examine your child internally and externally to check for any injury that might have been caused by the rape.

- A medical professional or trained technician may look for and take samples of the rapist's hair, skin, nails, or bodily fluids from your child's clothes or body.

- If you think your child has been given a rape drug, a doctor or technician can test for this, too.

- Pictures of any injuries may be taken for documentation purposes.

If your child has not yet gone through puberty:

- A medical professional may test for STDs, including HIV/AIDS. These tests may involve taking blood or saliva samples. Although the thought of having an STD after a rape is extremely scary, the quicker one is diagnosed, the more effectively it can be treated.

- A medical professional will perform an external examination on your child to check for any injury that might have been caused by the rape.

- A medical professional or trained technician may look for and take samples of the rapist's hair, skin, nails, or bodily fluids from your child's clothes or body.

- If you think your child has been given a rape drug, a doctor or technician can test for this, too.

- Pictures of any injuries may be taken for documentation purposes.

Even if your child doesn't get examined right away, it doesn't mean that he or she can't get a checkup later. A person can still go to a doctor or local clinic to get checked out for STDs, pregnancy, or injuries any time after being raped. In some cases, doctors can even gather evidence several days after a rape has occurred.

Exams Important for Prosecuting a Crime

Getting medical attention is recommended not just to ensure your child's health and safety, but also to provide documentation for any future criminal investigations. Medical centers and hospitals often report a sexual assault (or suspected sexual assault) to the police.

If a criminal case is pursued by authorities, medical tests may help provide the evidence needed to prosecute the rapist. Keep in mind, the statutes of limitations on rape give a person only a certain amount of time to pursue legal action, so be sure you know how long you have to report the rape. A local rape crisis center can advise you of the laws in your state.

Addressing Emotional Health

Those who have been raped sometimes avoid seeking help because they're afraid that talking about it will bring back memories or feelings that are too painful. But this can actually do more harm than good.

Seeking help and emotional support from a trained professional is the best way to ensure long-term healing. Working through the pain sooner rather than later can help reduce symptoms like nightmares and flashbacks. It also can help someone avoid potentially harmful behaviors and emotions, like major depression or self-injury.

How rape survivors work through feelings can vary. Ask your child what sort of counseling is preferable: Some people feel most comfortable talking one-on-one with a therapist. Others find that joining a support group where they can be with other survivors helps them to feel better, get their power back, and move on with their lives. In a support group, they can get help and might help others heal by sharing their own experiences and ideas.

Chapter 18

Extraterritorial Sexual Exploitation of Children

What Extraterritorial Sexual Exploitation of Children Mean

The extraterritorial sexual exploitation of children is the act of traveling to a foreign country and engaging in sexual activity with a child in that country. Federal law prohibits an American citizen or resident to travel to a foreign country with intent to engage in any form of sexual conduct with a minor (defined as persons under 18 years of age). It is also illegal to help organize or assist another person to travel for these purposes. This crime is a form of human trafficking, also referred to as child sex tourism. Convicted offenders face fines and up to 30 years of imprisonment.

The Crime Today

The relative ease of international travel in modern-day society has led to the growth of a dark, more clandestine phenomenon–the extraterritorial sexual exploitation of children. The various modes of international travel provide easier means and more opportunities for individuals to travel abroad and engage in sexual activity with children.

This chapter includes text excerpted from "Extraterritorial Sexual Exploitation of Children," U.S. Department of Justice (DOJ), January 25, 2016.

143

In addition, technological advances have revolutionized the travel industry. The Internet allows individuals to quickly and easily exchange information about how and where to find child victims in foreign locations. Violators are also finding it easier to organize and navigate travel to foreign countries for these purposes online. Moreover, the utilization of the Internet may promote or encourage others to become involved in this form of child sexual exploitation.

American Offenders

Each year, Americans are convicted of committing this crime against children. While some offenders are pedophiles who preferentially seek out children for sexual relationships, others are situational abusers. These individuals do not consistently seek out children as sexual partners, but do occasionally engage in sexual acts with children when the opportunity presents itself. Children from developing countries are seen as easy targets by American perpetrators because they are often disadvantaged by unstable or unfavorable economic, social, or political conditions, or their home country lacks effective law enforcement against this crime. However, incidents of the extraterritorial sexual exploitation of children involving American perpetrators are reported and occur all over the world, including less developed areas in Southeast Asia, Central and South America, to more developed areas in Europe.

Some perpetrators rationalize their sexual encounters with children with the idea that they are helping the children financially better themselves and their families. Other perpetrators are drawn towards this crime because they enjoy the anonymity that comes with being in a foreign land. Racism, gender discrimination, and cultural differences are among other justifications. However, the reason for travel makes no difference under the law; any American citizen or resident who engages in sexual conduct with a minor in a foreign land is subject to federal prosecution.

CEOS's Role

Child Exploitation and Obscenity Section (CEOS) attorneys work with the High Technology Investigative Unit (HTIU), the Federal Bureau of Investigation (FBI), Immigration and Customs Enforcement/Homeland Security Investigations (ICE), United States Attorney's Offices around the country, as well as foreign governments and law enforcement personnel to investigate and prosecute cases arising under federal statutes prohibiting the extraterritorial sexual exploitation of children.

CEOS is dedicated to developing strategies and long-lasting relationships with foreign governments, law enforcement agencies, and prosecutors to more efficiently and effectively prosecute Americans sexually exploiting children in foreign countries. The enforcement of these laws abroad is part of the United States' effort to eradicate the sexual exploitation of children. Offenders prosecuted in the United States often face more appropriate penalties than if they were prosecuted in the country where the sexual abuse occurred.

In addition, CEOS attorneys travel all over the country to conduct trainings for investigators, law enforcement personnel and others involved in efforts to investigate and prosecute this crime. Moreover, CEOS designs, implements, and supports law enforcement strategies, legislative proposals, and policy initiatives relating to federal laws on the extraterritorial sexual exploitation of children.

Part Three

Child Neglect and Emotional Abuse

Chapter 19

Child Neglect

Chapter Contents

Section 19.1

Definition and Scope of Neglect

This section includes text excerpted from "Acts of Omission: An Overview of Child Neglect," U.S. Department of Health and Human Services (HHS), August 2012. Reviewed May 2016.

An Overview of Child Neglect

Neglect accounts for over three-quarters of confirmed cases of child maltreatment in the United States—far more than physical or sexual abuse—but it continues to receive less attention from practitioners, researchers, and the media. Some reasons may be that neglect is not well understood and is difficult to identify, prevent, and treat effectively. This bulletin for professionals addresses the scope of the problem of child neglect as well as its consequences, reviews definitions and strategies for assessing neglect, presents lessons learned about prevention and intervention, and suggests sources of training and informational support.

Scope of the Problem

- Neglect is by far the most common form of maltreatment. More than 538,000 children were neglected in 2010, accounting for about 78 percent of all unique victims of child maltreatment. In addition, neglect was either the sole cause or one of the contributors to over 68 percent of the 1,560 child maltreatment-related deaths in 2010.

These statistics include only children who came to the attention of State child protective services (CPS) agencies. The National Incidence Study (NIS) of Child Abuse and Neglect, which generates broader estimates by gathering data from multiple sources, generally shows higher numbers of maltreatment. The NIS-4, which is the most recent version, uses data from 2005–2006 to show that more than 770,000 children were neglected, accounting for about 77 percent of all children harmed or endangered by maltreatment. While the incidence of other maltreatment types has declined in recent years, the persistently high rates of neglect point to the need for more effective prevention and intervention in cases of neglect.

Defining Child Neglect

Both Federal and State laws provide basic definitions of child abuse and neglect. The Federal Child Abuse Prevention and Treatment Act (CAPTA) (42 U.S.C.A. §5106g), as amended by the CAPTA Reauthorization Act of 2010, defines child abuse and neglect as, at minimum:

- Any recent act or failure to act on the part of a parent or caretaker which results in death, serious physical or emotional harm, sexual abuse or exploitation; or

- An act or failure to act which presents an imminent risk of serious harm.

Neglect is commonly defined in State law as the failure of a parent or other person with responsibility for the child to provide needed food, clothing, shelter, medical care, or supervision to the degree that the child's health, safety, and well-being are threatened with harm. Some States specifically mention types of neglect in their statutes, such as educational neglect, medical neglect, and abandonment; in addition, some States include exceptions for determining neglect, such as religious exemptions for medical neglect and financial considerations for physical neglect (Child Welfare Information Gateway, 2011b)

Neglect definitions are impacted by the accepted standards of care for children and the role of communities in families' lives. Some issues that are taken into account when defining neglect and standards of care include:

- Harm to the child

- Parent's ability or intent

- Family's concrete resources

- Community norms

- Availability of community resources

Difficulties in creating specific definitions of neglect contribute to the lack of consistency in research on neglect as well as CPS responses to neglect. The different ways children may be neglected, addressed below, also make it difficult to define such a complex issue.

Section 19.2

Types and Consequences of Neglect

This section includes text excerpted from "Acts of Omission:
An Overview of Child Neglect," U.S. Department of Health and
Human Services (HHS), August 2012. Reviewed May 2016.

Types of Neglect

Although State laws vary regarding the types of neglect included
in definitions, summarized below are the most commonly recognized
categories of neglect:

- **Physical neglect:** Abandoning the child or refusing to accept
  custody; not providing for basic needs like nutrition, hygiene, or
  appropriate clothing

- **Medical neglect:** Delaying or denying recommended health
  care for the child

- **Inadequate supervision:** Leaving the child unsupervised
  (depending on length of time and child's age/maturity); not protecting the child from safety hazards, providing inadequate caregivers, or engaging in harmful behavior

- **Emotional neglect:** Isolating the child; not providing affection
  or emotional support; exposing the child to domestic violence or
  substance abuse

- **Educational neglect:** Failing to enroll the child in school
  or homeschool; ignoring special education needs; permitting
  chronic absenteeism from school

Consequences of Neglect

Although the initial impact may not be as obvious as physical or
sexual abuse, the consequences of child neglect are just as serious.
Because the effects of neglect are cumulative, long-term research like
that being performed by the Longitudinal Studies of Child Abuse and
Neglect, funded by the Children's Bureau, helps us better understand
outcomes for children affected by neglect.

Research shows child neglect can have a negative impact in the following areas:

- Health and physical development—malnourishment, impaired brain development, delays in growth or failure to thrive

- Intellectual and cognitive development—poor academic performance, delayed or impaired language development

- Emotional and psychological development—deficiencies in self-esteem, attachment, or trust

- Social and behavioral development—interpersonal relationship problems, aggression, conduct disorders

The impacts in these areas are interrelated; problems in one developmental area may influence growth in another area. In addition, research indicates that experiencing neglect along with other forms of maltreatment worsens the impact. However, the impact of neglect can vary based on:

- The child's age

- The presence and strength of protective factors

- The frequency, duration, and severity of the neglect

- The relationship between the child and caregiver

Trauma and Neglect

While trauma is often discussed in terms of witnessing or being harmed by an intensely threatening event, one or multiple experiences of neglect can also have a traumatic effect, especially in severe cases. One recent study found that, similar to physical and sexual abuse, neglected children showed signs of posttraumatic stress disorder and other traumatic symptoms. Funded by the Federal Child Neglect Consortium, De Bellis (2005) summarized the results of numerous research studies that found that neglected children experienced adverse brain development and neuropsychological and psychosocial outcomes.

Fatal Neglect

A child's death is the most tragic consequence of neglect, and neglect causes or contributes to roughly two-thirds of all child maltreatment related deaths. Victims of fatal neglect are more likely to be age 7 or younger.

The most common reasons for fatal neglect are supervision neglect, chronic physical neglect, and medical neglect. Neglect fatalities can be difficult to identify due to lack of definitive evidence, limited investigative and training resources, and differing interpretations of child maltreatment definitions.

Section 19.3

Risk Factors and Special Considerations

This section includes text excerpted from "Acts of Omission: An Overview of Child Neglect," U.S. Department of Health and Human Services (HHS), August 2012. Reviewed May 2016.

Risk Factors

While the presence of a risk factor does not mean a child will be neglected, multiple risk factors are a cause for concern. Research indicates that the following factors place children at greater risk of being harmed or endangered by neglect:

Environmental Factors

- Poverty
- Lack of social support
- Neighborhood distress

Family Factors

- Single parent households
- Family stress or negative interactions
- Domestic violence

Parent Factors

- Unemployment or low socioeconomic status
- Young maternal age

- Health, mental illness, or substance use problems
- Parenting stress

Child Factors

- Age
- Developmental delays

Ultimately, as Straus and Kaufman (2005) caution, the only certain risk is that the more often a child experiences neglect, the more likely he or she will be harmed by it—which is why prevention and early identification of neglect are critical.

Protective Factors

Although a number of factors place children at greater risk of neglect, research shows that families with one or more of the following protective factors are less likely to experience abuse or neglect:

- Nurturing and attachment
- Knowledge of parenting and child development
- Parental resilience
- Social connections
- Concrete supports for parents
- Social and emotional competence of children

Protective factors are a key component of the Children's Bureau's national child abuse prevention initiative.

Special Considerations

Neglect rarely occurs in isolation; commonly related issues include poverty, substance abuse, and domestic violence. There are special considerations for addressing these issues with at-risk or neglected children and their families.

Poverty

Poverty is frequently linked to child neglect, but it is important to note that most poor families do not neglect their children. Poverty likely increases the risk of neglect by interacting with and worsening related risks like "parental stress, inadequate housing and homelessness, lack of basic needs, inadequate supervision, substance abuse, and domestic violence"

Caseworkers must differentiate between neglectful situations and poverty; in many States, definitions of neglect include considerations for a family's financial means. For example, if a family living in poverty was not providing adequate food for their children, it would be considered neglect only if the parents were aware of but chose not to use food assistance programs. Taking poverty into consideration can prevent unnecessary removals and place the focus on providing concrete services for families to protect and provide for their children.

Substance Abuse

Parental substance abuse is more closely related to child neglect than other forms of maltreatment. Parents who lose control under the influence of substances may have impaired reasoning abilities, leave the child in an unsafe situation, or neglect the child's basic needs. These parents may also have difficulty conforming to expected parenting roles and providing the child with emotional support. While treating the parent's substance abuse is a priority, treatment must be combined with services to address the child's needs and improve overall family functioning.

Substance-exposed newborns. When a woman abuses drugs or alcohol during her pregnancy, the unborn child is at greater risk for developmental delays. In addition, some substance-exposed newborns are left at the hospital by their parents; these infants, sometimes referred to as "boarder babies," usually require CPS intervention to place them in out-of-home care. Child welfare caseworkers and healthcare providers must work together to identify, assess, and develop a plan to care for affected infants and their families.

Domestic Violence

Some States include exposure to domestic violence in their legal definitions of child abuse or neglect due to its potential effects on children (Child Welfare Information Gateway, 2011c). An unintended consequence of these policies is that parents who are domestic violence victims sometimes are charged with a type of neglect termed "failure to protect," despite circumstances that may have impacted the victim's ability to prevent the child's exposure to violence. Child welfare caseworkers, in collaboration with domestic violence professionals, should consider the victim's access to resources or services outside the home as well as the victim's reasonable efforts to ensure the child had basic necessities and lived in the least detrimental environment possible.

A strong relationship with the victim parent is a protective factor that can increase the child's resilience, and research indicates one of the most effective ways to protect the child is to keep the victim safe. To address domestic violence cases involving children, workers should keep the victim parent and child together whenever possible; enhance the safety, stability, and well-being of all victims; and hold perpetrators of violence accountable through mechanisms such as batterer intervention programs.

Educational Neglect

Many States struggle to respond efficiently to reports of educational neglect due to overlapping responsibilities and lack of coordination between the departments of social services and education. A national review by Kelly (2010) found that nearly half of States neither define educational neglect in law nor hold one agency responsible for reporting it. There is inconsistency among the remaining States regarding which agency is responsible for enforcing neglect provisions, including the court, the school or school district, and the department of education.

Kelly (2010) recommends that the State's department of social services be primarily responsible for addressing educational neglect because it is better equipped to address the co-occurring problems families often face. He also cites promising programs in Missouri and Idaho that offer coordinated and flexible services through the department of social services to respond quickly to families in crisis and at risk of educational neglect.

Section 19.4

Recognizing Child Neglect

This section includes text excerpted from "Acts of Omission: An Overview of Child Neglect," U.S. Department of Health and Human Services (HHS), August 2012. Reviewed May 2016.

Investigation and Assessment

Identifying child neglect may seem more difficult than identifying other forms of maltreatment because neglect usually involves the absence of a certain behavior, rather than the presence. A thorough investigation of the child's safety and risk followed by a comprehensive family assessment can help determine what kinds of services and supports the family may need.

Consider the possibility of neglect when the child:

- Is frequently absent from school
- Begs or steals food or money
- Lacks needed medical or dental care, immunizations, or glasses
- Is consistently dirty and has severe body odor
- Lacks sufficient clothing for the weather
- Abuses alcohol or other drugs
- States that there is no one at home to provide care

Consider the possibility of neglect when the parent or other adult caregiver:

- Appears to be indifferent to the child
- Seems apathetic or depressed
- Behaves irrationally or in a bizarre manner
- Is abusing alcohol or other drugs

Investigation

The initial investigation should determine if neglect occurred and examine the child's safety and risk. Two of the most important factors to consider are (1) whether the child has any unmet cognitive, physical, or emotional needs and (2) whether the child receives adequate supervision.

Straus and Kaufman (2005) offer the following tips to assess neglect in families:

Gather information from multiple sources (child and parent self-reports; caseworker and neighbor observations)

- Ensure confidentiality to collect more honest and accurate reports

- Use nonjudgmental, open-ended questions that encourage diverse viewpoints on the situation

- Probe for signs of different types of neglect

- Consider contexts like the child's age, the home environment, and community resources

- Note the severity and frequency of neglect incidents and the length of time since the last incident and between multiple incidents

Safety. Determining the child's safety is as critical in the decision-making process in cases of possible neglect as it is in physical or sexual abuse cases. The determination should consider threats of danger in the family, the child's vulnerability, and the family's protective capacity. Lund and Renne (2009) encourage caseworkers to investigate the following key threats of danger:

- No adult in the home routinely performs basic and essential parenting duties and responsibilities

- The parent lacks sufficient resources, such as food and shelter, or parenting knowledge, skills, and motivation to meet the child's basic needs

- Living arrangements seriously endanger the child's physical health

- The parent refuses and/or fails to meet the child's needs or arrange care when the child:

  - Exhibits self-destructive behavior or serious emotional symptoms requiring immediate help

  - Has exceptional needs that can result in severe consequences to the child

- Has serious physical injuries or symptoms from maltreatment

The results of the investigation will inform whether the family requires additional assessment and intervention. A low-risk family may be referred for differential response, while the most severe cases may require placement in out-of-home care, preferably with relatives, to ensure the child's immediate safety while the family is assessed and a safety and service plan is developed.

Differential Response

Although one report or incident of neglect may not require CPS response, many families could still benefit from services. Particularly in cases of neglect, by the time the situation becomes serious enough for the child welfare system to respond, the family's issues are likely more complex and require intensive intervention.

To address this service gap, many States use differential response systems in which families with low risk are redirected to voluntary, often community-based, services to receive the supports they need.

Assessment

A comprehensive family assessment should help uncover the potential causes of neglect and underlying factors affecting the family's ability to care for the child. Because neglected children and their families often face complex issues, it is critical to use a holistic approach that looks at the child, family, and community context to identify strengths and the most effective ways to reduce risks and to engage the family in the assessment process.

The key purposes of assessment are:

- To **understand** the neglect and its impact on the child and family

- To **make decisions** to plan for the child's safety and connect the family to services

- To **engage** the family and its extended support network in services

Overarching categories for assessing child neglect include:

- The child's cognitive, physical, and emotional needs and capacities

- The parent's expectations and parenting abilities
- The family's circumstances, attitudes, and behaviors
- Family members' interactions and relationships in and outside the home.

To focus on strengths during the assessment process, the Children's Bureau's Preventing Child Maltreatment and Promoting Well Being: A Network for Action 2012 Resource Guide emphasizes identifying and enhancing the following protective factors in at-risk families:

- Nurturing and attachment
- Knowledge of parenting and child development
- Parental resilience
- Social connections
- Concrete supports for parents
- Social and emotional competence of children

The assessment process ultimately informs the level of intervention necessary for the family. Assessment should continue throughout the family's case to ensure progress toward goals.

Chapter 20

Neglect of Children's Health Care

Defining Neglected Health

Neglect of children's health is difficult to define in a precise way because this type of neglect can take many forms. Many different factors are considered when identifying neglect, including actual harm, the potential for harm, short-term and long-term consequences, physical and mental consequences, and availability of medical care. Health care neglect also covers the full spectrum of a child's condition, including physical, dental, and mental health.

One simple definition states that health care neglect occurs when a child's basic needs are not met, and when those unmet needs present substantial or life-threatening risk to the child. Under this definition, the determination of substantial risk is somewhat subjective and depends upon the opinion of an authority figure such as a health care provider or social worker. Another definition of child health neglect goes a step further and includes the probability that meeting the child's needs would result in a greatly improved quality of life and/or possibly saving the child's life. There is also a legal definition of neglect which requires evidence that parents failed to seek medical attention for their child.

"Neglect of Children's Health Care," © 2016 Omnigraphics, Inc. Reviewed May 2016.

Child health care neglect is also defined by severity. For example, lack of medical care for a bump or bruise might not be seen as neglect, but failure to seek medical attention for a broken are most likely would be seen as neglect. The frequency of potentially neglectful episodes is considered when defining child health neglect. Repeated or persistent absence of medical attention when needed is much more likely to be cited as neglect than a missed appointment or two.

Harm Caused by Neglect of Medical Health

Children can experience harm due to health care neglect in a variety of ways. Physical, mental, and behavioral problems can all arise from neglected health care, and children may suffer from problems in more than one area. Babies and toddlers without adequate health care can develop a low-weight condition known as failure to thrive. Lack of adequate health care in toddlers and young children can cause brain disorders, learning disabilities, and other developmental delays. Children can suffer from emotional problems such as depression and anxiety. In the absence of professional medical care, older children may turn to self-medicating behaviors for untreated physical or mental conditions. Self-medication often includes substance abuse, drug use, overeating, smoking, or other high-risk activities. These attempts to self-medicate can result in new health problems including cancer, addiction, or sexually transmitted diseases.

Factors Determining Neglected Health

Just as there is no single definition of child health neglect, there is also no single cause. Health neglect in children is often the result of a combination of issues at home, in the community, and in society at large. Poverty is a major contributing factor to health care neglect in children, as is the environment in which a child lives. Children are much more likely to experience health care neglect if they live in families affected by drug or alcohol abuse, chronic unemployment, eviction or homelessness, criminal activity, chronic or serious illness, domestic violence, or social isolation. The untreated physical and mental illnesses of caregivers can also be a factor in child health care neglect.

The intellectual ability of caregivers often plays a role in child health care neglect. In order for children to receive adequate health care, caregivers must be able to identify and understand the child's problem, respond appropriately to the problem, and implement recommended treatment. Other factors include a lack of understanding of the recommended treatment, perceived or actual adverse side effects of treatment, and the cost of treatment. Sometimes the child is also directly or indirectly responsible for his or her own health care neglect, such as in cases of older children refusing to comply with recommended treatment.

Incidence / Prevalence

Because health care neglect is difficult to define, it is difficult to measure the true extent of child health care neglect. It is generally understood that neglect of children's dental care is widespread, and it is also known that millions of children in the United States live without access to adequate health care and health insurance coverage.

Manifestations of Neglected Health Care

Child health care neglect manifests in several ways. The most common are not seeking medical attention when necessary, not following recommended treatment, missed appointments, and unfilled prescriptions for medication. Some health care neglect occurs when caregivers are aware of the need for treatment, but refuse treatment based on religious beliefs. In these cases, lack of medical care is often not labeled as neglect. Thirty U.S. states have religious exemptions from child abuse statutes where medical care is concerned.

Neglected health care can also manifest as environmental hazards. Examples include exposure to toxic materials such as lead paint in the home, exposure to dangerous objects such as unsecured weapons, exposure to domestic violence, failure to use a car seat or seat belt, failure to use a bicycle helmet, and prenatal drug or alcohol abuse by pregnant women.

Principles for Assessing Neglected Health Care

Child health care neglect manifests in several ways. The most common are not seeking medical attention when necessary, not following recommended treatment, missed appointments, and unfilled prescriptions for medication. Some health care neglect occurs when caregivers are aware of the need for treatment, but refuse treatment based on religious beliefs. In these cases, lack of medical care is often not labelled as neglect. Thirty U.S. states have religious exemptions from child abuse statutes where medical care is concerned.

Neglected health care can also manifest as environmental hazards. Examples include exposure to toxic materials such as lead paint in the home, exposure to dangerous objects such as unsecured weapons, exposure to domestic violence, failure to use a car seat or seat belt, failure to use a bicycle helmet, and prenatal drug or alcohol abuse by pregnant women.

References

1. Dubowitz, Howard. "Neglect of Children's Health Care." *The APSAC Handbook on Child Maltreatment, 3rd ed.* Edited by John E.B. Myers. Thousand Oaks, CA: Sage Publications, 2011.

2. "Long-Term Consequences of Child Abuse and Neglect." Child Welfare Information Gateway. July 2013.

3. "Medical Neglect." *Child Welfare Manual.* May 3, 2005.

Chapter 21

Educational Neglect and Truancy

Defining Educational Neglect

Educational neglect occurs when a child frequently misses school because of the direct or indirect actions of caregivers. This type of neglect includes failure to enroll children in school or to implement an adequate homeschooling program if allowed by law, and failure to ensure that children attend school as required by law. In many cases of excessive absence from school, educational neglect is considered to occur only when the caregiver refuses to work with the school in attempts to improve the child's attendance.

Characteristics of Educational Neglect

Educational neglect takes many forms, and each case varies according to individual circumstances. Educational neglect situations typically include more than one characteristic. When caregivers do not regard school attendance as important, children may not be prepared to attend school each day (e.g. child is not fed and dressed in time for school). Young children are often dependent upon the caregiver to ensure regular school attendance, and caregivers may fail to accomplish this. Once an attendance problem is identified by the school,

"Educational Neglect and Truancy," © 2016 Omnigraphics, Inc. Reviewed May 2016.

caregivers are typically contacted to participate in an intervention plan that will encourage children to attend school regularly. Educational neglect occurs when caregivers ignore attempts by the school to discuss and address the child's attendance problem and/or refuse to encourage or facilitate the child's school attendance. Caregivers may also fail to comply with special education or remedial instruction programs for the child when the child is not succeeding in school.

Children are at risk of educational neglect when they experience a chaotic or disorganized home life. Some children suffer from the family's lack of sufficient financial resources and are responsible for caring for other children while the caregiver is at work. In many cases of educational neglect, other indicators of child abuse or neglect are also present.

Different Types of Educational Neglect

There are several different types of educational neglect. Caregivers may fail to enroll children in school or establish a homeschooling program where permitted by law. Educational neglect occurs when this failure to enroll causes the child to miss at least one month of school without valid reasons. Caregivers may also fail to seek adequate education for children with special needs, or fail to comply with recommendations for special education. If the child has been diagnosed with a learning disability, educational neglect intersects with health care neglect.

School Truancy

Truancy is another type of educational neglect. A truant is generally defined as a child between the ages of six and 17 who is often absent from school without valid reasons. In addition to missing whole days of school, truancy can also apply to frequently arriving late or skipping classes. A distinction is often made between educational neglect and truancy. If a child misses school as a result of their own choices, that is generally considered truancy and not educational neglect.

Permitted truancy means that caregivers have been informed of the child's excessive absences and do nothing to resolve the problem. Habitual truancy applies to children between the ages of 12 and 17 who fail to comply with intervention plans developed and agreed upon by the school and caregivers, and who continues to miss school without valid reasons. Chronic truancy refers to children between the ages of 12 and 17 who receive a court order to attend school and continue to miss school without valid reasons.

Effects of School Truancy

School truancy affects children in many ways. Early effects include required participation in school-based intervention programs and increased monitoring by schools. If these programs are not successful, children may be referred to a government- or school-sponsored program in which a social worker or other caseworker attempts to resolve the truancy problem. Court intervention may be required, in which children and their parents must appear before a judge or other court official. At this stage, the court can set requirements for school attendance, often with strict consequences for non-compliance. A legal charge of truancy is a serious offense that can result in the child being removed from the home and placed under the jurisdiction of the court. Sometimes the court will order the family or caregiver to pay for the cost of intervention services for the child.

Longer-term effects of school truancy can also be quite serious. Missing many days of school usually results in poor performance when the child does attend classes. Children can then become discouraged and drop out of school entirely. Quitting school has been shown to greatly limit future career opportunities, while increasing the probability of engaging in criminal activity. Children who leave school are more likely to use alcohol and other drugs. Parents and caregivers also suffer the consequences of school truancy through lost income or work time to attend meetings, court hearing, counseling, or other intervention services.

Factors Responsible for School Truancy

There are many different factors that contribute to truancy. Some of the most common are issues associated with a troubled home life. This includes any problem that causes disruption at home, such as domestic violence, substance abuse, marital problems and divorce, a family that moves around a lot, or caregivers whose work schedules leave children frequently unsupervised. Medical issues with mental health or chronic illness of children or caregivers can also contribute to truancy. Children with learning disabilities sometimes find school too frustrating and discouraging, and choose not to attend for these reasons. A family history of school dropouts can lead to caregivers who do not value education.

Other potential causes of truancy are based on economic factors. Poverty may require caregivers to work multiple jobs, and older children may also be required to work to help support the family. A lack of transportation and/or affordable care for younger children also contribute to school truancy. The environment at school can also be a factor. Large schools, large class sizes, the behavior of other students, the attitudes of teachers and school administrators, and lack of individual attention can all result in truancy. Another issue in some schools is the lack of consequences for truancy, or inconsistent truancy policies.

References

1. "Educational Neglect." *Child Welfare Manual*. August 28, 2009.

2. "Educational Neglect and School Truancy: What Parents and Children Need to Know." Youth Assistance of Oakland County. n.d.

3. "Educational Neglect Statutes." Coalition for Responsible Home Education, 2015.

Chapter 22

Emotional Abuse of Children

Chapter Contents

Section 22.1

Understanding Emotional Abuse of Children

This section includes text excerpted from "Helping Students with Emotional Abuse: A Critical Area of Competence for School Counselors," U.S. Department of Education (ED), June 18, 2013.

Definition of Childhood Emotional Abuse

Childhood maltreatment refers to acts of commission or omission by an adult, which endanger the physical or psychological well-being of a child and violate social sanctions regarding proper parenting. Theorists and many state statutes categorized childhood maltreatment into four basic types: physical abuse, sexual abuse, emotional abuse, and neglect. The three types of abuse (i.e., physical, sexual, and emotional abuse) are generally understood to include acts of commission, or active 5 forms of maltreatment, which endanger the well-being of a child, while neglect includes acts of omission, or passive forms of maltreatment, which endanger the well-being of a child. In this section, we address the distinguishing characteristics of emotional abuse as well as cultural considerations pertinent to its identification.

Childhood emotional abuse is arguably the most challenging form of abuse to classify and define. Unlike physical abuse and sexual abuse, which include various forms of physical contact between a child and older person, emotional abuse is essentially a non-contact form of maltreatment. That is, emotional abuse does not involve physical contact between the abuser and child. Hence, markers of emotional abuse are less tangible, compared to other types of abuse.

Moreover, researchers grouped diverse behaviors under the construct of childhood emotional abuse—a practice which presents additional challenges in defining and differentiating emotional abuse. For example, Garbarino et al. defined childhood emotional abuse as a child's experience of being rejected (i.e., denied a sense of positive self-regard and worth), isolated (i.e., removed from relationships with others), terrorized (i.e., intimidated or frightened with threats of harm), ignored (i.e., denied responsiveness from others), or corrupted (i.e., encouraged to engage in deviant behavior) by an older person.

More recently, definitions of childhood emotional abuse emphasized hostile verbal communications, which attack a child's sense of psychological or physical well-being. Examples of hostile verbal communications include an adult's behavior of ridiculing a child's physical appearance or threatening the safety of a child. Emotional abuse may also include non-verbal, non-contact behaviors. Examples of nonverbal forms of childhood emotional abuse include isolating a child from relationships and solitary confinement of a child for extended periods of time.

Emotional Abuse as a Pattern of Behavior

There is consensus that childhood emotional abuse refers to a pattern of behaviors over time, rather than a single, isolated incident. As argued by various authors, many parents make the mistake of verbally demeaning or attacking their children at one time or another. In general, then, childhood emotional abuse pertains to parent-child relationships where non-contact forms of aggression (e.g., verbal assaults) become repetitive. As Romeo stated, "emotional abuse is not just a single event, but a systematic diminishment of the victim. It is the continuous behavior by the abuser that reduces a child's self-concept to the point where the child feels unworthy". Thus, school counselors are generally recommended to consider patterns of interaction over time when conceptualizing a case of suspected childhood emotional abuse. It should be noted, however, that emotional abuse may be understood as a single event in extreme situations. An example of extreme emotional abuse is the solitary confinement of a child in a closet for days. In such cases, the school counselor may not need to await the repetition of behaviors before reporting to a CPS agency.

Cultural Considerations in Defining Emotional Abuse

In further specifying the nature of childhood emotional abuse, consideration has been given to cultural standards of parenting conduct. Any definition of childhood emotional abuse—as is the case with other forms of abuse— involves cultural assumptions about appropriate parenting and human development. The influence of these assumptions, however, is a complex issue. On the one hand, several authors noted that there is substantive agreement across cultures regarding the propriety of basic parental behaviors (e.g., providing a safe environment, responding to the child's emotional and physical needs, and refraining from having sexual intercourse with the child). In support

173

of this view, researchers observed similarities across cultural groups in definitions and experiences of child abuse. Likewise, Slep et al. cited an international agreement on child rights by member states of the United Nation as evidence of cross-cultural overlap in assumptions about proper parenting and child abuse.

On the other hand, numerous authors argued that assumptions about parenting might differ by cultural 8 group, thereby yielding dissimilar conceptions of childhood abuse across groups. Gough, for example, recorded the views of Japanese individuals, who perceived cruelty in Westerners' practice of leaving infants by themselves at night to sleep. Relatedly, Elliott et al. recruited participants from different cultural groups in Singapore (N = 401; 78.3% Chinese, 14.5% Malay, 5.5% Indian, 1.7% other) and found widespread disagreement on whether verbal threats of abandonment, name-calling, and constant criticisms constituted abuse. Furthermore, it is possible that the same parental behavior can have different outcomes for children in different cultures. Along this line, Deater-Deckard, Dodge, Bates, and Pettit found that a harsh parental discipline style (consisting of physically and verbally aggressive acts) was associated with adverse outcomes for children in some cultural groups but not others. In view of such cultural variations, Esteban and Slep et al. concluded that emotionally abusive behaviors must be considered within the context of cultural norms of parenting conduct.

For the purposes of this review, then, childhood emotional abuse is defined as a pattern of hostile verbal or nonverbal behaviors, apart from physical contact, which is directed toward a child by an adult, endangers the child's psychological and/or physical well-being, and violates cultural norms of parenting conduct. Within the cultural context of the United States, commonly recognized forms of emotional abuse include the repeated humiliation, derogation, and intimidation of children by adults. Given the focus of this section on reporting issues, we emphasize definitions of emotional abuse as encoded in state laws—despite the importance of understanding and exploring cultural variations presented by students and their families. As Wekerle argued, parents are ultimately accountable to laws and definitions of abuse in their current place of residence, even if these definitions vary from cultural traditions of their country of origin. Moreover, school counselors are legally protected from liability when making a report as long as the report was pursuant to state law.

Section 22.2

Need for Reporting Suspected Emotional Abuse

This section includes text excerpted from "Helping Students with Emotional Abuse: A Critical Area of Competence for School Counselors," U.S. Department of Education (ED), June 18, 2013.

Reporting Suspected Emotional Abuse

Researchers found that emotional abuse can have dire consequences for children; in fact, on some outcomes, emotional abuse appears to be more damaging than other forms of abuse. In this section, we begin with a discussion of how commonly cases of emotional abuse occur relative to other forms of abuse. Second, detail is provided on the relationships among emotional abuse and adverse psychosocial outcomes. We believe it is beneficial for school counselors to review thoroughly the empirical findings on this section, in order to discern the seriousness of this form of maltreatment.

Rates of Emotional Abuse

Studies yielded dissimilar pictures regarding the frequency of occurrence of emotional abuse cases—a divergence that may be attributable to differences in the measures of emotional abuse employed by researchers. For example, Sedlak et al. found a relatively low incidence of emotional abuse during a one-year period, after analyzing reports of child abuse made to CPS agencies and non-CPS professionals in a nationwide sample. In this section, researchers estimated that 4 children per 1,000 were victims of emotional abuse over a one-year period (based on the Endangerment Standard, which includes children currently harmed by maltreatment and those at risk for future harm as a result of maltreatment). Their findings further indicated that emotional abuse was less common than physical abuse but more common than sexual abuse: emotional abuse was involved in 36% of all child abuse cases; physical abuse, by comparison, was involved in 57% of all child abuse cases, and sexual abuse, 22% of all cases.

Numerous authors, however, commented that such studies, which are based fully or in part on reports to CPS agencies, may be misleading. As discussed above, school counselors have more difficulty in recognizing and reporting emotional abuse than other types of abuse. Moreover, Hamarman, Pope, and Czaja found that, compared to other types of abuse, emotional abuse has the highest variability in the number of cases reported from state to state. Thus, CPS agency records may not provide a very sensitive or reliable measure of the prevalence of emotional abuse.

A more accurate estimate of frequency may be based on retrospective reports by adults, who are asked to reflect on their childhood abusive experiences, or on self-reports of parents themselves. Along this line, Vissing, Straus, Gelles, and Harrop found that 63% of parents (N = 3,346; 63% female; no racial/ethnic information reported) recalled emotionally abusing a child in the previous year. The average number of emotionally abusive acts reported by parents was 12.6. In a retrospective study of 100 female college students (predominantly Caucasian; mean age = 21), Paivio and McCulloch reported that 44% of participants had experienced emotional abuse during childhood—a rate approximately twice that of physical abuse (23%) and sexual abuse (20%). Similarly, Tietjen et al. found that 38% of patients from a clinical sample (N = 1,348; mean age = 41) had a history of childhood emotional abuse, compared to 21% of participants who reported a history of physical abuse, and 25% of participants, who reported a history of sexual abuse. Thus, the prevalence of childhood emotional abuse may be, in fact, much higher than rates of sexual or physical abuse.

In regard to cultural differences in prevalence rates, the research in this area is relatively sparse, compared to the amount of research on cultural variables associated with physical or sexual abuse. Moreover, findings are somewhat mixed: Thombs et al., for example, analyzed retrospective self-report data from two randomly selected samples of adults (N = 832 and N = 967). After controlling for the influence of several demographic characteristics of participants (i.e., age, marital status, education level, and sex), these researchers found no difference between White and Black adults in childhood emotional abuse. In a similar research design (N = 967), however, Scher et al. reported that White participants were twice as likely as Black participants to have experienced emotional abuse, after controlling for the effects of education level and biological sex. In view of such disparate results, more research is needed to support comparisons of prevalence rates across cultural groups.

Childhood Emotional Abuse and Adverse Outcomes

It could be argued that the distress caused by emotional abuse is betrayed by the very existence of oft-repeated adages, which implore us to believe that "words will never hurt me". In fact, emotional abuse may be especially damaging to children. In some studies, researchers found that emotional abuse is more strongly related than physical or sexual abuse to psychological difficulties, such as self-injurious behaviors, bipolar disorder, emotional dysregulation, eating disorders, depression and anxiety, and personality disorders.

The preferential relationship between emotional abuse and adverse outcomes is perhaps most consistently seen in research on pessimistic explanatory style. Pessimistic explanatory style—a cognitive predictor of depression—refers to an individual's tendency to construe the causes of negative events as stable in duration (rather than temporary), global in their influence over multiple domains of life functioning (rather than impacting only a select few domains), and located within, or internal to, the person (rather than in the external environment). In several studies, researchers found that emotional abuse, but not sexual or physical abuse, was related to pessimistic explanatory style (or a conceptually similar variant of this construct, negative cognitive style). In view of such findings, school counselors must remain sensitive to the seriousness of this form of abuse, its potential impact on children, and the necessity for well-informed intervention efforts.

Chapter 23

Coping with an Alcoholic Parent

Why Do People Drink Too Much?

Lots of people live with a parent or caregiver who is an alcoholic or who drinks too much. Alcoholism has been around for centuries, yet no one has discovered an easy way to prevent it.

Alcohol can affect people's health and also how they act. People who are drunk might be more aggressive or have mood swings. They may act in a way that is embarrassing to them or other people.

Alcoholism is a disease. Like any disease, it needs to be treated. Without professional help, a person with alcoholism will probably continue to drink and may even become worse over time.

Diseases like alcoholism are no one's fault. Some people are more susceptible to wanting to drink too much. Scientists think it has to do with genetics, as well as things like family history, and life events.

Sometimes what starts as a bad habit can become a very big problem. For example, people may drink to cope with problems like boredom, stress, or money troubles. Maybe there's an illness in the family, or parents are having marriage problems.

No matter what anyone says, people don't drink because of someone else's behavior. So if you live with someone who has a drinking problem, don't blame yourself.

This chapter includes text excerpted from "Coping With an Alcoholic Parent," © 1995–2016. The Nemours Foundation/KidsHealth®. Reprinted with permission.

How Does Alcoholism Affect Families?

If you live with a parent who drinks, you may feel embarrassed, angry, sad, hurt, or any number of emotions. You may feel helpless: When parents promise to stop drinking, for example, it can end in frustration when they don't keep their promises.

Problem drinking can change how families function. A parent may have trouble keeping a job and problems paying the bills. Older kids may have to take care of younger siblings.

Some parents with alcohol problems might mistreat or abuse their children emotionally or physically. Others may neglect their kids by not providing sufficient care and guidance. Parents with alcohol problems might also use other drugs.

Despite what happens, most children of alcoholics love their parents and worry about something bad happening to them. Kids who live with problem drinkers often try all kinds of ways to prevent them from drinking. But, just as family members don't cause the addiction, they can't stop it either.

The person with the drinking problem has to take charge. Someone who has a bad habit or an addiction to alcohol needs to get help from a treatment center.

Alcoholism affects family members just as much as it affects the person drinking. Because of this, there are lots of support groups to help children of alcoholics cope with the problem.

What If a Parent Doesn't See a Problem?

Drinking too much can be a problem that nobody likes to talk about. In fact, lots of parents may become enraged at the slightest suggestion that they are drinking too much.

Sometimes, parents deny that they have a problem. A person in denial refuses to believe the truth about a situation. So problem drinkers may try to blame someone else because it is easier than taking responsibility for their own drinking.

Some parents make their families feel bad by saying stuff like, "You're driving me crazy!" or "I can't take this anymore." That can be harmful, especially to kids. Most young children don't know that the problem has nothing to do with their actions and that it's all in the drinker's mind.

Some parents do acknowledge their drinking, but deny that it's a problem. They may say stuff like, "I can stop anytime I want to," "Everyone drinks to unwind sometimes," or "My drinking is not a problem."

Lots of people fall into the trap of thinking that a parent's drinking is only temporary. They tell themselves that, when a particular problem is over, like having a rough time at work, the drinking will stop. But even if a parent who drinks too much has other problems, drinking is a separate problem. And that problem won't go away unless the drinker gets help.

Why Do I Feel So Bad?

If you're like most teens, your life is probably filled with emotional ups and downs, regardless of what's happening at home. Add a parent with a drinking problem to the mix, and it can all seem like too much.

There are many reasons why a parent's drinking can contribute to feelings of anger, frustration, disappointment, sadness, embarrassment, worry, loneliness, and helplessness. For example:

- **You might be subjected to a parent's changing moods**. People who drink can behave unpredictably. Kids who grow up around them may spend a lot of energy trying to figure out a parent's mood or guess what that parent wants. One day you might walk on eggshells to avoid an outburst because the dishes aren't done or the lawn isn't mowed. The next day, you may find yourself comforting a parent who promises that things will be better.

- **It may be hard to do things with friends or other people.** For some people, it feels like too much trouble to have a friend over or do the things that everyone else does. You just never know how your parent will act. Will your mom or dad show up drunk for school events or drive you (and your friends) home drunk?

- **You might be stressed or worried.** It can be scary to listen to adults in the house yell, fight, or break things by accident. Worrying about a parent just adds to all the other emotions you may be feeling. Are you lying awake waiting for mom or dad to get home safely? Do you feel it's not fair that you have to be the grown up and take care of things around the house? These are all normal reactions.

Although each family is different, people who grow up with alcoholic parents often feel alone, unloved, depressed, or burdened by the secret life they lead at home.

You know it's not possible to cause or stop the behavior of an alcoholic. So what can you do to feel better (or help a friend feel better)?

What Can I Do?

Acknowledge the problem. Many kids of parents who drink too much try to protect their parents or hide the problem. Admitting that your parent has a problem—even if he or she won't—is the first step in taking control. Start by talking to a friend, teacher, counselor, or coach. If you can't face telling someone you know, call an organization like Al-Anon/Alateen (they have a 24-hour hotline at 1-800-344-2666) or go online for help.

Be informed. Being aware of how your parent's drinking affects you can help put things in perspective. For example, some teens who live with alcoholic adults become afraid to speak out or show any normal anger or emotion because they worry it may trigger a parent's drinking. Remind yourself that you are not responsible for your parent drinking too much, and that you cannot cause it or stop it.

Be aware of your emotions. When you feel things like anger or resentment, try to identify those feelings. Talk to a close friend or write down how you are feeling. Recognizing how a parent's problem drinking makes you feel can help you from burying your feelings and pretending that everything's OK.

Learn healthy coping strategies. When we grow up around people who turn to alcohol or other unhealthy ways of dealing with problems, they become our example. Watching new role models can help people learn healthy coping mechanisms and ways of making good decisions.

Coaches, aunts, uncles, parents of friends, or teachers all have to deal with things like frustration or disappointment. Watch how they do it. School counselors can be a great resource here. Next time you have a problem, ask someone you trust for help.

Find support. It's good to share your feelings with a friend, but it's equally important to talk to an adult you trust. A school counselor, favorite teacher, or coach may be able to help. Some teens turn to their school D.A.R.E. (Drug and Alcohol Resistance Education) officer. Others prefer to talk to a family member or parents of a close friend.

Because alcoholism is such a widespread problem, several organizations offer confidential support groups and meetings for people living with alcoholics. Alateen is a group specifically geared to young people living with adults who have drinking problems. Alateen can also help teens whose parents may already be in treatment or recovery. The group Alcoholics Anonymous (AA) also offers resources for people living with alcoholics.

Find a safe environment. Do you find yourself avoiding your house as much as possible? Are you thinking about running away? If you feel that the situation at home is becoming dangerous, you can call the National Domestic Violence Hotline at 1-800-799-SAFE (1-800-799-7233). And don't hesitate to dial 911 if you think you or another family member is in immediate danger.

Stop the cycle. Teenage children of alcoholics are at higher risk of becoming alcoholics themselves. Scientists think this is because of genetics and the environment that kids grow up in. For example, people might learn to drink as a way to avoid fear, boredom, anxiety, sadness, or other unpleasant feelings. Understanding that there could be a problem and finding adults and peers to help you can be the most important thing you do to reduce the risk of problem drinking.

Alcoholism is a disease. You can show your love and support, but you won't be able to stop someone from drinking. Talking about the problem, finding support, and choosing healthy ways to cope are choices you can make to feel more in control of the situation. Above all, don't give up!

Chapter 24

Abusive Relationships

Healthy Relationships = Respect and Trust

When Brian and Sarah began dating, her friends were envious. Brian was smart, sensitive, funny, athletic, and good-looking. Even her mom loved him.

For the first couple of months, Sarah seemed happy. She started to miss her friends and family, though, because she was spending more time with Brian and less time with everyone else. That seemed easier than dealing with Brian's endless questions. He worried about what she was doing at every moment of the day.

But Sarah's friends became concerned when her behavior started to change. She lost interest in the things she once enjoyed, like swim meets and going to the mall. She became secretive and moody. When her friends asked if she was having trouble with Brian, she told them nothing was wrong.

Healthy relationships involve respect, trust, and consideration for the other person. Sadly, some relationships can turn bad. In fact, 1 in 11 high school students report being physically hurt by a date.

People in these relationships sometimes mistake the abuse for intense feelings of caring or concern. It can even seem flattering. Think of a friend whose boyfriend or girlfriend is very jealous: Maybe it seems like your friend's partner really cares. But actually, excessive jealousy and controlling behavior are not signs of affection at all.

This chapter includes text excerpted from "Abusive Relationships," © 1995–2016. The Nemours Foundation/KidsHealth®. Reprinted with permission.

Love involves respect and trust; it doesn't mean constantly worrying about the possible end of the relationship. If you feel nervous or insecure about your relationship, it's important to talk it through with your boyfriend or girlfriend, rather than try to control your partner's behavior.

What Is Abuse?

Abuse can be physical, emotional, or sexual. Physical abuse means any form of violence, such as hitting, punching, pulling hair, and kicking. Abuse can happen in both dating relationships and friendships.

Emotional abuse (stuff like teasing, bullying, and humiliating others) can be difficult to recognize because it doesn't leave any visible scars. Threats, intimidation, putdowns, and betrayal are all harmful forms of emotional abuse that can really hurt—not just during the time it's happening, but long afterward, too.

Sexual abuse can happen to anyone, guy or girl. It's never right to be forced into any type of sexual experience that you don't want.

The first step in getting out of an abusive relationship is to realize that you have the right to be treated with respect and not be physically or emotionally harmed by another person.

Signs of Abusive Relationships

Important warning signs that you may be involved in an abusive relationship include when someone:

- harms you physically in any way, including slapping, pushing, grabbing, shaking, smacking, kicking, and punching

- tries to control different aspects of your life, such as how you dress, who you hang out with, and what you say

- frequently humiliates you or makes you feel unworthy (for example, if a partner puts you down but tells you that he or she loves you)

- threatens to harm you, or self-harm, if you leave the relationship

- twists the truth to make you feel you are to blame for your partner's actions

- demands to know where you are at all times

- constantly becomes jealous or angry when you want to spend time with your friends

Unwanted sexual advances that make you uncomfortable are also red flags that the relationship needs to focus more on respect. When someone says stuff like "If you loved me, you would . . . " that's also a warning of possible abuse, and is a sign that your partner is trying to manipulate you. A statement like this is controlling and is used by people who are only concerned about getting what they want—not caring about what you want. Trust your intuition. If something doesn't feel right, it probably isn't.

Signs That a Friend Is Being Abused

In addition to the signs listed above, here are some signs a friend might be being abused by a partner:

- unexplained bruises, broken bones, sprains, or marks

- excessive guilt or shame for no apparent reason

- secrecy or withdrawal from friends and family

- avoidance of school or social events with excuses that don't seem to make any sense

A person who is being abused needs someone to hear and believe him or her. Maybe your friend is afraid to tell a parent because that will bring pressure to end the relationship. People who are abused often feel like it's their fault—that they "asked for it" or that they don't deserve any better. But abuse is never deserved. Help your friend understand that it is not his or her fault. Your friend is not a bad person. The person who is being abusive has a serious problem and needs professional help.

A friend who is being abused needs your patience, love, and understanding. Your friend also needs your encouragement to get help immediately from an adult, such as a parent, family member, or guidance counselor. Most of all, your friend needs you to listen without judging. It takes a lot of courage to admit being abused; let your friend know that you're offering your full support.

How You Can Help Yourself

What should you do if you think someone might be abusing you? If you feel that you love someone but often feel afraid, it's time to get out of the relationship—fast. You're worth being treated with respect and you can get help.

First, make sure you're safe. A trusted adult or friend can help. If the person has physically attacked you, don't wait to get medical attention or to call the police. Assault is illegal, and so is rape—even if it's done by someone you are dating.

Avoid the tendency to isolate yourself from your friends and family. You might feel like you have nowhere to turn, or you might be embarrassed about what's been going on, but this is when you need support most. People like counselors, doctors, teachers, coaches, and friends will want to help you, so let them.

Don't rely on yourself alone to get out of the situation. Friends and family who love and care about you can help you break away. It's important to know that asking for help isn't a sign of weakness. It actually shows that you have a lot of courage and are willing to stand up for yourself. It's also likely you will need help to break out of a cycle of abuse, especially if you still love the person who has hurt you, or feel guilty about leaving.

Where to Get Help

Ending abuse and violence in teen relationships is a community effort with plenty of people ready to help. Your local phone book or the Internet will list crisis centers, teen help lines, and abuse hotlines. These organizations have professionally trained staff to listen, understand, and help. In addition, religious leaders, school nurses, teachers, school counselors, doctors, and other health professionals can be sources of support and information.

You can also get involved at a school or community level as an advocate to help prevent future dating abuse. One example of a school-based program is Safe Dates. Talk to your school guidance counselor about starting a group or other ways to get involved in making sure dating abuse doesn't happen to people in your school.

Chapter 25

Sexual Harassment and Sexual Bullying

What Are Sexual Bullying and Harassment?

Just like other kinds of bullying, sexual harassment can involve comments, gestures, actions, or attention that is intended to hurt, offend, or intimidate another person. With sexual harassment, the focus is on things like a person's appearance, body parts, sexual orientation, or sexual activity.

Sexual harassment may be verbal (like making comments about someone), but it doesn't have to be spoken. Bullies may use technology to harass someone sexually (like sending inappropriate text messages, pictures, or videos). Sometimes sexual harassment can even get physical when someone tries to kiss or touch someone that does not want to be touched.

Sexual harassment doesn't just happen to girls. Boys can harass girls, but girls also can harass guys, guys may harass other guys, and girls may harass other girls. Sexual harassment isn't limited to people of the same age, either. Adults sometimes sexually harass young people (and, occasionally, teens may harass adults, though that's pretty rare). But most of the time, when sexual harassment happens to teens, it's being done by people in the same age group.

This chapter includes text excerpted from "Sexual Harassment and Sexual Bullying," © 1995–2016. The Nemours Foundation/KidsHealth®. Reprinted with permission.

Sexual harassment and bullying are very similar—they both involve unwelcome or unwanted sexual comments, attention, or physical contact. So why call one thing by two different names?

Sometimes schools and other places use one term or the other for legal reasons. For instance, a school document may use the term "bullying" to describe what's against school policy, while a law might use the term "harassment" to define what's against the law. Some behaviors might be against school policy and also against the law.

For the person who is being targeted, though, it doesn't make much difference if something is called bullying or harassment. This kind of behavior is upsetting no matter what it's called. Like anyone who's being bullied, people who are sexually harassed can feel threatened and scared and experience a great deal of emotional stress.

What Behaviors Count?

Some pictures, images, jokes, language, and contact are called "inappropriate" for a reason. **If a behavior or interaction makes you uncomfortable or upset, talk to a trusted adult.** It may fall into the sexual harassment or bullying category.

Sexual harassment or bullying can include:

- making sexual jokes, comments, or gestures to or about someone

- spreading sexual rumors (in person, by text, or online)

- writing sexual messages about people on bathroom stalls or in other public places

- showing someone inappropriate sexual pictures or videos

- asking someone to send you naked pictures of herself or himself ("nudes")

- posting sexual comments, pictures, or videos on social networks like Facebook, or sending explicit text messages

- making sexual comments or offers while pretending to be someone else online

- touching, grabbing, or pinching someone in a deliberately sexual way

- pulling at someone's clothing and brushing up against them in a purposefully sexual way

- asking someone to go out over and over again, even after the person has said no

Sending sexual messages or images by text, or "sexting," is not a good idea for many reasons. Sexting can lead to problems for you and the person getting the text, even when you are dating or in a relationship with that person. In some cases these messages can be considered harassment or bullying and can bring very serious consequences. Also, messages or images you intend to be private can get into the wrong hands and be used to embarrass, intimidate, or humiliate. Even if you send someone's picture just to one other person, it can be forwarded to many other people or posted online for the world to see.

Forcing another person into doing things he or she doesn't want to do, such as kissing, oral sex, or intercourse, goes beyond sexual harassment or bullying. **Forcing someone to do sexual things is sexual assault or rape, and it's a serious crime.**

Flirting or Harassment?

Sometimes people who make sexual jokes or comments laugh off their behavior as flirting, and you might be tempted to do the same. So what's the difference between flirting and sexual harassment? Here are three examples of flirting versus harassment:

1. **You and your crush have been flirting and you both start making jokes about sexting.** Your crush asks if you'd ever do that. You say, "No way!" With normal flirting, that's the end of it. But if your crush starts pressuring you to send sexual pictures, then it's getting into harassment territory

2. **Someone in class says your new jeans look great.** That's a compliment. But if they say your new jeans make your butt look great, or they make comments about specific body parts, that's crossing the line.

3. **Someone you're not attracted to asks you to go to a dance.** It seems harsh to say you're not interested, so you make up an excuse. The person asks a couple more times but eventually gets the hint. This is a normal social interaction. But if the person hits on you in a creepy way—like making references to sex or your body, sending sexual messages, always showing up wherever you happen to be, or trying to touch you, hug you, or bother you—that's harassment.

Some things may be awkward, but they don't count as harassment. A guy who blurts out a sex-related swearword because he spills his lunch tray isn't likely to be trying to harass or bother you. But if someone is deliberately doing or saying sexual things that make you uncomfortable, it's probably sexual harassment.

Not sure? Ask yourself, "Is this something I wanted to happen or I want to continue happening? How does it make me feel?" If it doesn't feel right, talk to a parent, teacher, guidance counselor, or someone else you trust.

How to Handle Sexual Harassment

If you think you're being harassed, don't blame yourself. People who harass or bully can be very manipulative. They are often good at blaming the other person—and even at making victims blame themselves. But no one has the right to sexually harass or bully anyone else, no matter what. There is no such thing as "asking for it."

There's no single "right" way to respond to sexual harassment. Each situation is unique. It often can be helpful to start by telling the person doing the harassing to stop. Let him or her know that this behavior is not OK with you. Sometimes that will be enough, but not always. The harasser may not stop. He or she might even laugh off your request, tease you, or bother you more.

That's why it's important to share what's happening with an adult you trust. Is there a parent, relative, coach, or teacher you can talk to? More and more schools have a designated person who's there to talk about bullying issues, so find out if there's someone at your school.

Most schools have a sexual harassment policy or a bullying policy to protect you. Ask a guidance counselor, school nurse, or administrator about your school's policy. If you find the adult you talk to doesn't take your complaints seriously at first, you may have to repeat yourself or find someone else who will listen.

There's no doubt it can feel embarrassing to talk about sexual harassment at first. But that uncomfortable feeling quickly wears off after a minute or so of conversation. In most cases, telling someone sooner leads to faster results and fewer problems down the line, so it's worth it.

It can help to keep a record of the events that have happened. Write down dates and short descriptions in a journal. Save any offensive pictures, videos, texts, or IMs as evidence. That way you'll have them if your school or family has to take legal action. To avoid going through feeling upset all over again, save this evidence someplace where you don't have to see it every day.

If You See Something, Say Something

Bystanders play an important role in stopping bullying and sexual harassment. If you see someone who is being harassed, take action. If it feels safe and natural to speak up, say, "Come on, let's get out of here" to the person you see getting bullied or bothered. You probably shouldn't try to change the bully's behavior by yourself, but it is OK to let the bully know people are watching and will be getting involved.

If you don't feel you can say something at the time you see the incident, report the event to a teacher or principal. This isn't snitching. It's standing up for what's right. No one deserves to be harassed. You could also talk to the victim afterward and offer support. Say that you think what happened is not OK and offer some ideas for dealing with harassment.

If You Suspect Something

You won't always see sexual harassment or bullying happening. A friend who is going through it might not talk about it.

Sometimes people show signs that something's wrong even if they don't talk about it. Maybe a normally upbeat friend seems sad, worried, or distracted. Perhaps a friend has lost interest in hanging out or doing stuff. Maybe someone you know avoids school or has falling grades. Changes like these are often signs that something's going on. It may not be sexual harassment or bullying (things like mood swings or changes in eating habits can be signs of many different things). But it is a chance for you to ask if everything's OK.

Chapter 26

Technology and Abuse

Chapter Contents

Section 26.1

Understanding Youth Violence

This section includes text excerpted from "Youth Violence: Definitions," Centers for Disease Control and Prevention (CDC), March 5, 2015.

Youth Violence: Definitions

Interpersonal violence is defined as "the intentional use of physical force or power, threatened or actual, against another person or against a group or community that results in or has a high likelihood of resulting in injury, death, psychological harm, maldevelopment, or deprivation." Research and programs addressing youth violence typically include persons between the ages of 10 and 24, although patterns of youth violence can begin in early childhood.

This definition associates intent with committing the act-no matter the outcome. In other words, intent to use force does not necessarily mean intent to cause damage. Indeed, there may be a considerable disparity between intended behavior and intended consequence. A perpetrator may commit a seemingly dangerous act that will likely result in adverse health effects, but the perpetrator may not perceive it as such. For example, a youth may get in a physical fight with another youth. The use of a fist against the head or the use of a weapon in the dispute certainly increases the risk of serious injury or death, though neither outcome may be intended.

Other aspects of violence are implied in this definition. For example, it includes all acts of violence, whether public or private, reactive (in response to previous events such as provocation), proactive (instrumental for or anticipating more self-serving outcomes), or criminal or noncriminal. Each of these aspects is important to understanding the causes of violence and in designing prevention programs.

Risk Factors for the Perpetration of Youth Violence

Research on youth violence has increased our understanding of factors that make some populations more vulnerable to victimization and perpetration. Risk factors increase the likelihood that a young person will become violent. However, risk factors are not direct causes of youth violence; instead, risk factors contribute to youth violence

Research associates the following risk factors with perpetration of youth violence:

Individual Risk Factors

- History of violent victimization

- Attention deficits, hyperactivity or learning disorders

- History of early aggressive behavior

- Involvement with drugs, alcohol or tobacco

- Low IQ

- Poor behavioral control

- Deficits in social cognitive or information-processing abilities

- High emotional distress

- History of treatment for emotional problems

- Antisocial beliefs and attitudes

- Exposure to violence and conflict in the family

Family Risk Factors

- Authoritarian childrearing attitudes

- Harsh, lax or inconsistent disciplinary practices

- Low parental involvement

- Low emotional attachment to parents or caregivers

- Low parental education and income

- Parental substance abuse or criminality

- Poor family functioning

- Poor monitoring and supervision of children

Peer and Social Risk Factors

- Association with delinquent peers

- Involvement in gangs

- Social rejection by peers

- Lack of involvement in conventional activities
- Poor academic performance
- Low commitment to school and school failure

Community Risk Factors

- Diminished economic opportunities
- High concentrations of poor residents
- High level of transiency
- High level of family disruption
- Low levels of community participation
- Socially disorganized neighborhoods

Section 26.2

Electronic Devices and Aggression

This section includes text excerpted from "Electronic Aggression," Centers for Disease Control and Prevention (CDC), December 10, 2015.

Electronic Aggression

Technology and Youth Violence

Young people are using media technology, including cell phones, personal data assistants, and the Internet, to communicate with others in the United States and throughout the world. Communication avenues, such as text messaging, chat rooms, and social networking websites (e.g., MySpace and Facebook), have allowed youth to easily develop relationships, some with people they have never met in person.

Media technology has many potential benefits for youth. It allows young people to communicate with family and friends on a regular basis. This technology also provides opportunities to make rewarding social connections for those teens and pre-teens who have difficulty developing friendships in traditional social settings or because of limited contact with same-aged peers. In addition, regular Internet access allows young people to quickly increase their knowledge on a wide variety of topics.

However, the explosion in communication tools and avenues does not come without possible risks. Youth can use electronic media to embarrass, harass or threaten their peers. Increasing numbers of teens and pre-teens are becoming victims of this new form of violence. Although many different terms—such as cyberbullying, Internet harassment, and Internet bullying—have been used to describe this type of violence, electronic aggression is the term that most accurately captures all types of violence that occur electronically. Like traditional forms of youth violence, electronic aggression is associated with emotional distress and conduct problems at school. In fact, recent research suggests that youth who are victimized electronically are also very likely to also be victimized offline (i.e., sexually harassed, psychological or emotional abuse by a caregiver, witnessing an assault with a weapon, and being raped).

Violence Prevention and Social Media

Using Facebook and Twitter to Raise Awareness about Violence Prevention

As a part of CDC's Injury Center, the Division of Violence Prevention works to prevent violence and its consequences, which includes sharing the importance of prevention to all of our audiences where they engage in discussions. Social media, like Facebook and Twitter, plays an important role in our outreach and interactions.

Our fans and followers can keep up with our most recent research, new articles, and prevention resources on social media. Fans also have opportunities to interact with our experts in real time, through coordinated events and chats. In recognition of national violence prevention observances, we have opened up our **VetoViolence** Facebook page to **Ask the Expert Forums** and participate in national conversations through the Injury Center's @CDCInjury Twitter account. We encourage you to follow us on social media and join in conversations with others interested in effective violence prevention.

The **VetoViolence** Facebook page also spotlights a partner working in the field of violence prevention each month. This feature provides our fans with instant access to other organizations that also work to help us all live safer, healthier lives.

To share your commitment to violence prevention, you can pledge to prevent violence with the interactive **VetoViolence Pledge** app, which allows you to create a custom badge that will appear on your own Facebook profile page. Fans of the page can also listen to violence prevention experts talk about a variety of topics through violence prevention podcasts.

Section 26.3

Cyberbullying

This section includes text excerpted from "Cyberbullying," Stopbullying.gov, U.S. Department of Health and Human Services (HHS), September 30, 2014.

What Is Cyberbullying

Cyberbullying is bullying that takes place using electronic technology. Electronic technology includes devices and equipment such as cell phones, computers, and tablets as well as communication tools including social media sites, text messages, chat, and websites.

Examples of cyberbullying include mean text messages or emails, rumors sent by email or posted on social networking sites, and embarrassing pictures, videos, websites, or fake profiles.

Why Cyberbullying is Different

Kids who are being cyberbullied are often bullied in person as well. Additionally, kids who are cyberbullied have a harder time getting away from the behavior.

- Cyberbullying can happen 24 hours a day, 7 days a week, and reach a kid even when he or she is alone. It can happen any time of the day or night.

- Cyberbullying messages and images can be posted anonymously and distributed quickly to a very wide audience. It can be difficult and sometimes impossible to trace the source.

- Deleting inappropriate or harassing messages, texts, and pictures is extremely difficult after they have been posted or sent.

Effects of Cyberbullying

Cell phones and computers themselves are not to blame for cyberbullying. Social media sites can be used for positive activities, like connecting kids with friends and family, helping students with school, and for entertainment. But these tools can also be used to hurt other people. Whether done in person or through technology, the effects of bullying are similar.

Kids who are cyberbullied are more likely to:

- Use alcohol and drugs

- Skip school

- Experience in-person bullying

- Be unwilling to attend school

- Receive poor grades

- Have lower self-esteem

- Have more health problems

Frequency of Cyberbullying

The 2013-2014 School Crime Supplement (National Center for Education Statistics and Bureau of Justice Statistics) indicates that 7% of students in grades 6–12 experienced cyberbullying.

The 2013 Youth Risk Behavior Surveillance Survey finds that 15% of high school students (grades 9-12) were electronically bullied in the past year.

Research on cyberbullying is growing. However, because kids' technology use changes rapidly, it is difficult to design surveys that accurately capture trends.

Prevent Cyberbullying

Parents and kids can prevent cyberbullying. Together, they can explore safe ways to use technology.

- Be Aware of What Your Kids are Doing Online

- Establish Rules about Technology Use

- Understand School Rules

Be Aware of What Your Kids are Doing Online

Talk with your kids about cyberbullying and other online issues regularly.

- Know the sites your kids visit and their online activities. Ask where they're going, what they're doing, and who they're doing it with.

- Tell your kids that as a responsible parent you may review their online communications if you think there is reason for concern. Installing parental control filtering software or monitoring programs are one option for monitoring your child's online behavior, but do not rely solely on these tools.

- Have a sense of what they do online and in texts. Learn about the sites they like. Try out the devices they use.

- Ask for their passwords, but tell them you'll only use them in case of emergency.

- Ask to "friend" or "follow" your kids on social media sites or ask another trusted adult to do so.

- Encourage your kids to tell you immediately if they, or someone they know, is being cyberbullied. Explain that you will not take away their computers or cell phones if they confide in you about a problem they are having.

Establish Rules about Technology Use

Establish rules about appropriate use of computers, cell phones, and other technology. For example, be clear about what sites they can visit and what they are permitted to do when they're online. Show them how to be safe online.

Help them be smart about what they post or say. Tell them not to share anything that could hurt or embarrass themselves or others. Once something is posted, it is out of their control whether someone else will forward it.

Encourage kids to think about who they want to see the information and pictures they post online. Should complete strangers see it? Real friends only? Friends of friends? Think about how people who aren't friends could use it.

Tell kids to keep their passwords safe and not share them with friends. Sharing passwords can compromise their control over their online identities and activities.

Understand School Rules

Some schools have developed policies on uses of technology that may affect the child's online behavior in and out of the classroom. Ask the school if they have developed a policy.

Report Cyberbullying

When cyberbullying happens, it is important to document and report the behavior so it can be addressed.

- Steps to Take Immediately
- Report Cyberbullying to Online Service Providers
- Report Cyberbullying to Law Enforcement
- Report Cyberbullying to Schools

Steps to Take Immediately

- Don't respond to and don't forward cyberbullying messages.
- Keep evidence of cyberbullying. Record the dates, times, and descriptions of instances when cyberbullying has occurred. Save and print screenshots, emails, and text messages. Use this evidence to report cyberbullying to web and cell phone service providers.
- Block the person who is cyberbullying.

Report Cyberbullying to Online Service Providers

Cyberbullying often violates the terms of service established by social media sites and Internet service providers.

- Review their terms and conditions or rights and responsibilities sections. These describe content that is or is not appropriate.
- Visit social media safety centers to learn how to block users and change settings to control who can contact you.
- Report cyberbullying to the social media site so they can take action against users abusing the terms of service.

Report Cyberbullying to Law Enforcement

When cyberbullying involves these activities it is considered a crime and should be reported to law enforcement:

- Threats of violence

- Child pornography or sending sexually explicit messages or photos

- Taking a photo or video of someone in a place where he or she would expect privacy

- Stalking and hate crimes

Some states consider other forms of cyberbullying criminal. Consult your state's laws and law enforcement for additional guidance.

Report Cyberbullying to Schools

- Cyberbullying can create a disruptive environment at school and is often related to in-person bullying. The school can use the information to help inform prevention and response strategies.

- In many states, schools are required to address cyberbullying in their anti-bullying policy. Some state laws also cover off-campus behavior that creates a hostile school environment.

Section 26.4

Protecting Your Online Identity and Reputation

This section includes text excerpted from "Protecting Your Online Identity and Reputation," © 1995–2016. The Nemours Foundation/KidsHealth®. Reprinted with permission.

Creating Your Online Identity

From the first time you log on to a social networking site, pick a screen name for instant messaging (IM), or post to a blog on your favorite band, you're creating an online identity.

Your online identity may be different from your real-world identity—the way your friends, parents, and teachers think of you—and some parts of it may be entirely made up. Maybe you're a little shy in real life, but online you're a jokester and your avatar is a famous comedian. Maybe your classmates think of you as a soccer star, but online you indulge your passion for chess and environmentalism.

Playing around and trying on different characteristics are part of the fun of an online life. You can change your look or the way you act and present yourself to others, and you can learn more about things that interest you. And, just as in real life, you can take steps to help make sure you stay in control.

Things to Consider

Here are some things to consider to safeguard your online identity and reputation:

Remember that nothing is temporary online. The virtual world is full of opportunities to interact and share with people around the world. It's also a place where nothing is temporary and there are no "take-backs." A lot of what you do and say online can be retrieved online even if you delete it—and it's a breeze for others to copy, save, and forward your information.

Mark your profiles as private. Anyone who accesses your profile on a social networking site can copy or screen-capture information and photos that you may not want the world to see. Don't rely on the site's default settings. Read each site's instructions or guidelines to make sure you're doing everything you can to keep your material private.

Safeguard your passwords and change them frequently. If someone logs on to a site and pretends to be you, they can trash your identity. Pick passwords that no one will guess (don't use your favorite band or your dog's birthday; try thinking of two utterly random nouns and mixing in a random number), and change them often. Never share them with anyone other than your parents or a trusted adult. Not even your best friend, boyfriend, or girlfriend should know your private passwords!

Don't post inappropriate or sexually provocative pictures or comments. Things that seem funny or cool to you right now might not seem so cool years from now—or when a teacher, admissions officer, or potential employer sees them. A good rule of thumb is: if you'd feel weird if your grandmother, coach, or best friend's parents saw it, it's probably not a good thing to post. Even if it's on a private site, it could be hacked or copied and forwarded.

Don't respond to inappropriate requests. Research shows that a high percentage of teens receive inappropriate messages and solicitations when they're online. These can be scary, strange, and even embarrassing. If you feel harassed by a stranger or a friend online, tell an adult you trust immediately. It is never a good idea to respond. Responding is only likely to make things worse, and might result in you saying something you wish you hadn't.

You can report inappropriate behavior or concerns at www.cybertipline.org.

Take a breather to avoid "flaming". File this one under "nothing's temporary online": If you get the urge to fire off an angry IM or comment on a message board or blog, it's a good idea to wait a few minutes, calm down, and remember that the comments may stay up (with your screen name right there) long after you've regained your temper and maybe changed your mind.

You might feel anonymous or disguised in chat rooms, social networks, or other sites—and this could lead to mean, insulting, or abusive comments toward someone else, or sharing pictures and comments you may later regret. We've all heard of cyberbullying, but most people think online bullying is something people do intentionally. But sharing stuff or dropping random comments when we're not face to face with someone can hurt just as much, if not more. And it can damage how others see you if they find out. A good rule to remember: if you wouldn't say it, show it, or do it in person, you probably don't want to online.

Learn about copyrights. It's a good idea to learn about copyright laws and make sure you don't post, share, or distribute copyrighted images, songs, or files. Sure, you want to share them, but you don't want to accidentally do anything illegal that can come back to haunt you later.

Check yourself. Chances are, you've already checked your "digital footprint"—nearly half of all online users do. Try typing your screen name or email address into a search engine and see what comes up. That's one way to get a sense of what others see as your online identity.

Take it offline. In general, if you have questions about the trail you're leaving online, don't be afraid to ask a trusted adult. Sure, you might know more about the online world than a lot of adults do, but they have life experience that can help.

Your online identity and reputation are shaped in much the same way as your real-life identity, except that when you're online you don't always get a chance to explain your tone or what you mean. Thinking before you post and following the same rules for responsible behavior online as you do offline can help you avoid leaving an online identity trail you regret.

Section 26.5

Child Pornography

This section includes text excerpted from "Child Pornography," U.S. Department of Justice (DOJ), June 3, 2015.

Defining Child Pornography

Child pornography is a form of child sexual exploitation. Federal law defines child pornography as any visual depiction of sexually explicit conduct involving a minor (persons less than 18 years old). Images of child pornography are also referred to as child sexual abuse images.

Federal law prohibits the production, distribution, importation, reception, or possession of any image of child pornography. A violation of federal child pornography laws is a serious crime, and convicted offenders face fines severe statutory penalties

Child Pornography Today

By the mid-1980's, the trafficking of child pornography within the United States was almost completely eradicated through a series of successful campaigns waged by law enforcement. Producing and reproducing child sexual abuse images was difficult and expensive.

Anonymous distribution and receipt was not possible, and it was difficult for pedophiles to find and interact with each other. For these reason, child pornographers became lonely and hunted individuals because the purchasing and trading of such images was extremely risky.

Unfortunately, the child pornography market exploded in the advent of the Internet and advanced digital technology. The Internet provides ground for individuals to create, access, and share child sexual abuse images worldwide at the click of a button. Child pornography images are readily available through virtually every Internet technology including websites, email, instant messaging/ICQ, Internet Relay Chat (IRC), newsgroups, bulletin boards, peer-to-peer networks, and social networking sites. Child pornography offenders can connect on Internet forums and networks to share their interests, desires, and experiences abusing children in addition to selling, sharing, and trading images.

Moreover, these online communities have promoted communication between child pornography offenders, both normalizing their interest in children and desensitizing them to the physical and psychological damages inflicted on child victims. Online communities may also attract or promote new individuals to get involved in the sexual exploitation of children.

Victims of Child Pornography

It is important to distinguish child pornography from the more conventional understanding of the term pornography. Child pornography is a form of child sexual exploitation, and each image graphically memorializes the sexual abuse of that child. Each child involved in the production of an image is a victim of sexual abuse.

While some child sexual abuse images depict children in great distress and the sexual abuse is self-evident, other images may depict children that appear complacent. However, just because a child appears complacent does not mean that sexual abuse did not occur. In most child pornography cases, the abuse is not a one-time event, but rather ongoing victimization that progresses over months or years. It is common for producers of child pornography to groom victims, or cultivate a relationship with a child and gradually sexualize the contact over time. The grooming process fosters a false sense of trust and authority over a child in order to desensitize or break down a child's resistance to sexual abuse. Therefore, even if a child appears complacent in a particular image, it is important to remember that the abuse may have started years before that image was created.

Furthermore, victims of child pornography suffer not just from the sexual abuse inflicted upon them to produce child pornography, but also from knowing that their images can be traded and viewed by others worldwide. Once an image is on the Internet, it is irretrievable and can continue to circulate forever. The permanent record of a child's sexual abuse can alter his or her live forever. Many victims of child pornography suffer from feelings of helplessness, fear, humiliation, and lack of control given that their images are available for others to view in perpetuity.

Unfortunately, emerging trends reveal an increase in the number of images depicting sadistic and violent child sexual abuse, and an increase in the number of images depicting very young children, including toddlers and infants.

CEOS' Role

CEOS works to deter and eradicate the production, distribution and possession of child pornography. CEOS attorneys work with the High Technology Investigative Unit (HTIU), the Federal Bureau of Investigation (FBI), United States Attorney's Offices throughout the country, and the National Center for Missing and Exploited Children (NCMEC) to vigorously combat this growing problem by investigating and prosecuting violators of federal child pornography laws. In addition, CEOS attorneys work with law enforcement personnel to identify and rescue victims of child pornography from continued abuse.

The use of the Internet to commit child pornography offenses has blurred traditional notions of jurisdiction. CEOS maintains a coordinated, national-level law enforcement focus to help coordinate nationwide and international investigations and initiatives.

Furthermore, CEOS attorneys and HTIU computer forensic specialists travel all over the world to conduct and participate in trainings for investigators, law enforcement personnel, and others involved in efforts to investigate and prosecute child pornography offenders. CEOS also designs, implements, and supports law enforcement strategies, legislative proposals, and policy initiatives relating to federal child pornography laws.

Chapter 27

International Parental Kidnapping

Defining International Parental Kidnapping

Federal law prohibits a parent from removing a child from the United States or retaining a child in another country with intent to obstruct another parent's custodial rights. This crime is known as international parental kidnapping. For example, consider that a married couple had a son together in the United States. During a martial dispute, the father moves with his son to another country in order to keep him away from the mother with no intent of return. In this situation, the father has committed the federal crime of international parental kidnapping. Convicted offenders of this crime can face up to three years of imprisonment.

Child Victims of International Parental Kidnapping

Every year, situations of international parental kidnapping are reported in the United States. It is common for the removal of a child to occur during a heated or emotional marital dispute, in the early stages of separation or divorce, or in the waiting period for a court custody order or agreement. International parental kidnappings of U.S. children have been reported in countries all over the world, including

This chapter includes text excerpted from "International Parental Kidnapping," U.S Department of Justice (DOJ), June 3, 2015.

Australia, Brazil, Canada, Colombia, Germany, India, Japan, Mexico, Philippines, and the United Kingdom.

Child victims of international parental kidnapping are often taken from a familiar environment and suddenly isolated from their community, family, and friends. They may miss months or even years of schooling. The child may be moved to multiple locations in order to stay hidden or out of reach of the parent remaining in the United States. In some cases, the child's name, birth date, and physical appearance are altered or concealed to hide identity.

In addition, the tense and unfavorable situation between the parents may be emotionally troubling to a child. Kidnapped children are at high risk for long-term psychological problems including anxiety, eating disorders, nightmares, mood swings, sleep disturbances, and aggressive behavior. As adults, child victims of international parental kidnapping may struggle with identity, relationship, and family issues.

Legal Hurdles and the Return of a Kidnapped Child to the United States

Under federal law, prosecutors may investigate and prosecute the parent who kidnapped the child, however, prosecutors generally have no control over the custodial decisions affecting the child or whether foreign authorities will order the return of the child.

The return of kidnapped children is often settled through negotiation. The U.S. Department of State handles the coordination of efforts with foreign officials and law enforcement agencies to effectuate the return of children to the United States. In some circumstances, the return may be governed by the *Hague Convention on the Civil Aspects of International Parental Child Abduction (1980)*. This Convention was established to facilitate the return of children abducted to foreign countries. However, it only applies if both countries involved in the international parental kidnapping situation are signatories to the Convention. The United States is a signatory state.

Adhering to the provisions of the Convention, when applicable, and working with the U.S. Department of State are the best methods to legally and safely return a kidnapped child to the United States. In acts of desperation, some parents will attempt to use extra-judicial forms of recovery, such as personally traveling to the foreign country to recover a child. Although it may seem easier and faster to use extra-judicial methods, they often violate U.S. federal laws and the laws of the foreign country involved, and may potentially exacerbate the situation. For example, the parent who kidnapped the child may have sought assistance from a foreign court or obtained a foreign custody order. In such circumstances, the other parent's direct removal of a child from the foreign jurisdiction, without the assistance of the U.S. Department of State, could result in his or her arrest or even imprisonment in that foreign country. Furthermore, any unlawful attempt to recover a child may adversely impact a have a petition for return under the *Hague Convention.*

CEOS's Role

The Child Exploitation and Obscenity Section (CEOS) provides advice and litigation support to United States Attorney's Offices throughout the country regarding international parental kidnapping prosecutions. While CEOS does not have the authority to intervene in the return of children, the section works directly with the U.S. Department of State and the National Center for Missing and Exploited Children (NCMEC) to monitor active international parental kidnapping cases and provide legal assistance.

In addition, CEOS conducts trainings for federal prosecutors and law enforcement personnel on federal international parental kidnapping law and its interplay with the *Hague Convention on the Civil Aspects of International Parental Child Abduction (1980).*

Child Custody and Visitation Matters

With the exception of international parental kidnapping, child custody and visitation matters are handled by local and states authorities, and not by the federal government. The matters are governed by the relevant state family court system and human services agency. Therefore, child custody or visitation issues should be reported to state or local law enforcement authorities or a state judicial officer.

Chapter 28

Childhood Maltreatment among Children with Disabilities

Children with disabilities may be at higher risk for abuse or neglect than children without disabilities. There are steps that parents can take to protect children with disabilities from abuse or neglect.

What We Know about Disability and Maltreatment

- Parents can more easily become stressed with the demands placed on them by parenting a child with a disability.

- Kids with behavior problems, like, Attention-Deficit/Hyperactivity Disorder (ADHD) or other conduct problems, may be more likely to experience physical abuse because parents can become frustrated by the child's difficult behavior and respond harshly.

- Kids who are less able to do things independently rely more on adults for their care. These children may be more likely to be sexually abused or neglected by adults.

This chapter includes text excerpted from "Childhood Maltreatment among Children with Disabilities," Centers for Disease Control and Prevention (CDC), March 15, 2016.

- Abusers may take advantage of kids who have problems speaking, hearing or who don't understand social situations very well. These children may be more likely to experience sexual abuse.

What Can You Do?

Safe stable nurturing relationships between parents and children and between parents and other adults are an important way to protect your child from harm.

Be Informed

Parents can prevent abuse and neglect of children:

- Know the signs of possible abuse, such as

  - Sudden changes in, or unusual behavior

  - Cuts and bruises

  - Broken bones (not due to a medical condition)

  - Burns

  - Complaints about painful genitals

- Know the signs of possible neglect, such as

  - Constant hunger or thirst (not due to a medical condition)

  - Dirty hair or skin

  - Chronic diaper rash (not due to a medical condition)

- Know where your child is and what he or she is doing when he or she is not at home.

- Get to know the people who take care of your child. Only leave your child with someone you know and who can take care of your child in place where your child will be safe from harm and danger.

- Know that your child's school must treat your child with dignity. Your child should not be punished by being mistreated, restrained, or secluded.

- Take steps to make sure your house is a safe place for your child so he or she will not get injured.

- Talk to your child about behavior and situations that are safe and not safe.

- Identify and remind your child of safe adults that he or she can turn to. Role playing and practicing how to find a safe adult can help young children learn where to go.

If you think your child has been abused or neglected you can:

- Talk to your child's doctor about your concerns
- Take your child to a hospital or doctor's office to be examined
- Call the police (dial 911 on your phone)
- Call the Childhelp National Child Abuse Hotline: 1-800-4-A-CHILD (1-800-422-4453)

Take Care of Yourself

Being a parent is the hardest job you will ever love. It is easy to become overwhelmed, especially if you have a child who has a disability or other special health care needs.

Here are some things to remember when parenting gets stressful or difficult:

- Be realistic about what your child can and cannot do.
- If you are frustrated, give yourself a time-out to calm down and refocus!
- Ask people who you trust to help you.
- Focus on the positive.
- Make time for yourself.
- Talk to a healthcare professional like your doctor or a therapist if you don't know how to handle your child's behavior.

Part Four

Adult Survivors of Child Abuse

Chapter 29

Adverse Childhood Experiences and Adult Survivors

Chapter Contents

Section 29.1

Prevalence of Individual Adverse Childhood Experiences

This section includes text excerpted from "Adverse Childhood Experiences," Substance Abuse and Mental Health Services Administration (SAMHSA), March 7, 2016.

Adverse Childhood Experiences

Adverse childhood experiences (ACEs) are a significant risk factor for substance use disorders and can impact prevention efforts.

Adverse childhood experiences (ACEs) are stressful or traumatic events, including abuse and neglect. They may also include household dysfunction such as witnessing domestic violence or growing up with family members who have substance use disorders. ACEs are strongly related to the development and prevalence of a wide range of health problems throughout a person's lifespan, including those associated with substance misuse.

ACEs include:

- Physical abuse
- Sexual abuse
- Emotional abuse
- Physical neglect
- Emotional neglect
- Mother treated violently
- Substance misuse within household
- Household mental illness
- Parental separation or divorce
- Incarcerated household member

ACEs are a good example of the types of complex issues that the prevention workforce often faces. The negative effects of ACEs are felt throughout the nation and can affect people of all backgrounds. Successfully addressing their impact requires:

- Assessing prevention needs and gathering data
- Effective and sustainable prevention approaches guided by applying the Strategic Prevention Framework (SPF)
- Prevention efforts aligned with the widespread occurrence of ACEs
- Building relationships with appropriate community partners through strong collaboration

Many studies have examined the relationship between ACEs and a variety of known risk factors for disease, disability, and early mortality. The Division of Violence Prevention at the Centers for Disease Control and Prevention (CDC), in partnership with Kaiser Permanente, conducted a landmark ACE study from 1995 to 1997 with more than 17,000 participants. The study found:

- **ACEs are common.** For example, 28% of study participants reported physical abuse and 21% reported sexual abuse. Many also reported experiencing a divorce or parental separation, or having a parent with a mental and/or substance use disorder.
- **ACEs cluster/strong.** Almost 40% of the Kaiser sample reported two or more ACEs and 12.5% experienced four or more. Because ACEs cluster, many subsequent studies now look at the cumulative effects of ACEs rather than the individual effects of each.
- **ACEs have a dose-response relationship with many health problems**. As researchers followed participants over time, they discovered that a person's cumulative ACEs score has a strong, graded relationship to numerous health, social, and behavioral problems throughout their lifespan, including substance use disorders. Furthermore, many problems related to ACEs tend to be comorbid or co-occurring.

ACEs and Prevention Efforts

Preventing ACEs and engaging in early identification of people who have experienced them could have a significant impact on a range of critical health problems. You can strengthen your substance misuse prevention efforts by:

- Informing local decision-making by collecting state- and county-level ACEs data.

- Increasing awareness of ACEs among state- and community-level substance misuse prevention professionals, emphasizing the relevance of ACEs to behavioral health disciplines.

- Including ACEs among the primary risk and protective factors when engaging in prevention planning efforts.

- Selecting and implementing programs, policies, and strategies designed to address ACEs, including efforts focusing on reducing intergenerational transmission of ACEs.

- Using ACEs research and local ACEs data to identify groups of people who may be at higher risk for substance use disorders and to conduct targeted prevention.

ACEs Research and Behavioral Health

Research has demonstrated a strong relationship between ACEs, substance use disorders, and behavioral problems. When children are exposed to chronic stressful events, their neurodevelopment can be disrupted. As a result, the child's cognitive functioning or ability to cope with negative or disruptive emotions may be impaired. Over time, and often during adolescence, the child may adopt negative coping mechanisms, such as substance use or self-harm. Eventually, these unhealthy coping mechanisms can contribute to disease, disability, and social problems, as well as premature mortality.

ACEs and Substance Use Disorders

- Early initiation of alcohol use. Underage drinking prevention efforts may not be effective unless ACEs are addressed as a contributing factor. Underage drinking prevention programs may not work as intended unless they help youth recognize and cope with stressors of abuse, household dysfunction, and other adverse experiences.

- Higher risk of alcohol abuse as an adult. ACEs such as child abuse, parental alcoholism, and family dysfunction correlate with a higher risk of problem drinking behavior in adulthood.

- Continued tobacco use during adulthood. Prevalence ratios for current and ever smoking increased as ACEs scores increased, a 2011 study on ACEs and smoking status found.

- Prescription drug use. Prescription drug use increased as ACEs scores increased, according to a 2008 study of adverse childhood experiences and prescription drug use.

- Lifetime illicit drug use, drug dependency, and self-reported addiction. Each ACE increased the likelihood of early initiation into illicit drug use by 2- to 4-fold, according to a 2003 study on childhood abuse, neglect, and household dysfunction and the risk of illicit drug use.

ACEs and Behavioral Problems

- **Increased risk of suicide attempts.** ACEs in any category increased the risk of attempted suicide by 2- to 5-fold throughout a person's lifespan.

- **Lifetime depressive episodes.** Exposure to ACEs may increase the risk of experiencing depressive disorders well into adulthood—sometimes decades after ACEs occur.

- **Sleep disturbances in adults.** People with a history of ACEs have a higher likelihood of experiencing self-reported sleep disorders, according to a 2011 study on ACEs and sleep disturbances in adults.

- **High-risk sexual behaviors.** Women with ACEs have reported risky sexual behaviors, including early intercourse, having had 30 or more sexual partners, and perceiving themselves to be at risk for HIV/AIDS.

- **Fetal mortality.** Fetal deaths attributed to adolescent pregnancy may result from underlying ACEs rather than adolescent pregnancy, according to a 2004 study of the association between ACEs and adolescent pregnancy.

Section 29.2

Adverse Childhood Experiences (ACE) Study

This section includes text excerpted from "ACE Study,"
Centers for Disease Control and Prevention (CDC), April 1, 2016.

Overview

Childhood experiences, both positive and negative, have a tremendous impact on future violence victimization and perpetration, and lifelong health and opportunity. As such, early experiences are an important public health issue. Much of the foundational research in this area has been referred to as Adverse Childhood Experiences (ACEs).

Adverse Childhood Experiences have been linked to

• risky health behaviors,

• chronic health conditions,

• low life potential, and

• early death.

As the number of ACEs increases, so does the risk for these outcomes.

The wide-ranging health and social consequences of ACEs underscore the importance of preventing them before they happen.

The ACE Pyramid

The ACE Pyramid represents the conceptual framework for the study. During the time period of the 1980s and early 1990s information about risk factors for disease had been widely researched and merged into public education and prevention programs. However, it was also clear that risk factors, such as smoking, alcohol abuse, and sexual behaviors for many common diseases were not randomly distributed in the population. In fact, it was known that risk factors for many chronic diseases tended to cluster, that is, persons who had one risk factor tended to have one or more other risk factors too.

Because of this knowledge, the ACE Study was designed to assess what we considered to be "scientific gaps" about the origins of risk factors. These gaps are depicted as the two arrows linking Adverse Childhood Experiences to risk factors that lead to the health and social consequences higher up the pyramid. Specifically, the study was designed to provide data that would help answer the question: "If risk factors for disease, disability, and early mortality are not randomly distributed, what influences precede the adoption or development of them?" By providing information to answer this question, we hoped to provide scientific information that would be useful for developing new and more effective prevention programs.

The ACE Study takes a whole life perspective, as indicated on the orange arrow leading from conception to death. By working within this framework, the ACE Study began to progressively uncover how adverse childhood experiences (ACE) are strongly related to development and prevalence of risk factors for disease and health and social well-being throughout the lifespan.

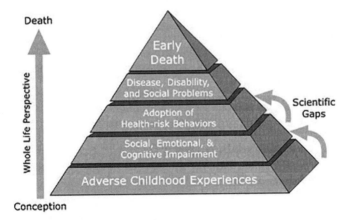

Figure 29.1. *ACE Pyramid*

Major Findings

Childhood abuse, neglect, and exposure to other traumatic stressors which we term *adverse childhood experiences* (ACE) are common. Almost two-thirds of our study participants reported at least one ACE, and more than one of five reported three or more ACE. The short- and long-term outcomes of these childhood exposures include a multitude of health and social problems.

The ACE Study uses the ACE Score, which is a total count of the number of ACEs reported by respondents. The ACE Score is used to assess the total amount of stress during childhood and has demonstrated that as the number of ACE increase, the risk for the following health problems increases in a strong and graded fashion:

- Alcoholism and alcohol abuse

- Chronic obstructive pulmonary disease (COPD)

- Depression

- Fetal death

- Health-related quality of life

- Illicit drug use

- Ischemic heart disease (IHD)

- Liver disease

- Risk for intimate partner violence

- Multiple sexual partners

- Sexually transmitted diseases (STDs)

- Smoking

- Suicide attempts

- Unintended pregnancies

- Early initiation of smoking

- Early initiation of sexual activity

- Adolescent pregnancy

Chapter 30

Early Life Stress and Adult CFS

Early Life Stress and Adult CFS

It is a well-established fact that experiences during early life shape the development of the brain, particularly during sensitive periods. Adverse experiences can 'program' the development of certain brain regions that are involved in the regulation and integration of hormonal, autonomic and immune responses to challenges later in life. Such challenges may encompass infections, physical stresses or emotional challenges.

Approximately 14% of children in the United States are subjected to some form of maltreatment, and in 2007, over 3 million reports of childhood abuse and neglect were investigated. Childhood trauma, defined as abuse, neglect, or loss, is a stressor that affects the physical and mental well-being of humans from infancy throughout the lifespan. In various animal and human studies childhood trauma has been associated with low resting cortisol levels, altered stress response, increased inflammatory markers, and cognitive impairment.

Childhood abuse has been connected to a wide range of disorders, such as depression, anxiety disorders, and substance abuse problems, but also more classic medical diseases such as cardiovascular

This chapter includes text excerpted from "Chronic Fatigue Syndrome (CFS)," Centers for Disease Control and Prevention (CDC), November 5, 2014.

disease. Of note, markedly elevated levels of pain and fatigue have been reported in studies of survivors of childhood abuse.

Chronic fatigue syndrome (CFS) is a debilitating illness that can sometimes occur in response to a stressor or a challenge. For example, there have been reports of people developing CFS after being in a serious car accident. Other examples of challenges are increased rates of CFS in Gulf war veterans and triggered relapses of CFS in persons affected by Hurricane Andrew.

Upon stress exposure, our central nervous system will activate hormone and immune responses that help the body to maintain balance during stress. There is evidence that childhood maltreatment may alter the way how the body's regulatory systems respond to stress. Early adversity may thus increase a person's risk to develop adult CFS, particularly in response to challenges. Therefore, childhood trauma may be an important risk factor for adult CFS. Research has shown that when adults with CFS and without CFS were asked about childhood trauma, those with CFS self-reported higher levels of childhood maltreatment. In particular, for women, emotional and sexual abuse during childhood was associated with a greater risk of developing CFS later in life.

Of note, a risk factor is not "the cause" of a disorder; it increases the relative risk, but is not present in all cases. The cause of CFS is still unknown, but childhood trauma might be factor that contributes to adult CFS risk in a subset of people. While these findings are important and have the potential to help many people, it is important to realize that not all persons with adult CFS experienced maltreatment as a child. Childhood maltreatment is just one risk factor for CFS and does not explain how other people with CFS (who did not experience such trauma) developed the illness.

The results from this research are important because healthcare providers can help people with a history of childhood maltreatment. For some people that have both a past of childhood maltreatment and CFS, talk therapy may be beneficial. While more research is needed on CFS and childhood maltreatment, patients are encouraged to talk to their healthcare provider about their physical and mental health history.

Helping Your Child Manage Chronic Fatigue Syndrome (CFS)

Chronic fatigue syndrome (CFS) is a complex illness that can be challenging for parents and children. Following are some tips to help you in dealing with this illness, whether it affects you or your child.

Be an Advocate for Your Child

Take an active role in managing your child's illness and encourage him or her to do the same. This can allow you to make the best possible choices for his or her health.

- Learn as much as you can about CFS and how it affects your child.

- Talk with your child's healthcare provider about your questions and concerns.

- Speak with school staff, such as teachers, guidance counselors, and school nurses, about concerns you have with your child in school.

- Work closely with teachers, counselors, and other school staff to develop an action plan and find resources to help your child succeed in school.

- Educate others involved in your child's life about CFS, such as school staff, other family members, and your child's peers. When people know more about this illness, they may be better able to help and accommodate your child. This is particularly important at your child's school.

Be Familiar with School Resources

CFS can affect a child or adolescent's experience at school. Fatigue, pain, and concentration or memory problems can make it hard for a child to complete homework assignments. It may also be difficult for them to participate in the classroom, or attend school on a regular basis. With some planning, teachers and parents can help a child or adolescent with CFS to have a successful school experience.

Evaluation is an important part of identifying the needs of a student with CFS. It can guide the development of programs to help them succeed in school. It is important to know that:

- Receiving a CFS diagnosis will not immediately qualify a child for services. A child will need to be further evaluated and identified as needing services at school.

- Evaluations will need to be conducted by a team from the school. This team will assess the student through in-class observations, tests, interviews, and conversations with teachers and parents.

- Parents will need to give consent before a student undergoes an evaluation.

Additional services could include an Individualized Education Plan (IEP) or a 504 Plan. A 504 plan lists your child's disability and how the school can help. An IEP is a legal document that tells the school what it must do to help meet your child's needs. These programs are developed with help from administrators, teachers, and parents.

Participate in Family and Social Activities

Having a chance to socialize is just as important for your child as having a chance to succeed in school. With limited social involvement inside and outside of school, students with CFS may feel isolated from their friends and peers. It can be challenging for families to be involved in social events or family activities. However, these activities are essential for the well-being of the child and family. Some families may find it helpful to connect with support groups to talk with other families who have a child with CFS.

Children with CFS may not be able to attend classes on a regular basis or stay for a full school day. Therefore, it's important to talk to your child's school about opportunities for your child to interact with peers. For example, the school could allow your child to participate in after-school activities or attend lunch periods.

Chapter 31

Factors Affecting the Consequences of Child Abuse and Neglect

Individual outcomes vary widely and are affected by a combination of factors, including:

- The child's age and developmental status when the abuse or neglect occurred

- The type of maltreatment (physical abuse, neglect, sexual abuse, etc.)

- The frequency, duration, and severity of the maltreatment

- The relationship between the child and the perpetrator

Researchers also have begun to explore why, given similar conditions, some children experience long-term consequences of abuse and neglect while others emerge relatively unscathed. The ability to cope, and even thrive, following a negative experience is often referred to as "resilience." It is important to note that resilience is not an inherent

---

This chapter includes text excerpted from "Long-Term Consequences of Child Abuse and Neglect," U.S. Department of Health and Human Services (HHS), July 2013.

trait in children but results from a mixture of both risk and protective factors that cause a child's positive or negative reaction to adverse experiences. A number of protective and promotive factors—individually, within a family, or within a community—may contribute to an abused or neglected child's resilience. These include positive attachment, self-esteem, intelligence, emotion regulation, humor, and independence.

Physical Health Consequences

The immediate physical effects of abuse or neglect can be relatively minor (bruises or cuts) or severe (broken bones, hemorrhage, or even death). In some cases, the physical effects are temporary; however, the pain and suffering they cause a child should not be discounted.

Child abuse and neglect can have a multitude of long-term effects on physical health. NSCAW researchers found that, at some point during the 3 years following a maltreatment investigation, 28 percent of children had a chronic health. Below are some outcomes other researchers have identified:

Abusive head trauma. Abusive head trauma, an inflicted injury to the head and its contents caused by shaking and blunt impact, is the most common cause of traumatic death for infants. The injuries may not be immediately noticeable and may include bleeding in the eye or brain and damage to the spinal cord and neck. Significant brain development takes place during infancy, and this important development is compromised in maltreated children. One in every four victims of shaken baby syndrome dies, and nearly all victims experience serious health consequences.

Impaired brain development. Child abuse and neglect have been shown to cause important regions of the brain to fail to form or grow properly, resulting in impaired development. These alterations in brain maturation have long-term consequences for cognitive, language, and academic abilities and are connected with mental health disorders. Disrupted neurodevelopment as a result of maltreatment can cause children to adopt a persistent fear state as well as attributes that are normally helpful during threatening moments but counterproductive in the absence of threats, such as hypervigilance, anxiety, and behavior impulsivity. Child Welfare Information Gateway has produced two publications on the impact of maltreatment on brain development.

Poor physical health. Several studies have shown a relationship between various forms of child maltreatment and poor health. Adults who experienced abuse or neglect during childhood are more likely to suffer from cardiovascular disease, lung and liver disease, hypertension, diabetes, asthma, and obesity. Specific physical health conditions are also connected to maltreatment type. One study showed that children who experienced neglect were at increased risk for diabetes and poorer lung functioning, while physical abuse was shown to increase the risk for diabetes and malnutrition. Additionally, child maltreatment has been shown to increase adolescent obesity. A longitudinal study found that children who experienced neglect had body mass indexes that grew at significantly faster rates compared to children who had not experienced neglect.

Psychological Consequences

The immediate emotional effects of abuse and neglect—isolation, fear, and an inability to trust—can translate into lifelong psychological consequences, including low self-esteem, depression, and relationship difficulties. Researchers have identified links between child abuse and neglect and the following:

Difficulties during infancy. Of children entering foster care in 2010, 16 percent were younger than 1 year. When infants and young children enter out-of-home care due to abuse or neglect, the trauma of a primary caregiver change negatively affects their attachments. Nearly half of infants in foster care who have experienced maltreatment exhibit some form of cognitive delay and have lower IQ scores, language difficulties, and neonatal challenges compared to children who have not been abused or neglected.

Poor mental and emotional health. Experiencing childhood trauma and adversity, such as physical or sexual abuse, is a risk factor for borderline personality disorder, depression, anxiety, and other psychiatric disorders. One study using ACE data found that roughly 54 percent of cases of depression and 58 percent of suicide attempts in women were connected to adverse childhood experiences. Child maltreatment also negatively impacts the development of emotion regulation, which often persists into adolescence or adulthood.

Cognitive difficulties. NSCAW researchers found that children with substantiated reports of maltreatment were at risk for severe developmental and cognitive problems, including grade repetition. In its final report on the second NSCAW study (NSCAW II), more than 10 percent of school-aged children and youth showed some risk of cognitive problems or low academic achievement, 43 percent had emotional or behavioral problems, and 13 percent had both.

Social difficulties. Children who experience neglect are more likely to develop antisocial traits as they grow up. Parental neglect is associated with borderline personality disorders, attachment issues or affectionate behaviors with unknown/little-known people, inappropriate modeling of adult behavior, and aggression.

Behavioral Consequences

Not all victims of child abuse and neglect will experience behavioral consequences. However, behavioral problems appear to be more likely among this group. According to NSCAW, more than half of youth reported for maltreatment are at risk for an emotional or behavioral problem. Child abuse and neglect appear to make the following more likely:

Difficulties during adolescence. NSCAW data show that more than half of youth with reports of maltreatment are at risk of grade repetition, substance abuse, delinquency, truancy, or pregnancy. Other studies suggest that abused or neglected children are more likely to engage in sexual risk-taking as they reach adolescence, thereby increasing their chances of contracting a sexually transmitted disease. Victims of child sexual abuse also are at a higher risk for rape in adulthood, and the rate of risk increases according to the severity of the child sexual abuse experience(s).

Juvenile delinquency and adult criminality. Several studies have documented the correlation between child abuse and future juvenile delinquency. Children who have experienced abuse are nine times more likely to become involved in criminal activities.

Alcohol and other drug abuse. Research consistently reflects an increased likelihood that children who have experienced abuse or neglect will smoke cigarettes, abuse alcohol, or take illicit drugs during their lifetime. In fact, male children with an ACE Score of 6 or more (having six or more adverse childhood experiences) had an increased likelihood—of more than 4,000 percent—to use intravenous drugs later in life.

Abusive behavior. Abusive parents often have experienced abuse during their own childhoods. Data from the Longitudinal Study of Adolescent Health showed that girls who experienced childhood physical abuse were 1–7 percent more likely to become perpetrators of youth violence and 8–10 percent more likely to be perpetrators of interpersonal violence (IPV). Boys who experienced childhood sexual violence were 3–12 percent more likely to commit youth violence and 1–17 percent more likely to commit IPV.

Societal Consequences

While child abuse and neglect usually occur within the family, the impact does not end there. Society as a whole pays a price for child abuse and neglect, in terms of both direct and indirect costs.

Direct costs. The lifetime cost of child maltreatment and related fatalities in 1 year totals $124 billion, according to a study funded by the CDC. Child maltreatment is more costly on an annual basis than the two leading health concerns, stroke and type 2 diabetes. On the other hand, programs that prevent maltreatment have shown to be cost effective. The U.S. Triple P System Trial, funded by the CDC, has a benefit/cost ratio of $47 in benefits to society for every $1 in program costs.

Indirect costs. Indirect costs represent the long-term economic consequences to society because of child abuse and neglect. These include costs associated with increased use of our health-care system, juvenile and adult criminal activity, mental illness, substance abuse, and domestic violence. Prevent Child Abuse America estimates that child abuse and neglect prevention strategies can save taxpayers $104 billion each year. According to the Schuyler Center for Analysis and Advocacy, every $1 spent on home visiting yields a $5.70 return on investment in New York, including reduced confirmed reports of abuse, reduced family enrollment in Temporary Assistance for Needy Families, decreased visits to emergency rooms, decreased arrest rates for mothers, and increased monthly earnings. One study found that all eight categories of adverse childhood experiences were associated with an increased likelihood of employment problems, financial problems, and absenteeism. The authors assert that these long-term costs—to the workforce and to society—are preventable.

Prevention Practice and Strategies

To break the cycle of maltreatment and reduce the likelihood of long-term consequences, communities across the country must continue to develop and implement strategies that prevent abuse or neglect from happening. While experts agree that the causes of child abuse and neglect are complex, it is possible to develop prevention initiatives that address known risk factors.

Trauma-Informed Practice

While the priority is to prevent child abuse and neglect from occurring, it is equally important to respond to those children and adults who have experienced abuse and neglect. Over the past 30 years, researchers and practitioners have developed a better understanding of the effects of trauma. More has been done in the way of developing supports to address these effects, build resiliency, and, hopefully, prevent further trauma.

Trauma-informed practice refers to the services and programs specifically designed to address and respond to the impact of traumatic stress. The importance of this approach has become especially evident in the child welfare system, as a majority of children and families involved with child welfare have experienced some form of past trauma. When human service systems recognize and respond to the impact of trauma and use this knowledge to adapt policies and practices, children, youth, and families benefit. The National Child Traumatic Stress Network strives to raise the standard of care and improve access to services for traumatized children, their families, and communities.

Chapter 32

Reactions to Trauma in Adult Survivors of Child Abuse

Chapter Contents

Section 32.1

Prevalence of Trauma-Related Difficulties among Persons Exposed to Violence

This section includes text excerpted from "Childhood Trauma and Its Effects: Implications for Police," U.S. Department of Justice (DOJ), July 2015.

The number of individuals who, as children, were repeatedly exposed to violent trauma in the absence of parental protection, and then went on to develop the cluster of psychiatric and neuropsychiatric difficulties, is difficult to determine. This is because there are no studies that have attempted to determine the overall prevalence of children exposed to one or more of the various types of violent trauma known to cause such psychiatric or neuropsychiatric difficulties. Nor are there any studies that followed the traumatized children to see what percentage actually develop such psychiatric or neuropsychiatric difficulties. However, studies that have tried to look at prevalence in subsets of these children suggest that the rate is alarmingly high. For example, it is estimated that 35 percent of children exposed to domestic violence will develop trauma-related difficulties.

A recent estimate puts the number of children exposed to domestic violence during 2012 at 266, 110—meaning that approximately 93, 139 children will develop trauma-related difficulties as a result of exposure to domestic violence during that year. Similarly, it is estimated that between 42 percent and 90 percent of child victims of sexual abuse will develop trauma-related difficulties. During 2012, an estimated 62,936 children were victims of sexual abuse—meaning that between 26,433 and 56,642 of those children will likely develop trauma-related difficulties as a result of being sexually abused.

Although these data give some indication of the scope of exposure to domestic violence and childhood sexual abuse, statistics related to both these issues are thought to be underestimates. It is, therefore, likely that the actual prevalence of PTSD stemming from both childhood sexual abuse and exposure to domestic violence is greater than stated above.

More difficult to estimate is the number of children repeatedly exposed to or even directly threatened by various forms of neighborhood violence. We know that, although domestic violence and child sexual abuse occur in all neighborhoods, children who are raised in poor, drug-infested, violent neighborhoods are at increased risk of exposure to street violence, increasing their risk of developing trauma-related difficulties. In addition, because these children are much less likely to be identified as needing treatment and have less access to medical care, their difficulties are more likely to continue unabated into adolescence and adulthood.

Section 32.2

Posttraumatic Stress Disorder

This section includes text excerpted from "Post-Traumatic Stress Disorder," National Institute of Mental Health (NIMH), February 2016.

What Is Posttraumatic Stress Disorder?

Posttraumatic stress disorder (PTSD) is a disorder that develops in some people who have seen or lived through a shocking, scary, or dangerous event.

It is natural to feel afraid during and after a traumatic situation. Fear triggers many split-second changes in the body to help defend against danger or to avoid it. This "fight-or-flight" response is a healthy reaction meant to protect a person from harm. Nearly everyone will experience a range of reactions after trauma, yet most people recover from initial symptoms naturally. Those who continue to experience problems may be diagnosed with PTSD. People who have PTSD may feel stressed or frightened even when they are not in danger.

Signs and Symptoms

Not every traumatized person develops ongoing (chronic) or even short-term (acute) PTSD. Symptoms usually begin early, within 3 months of the traumatic incident, but sometimes they begin years afterward. Symptoms must last more than a month to be considered PTSD. The course of the illness varies. Some people recover within 6 months, while others have symptoms that last much longer. In some people, the condition becomes chronic.

A doctor who has experience helping people with mental illnesses, such as a psychiatrist or psychologist, can diagnose PTSD.

To be diagnosed with PTSD, an adult must have all of the following for at least 1 month:

- At least one re-experiencing symptom

- At least one avoidance symptom

- At least two arousal and reactivity symptoms

- At least two cognition and mood symptoms

Re-experiencing symptoms include:

- Flashbacks—reliving the trauma over and over, including physical symptoms like a racing heart or sweating

- Bad dreams

- Frightening thoughts

Re-experiencing symptoms may cause problems in a person's everyday routine. The symptoms can start from the person's own thoughts and feelings. Words, objects, or situations that are reminders of the event can also trigger re-experiencing symptoms.

Avoidance symptoms include:

- Staying away from places, events, or objects that are reminders of the traumatic experience

- Feeling emotionally numb

- Feeling strong guilt, depression, or worry

- Losing interest in activities that were enjoyable in the past

- Having trouble remembering the dangerous event

Things that remind a person of the traumatic event can trigger avoidance symptoms. These symptoms may cause a person to change his or her personal routine. For example, after a bad car accident, a person who usually drives may avoid driving or riding in a car.

Arousal and reactivity symptoms include:

- Being easily startled

- Feeling tense or "on edge"

- Having difficulty sleeping

- Having angry outbursts

Arousal symptoms are usually constant, instead of being triggered by things that remind one of the traumatic events. These symptoms can make the person feel stressed and angry. They may make it hard to do daily tasks, such as sleeping, eating, or concentrating.

Cognition and mood symptoms include:

- Trouble remembering key features of the traumatic event

- Negative thoughts about oneself or the world

- Distorted feelings like guilt or blame

- Loss of interest in enjoyable activities

Cognition and mood symptoms can begin or worsen after the traumatic event, but are not due to injury or substance use. These symptoms can make the person feel alienated or detached from friends or family members.

It is natural to have some of these symptoms after a dangerous event. Sometimes people have very serious symptoms that go away after a few weeks. This is called acute stress disorder, or ASD. When the symptoms last more than a few weeks and become an ongoing problem, the person may have developed PTSD. Some people with PTSD don't show any symptoms for weeks or months. PTSD is often accompanied by depression, substance abuse, or one or more of the other anxiety disorders.

Do Children React Differently than Adults?

Children and teens can have extreme reactions to trauma, but their symptoms may not be the same as adults. In very young children (less than 6 years of age), these symptoms can include:

- Wetting the bed after having learned to use the toilet

- Forgetting how to or being unable to talk

- Acting out the scary event during playtime

- Being unusually clingy with a parent or other adult

Older children and teens are more likely to show symptoms similar to those seen in adults. They may also develop disruptive, disrespectful, or destructive behaviors. Older children and teens may feel guilty for not preventing injury or deaths. They may also have thoughts of revenge.

Risk Factors

Anyone can develop PTSD at any age. This includes war veterans, children, and people who have been through a physical or sexual assault, abuse, accident, disaster, or many other serious events. According to the National Center for PTSD, about 7 or 8 out of every 100 people will experience PTSD at some point in their lives. Women are more likely to develop PTSD than men, and genes may make some people more likely to develop PTSD than others.

Not everyone with PTSD has been through a dangerous event. Some people develop PTSD after a friend or family member experiences danger or harm. The sudden, unexpected death of a loved one can also lead to PTSD.

Why Do Some People Develop PTSD and Other People Do Not?

It is important to remember that not everyone who lives through a dangerous event gets PTSD. In fact, most people will not get the disorder.

Many factors play a part in whether a person will develop PTSD. Some examples are listed below. Risk factors make a person more likely to get PTSD. Other factors, called resilience factors, can help reduce the risk of the disorder.

Risk Factors and Resilience Factors for PTSD

Some factors that increase risk for PTSD include:

- Living through dangerous events and traumas

- Getting hurt

- Seeing another person hurt, or seeing a dead body

- Childhood trauma

- Feeling horror, helplessness, or extreme fear

- Having little or no social support after the event

- Dealing with extra stress after the event, such as loss of a loved one, pain and injury, or loss of a job or home

- Having a history of mental illness

  Some resilience factors that may reduce the risk of PTSD include:

- Seeking out support from other people, such as friends and family

- Finding a support group after a traumatic event

- Learning to feel good about one's own actions in the face of danger

- Having a positive coping strategy, or a way of getting through the bad event and learning from it

- Being able to act and respond effectively despite feeling fear

Researchers are studying the importance of these and other risk and resilience factors, including genetics and neurobiology. With more research, someday it may be possible to predict who is likely to get PTSD and to prevent it.

Section 32.3

Faqs about PTSD Assessment

This section includes text excerpted from "FAQs about PTSD Assessment," U.S. Department of Veterans Affairs (VA), August 13, 2015.

How Can I Tell If I Have PTSD?

Many people ask us how they can decide for themselves whether they have posttraumatic stress disorder (PTSD). It is natural to want to know why you are feeling or acting a certain way. However, trying to figure out on your own whether or not you have PTSD is difficult. Since many common reactions after trauma look like the symptoms of PTSD, a mental health provider must decide if you have PTSD.

Providers who have been trained to understand the thoughts and behaviors that go along with PTSD are best able to make that decision.

A provider must use his or her training and judgment to select the best test or set of questions to use. Then he or she must interpret the results of the test.

The American Psychological Association suggests that only trained professionals give tests to assess for PTSD. If you think you may have PTSD, talk to your doctor or a mental health provider.

How Can I Find out If a Mental Health Provider Is Able to Evaluate Me for PTSD?

You can ask questions about the provider's training and experience. Here are some questions you might ask:

"What Is Your Specialty Area?"

Many providers specialize in assessing and treating people who have experienced trauma. Providers who specialize in trauma will likely have expertise in evaluating PTSD. Some providers may specialize in working with certain kinds of trauma survivors. For example, a provider may work with adult survivors of childhood traumas. You may find a provider who specializes in a different trauma area than what you need, or who does not specialize at all. A provider who has experience assessing trauma survivors like you is most likely to have the expertise to do a good job on your assessment.

"How Many PTSD Assessments Have You Done?"

If possible, find a professional who has experience conducting PTSD assessments.

"What Formal Training Have You Had That Will Allow You to Evaluate Me for PTSD?"

If possible, find a professional who has completed training focused on PTSD assessment. Such providers are preferred over those trained only in general assessment.

"What Formal Training Have You Had That Will Allow You to Evaluate Me for PTSD?"

If possible, find a professional who has completed training focused on PTSD assessment. Such providers are preferred over those trained only in general assessment.

"Can You Tell Me a Little about How You Assess PTSD?"

You should feel comfortable with the assessment methods that a provider will use. A good assessment of PTSD can be done without the use of any special equipment. Most often, providers will have you fill out surveys or they will use a standard interview in which the provider will read a series of questions from a printed document.

Who Can Request a PTSD or Trauma Measure from the National Center for PTSD?

The American Psychological Association (APA) requires that anyone who gives and interprets psychological tests must have advanced training. That is why we only give out measures to people with at least a master's degree in psychology or a related clinical area.

What Is the Difference between an Evaluation That Measures Trauma Exposure and an Evaluation That Measures PTSD?

An evaluation that measures trauma exposure looks at whether you've gone through a traumatic event. Examples of traumatic events include combat, a car accident, or child sexual abuse. Sometimes, the evaluation asks when the event happened. For example, you might be asked your age at the time of the experience. A measure of trauma exposure may also assess how you felt at the time of the event. You might be asked if you felt your life or the life of someone else was in danger.

By contrast, an evaluation that measures PTSD looks at how you felt or acted after you went through the traumatic event. You might be asked about the effect the trauma has had on your life, or any symptoms you may have had since the trauma. Some PTSD evaluations also ask about other problems such as depression or relationship problems. These other problems do not lead to a PTSD diagnosis, however.

If an Organization Is Asking for Proof of a PTSD Diagnosis, What Should I Provide?

Only the results of a complete evaluation given by a professional can determine whether you have PTSD. Any organization with which you might be dealing will likely need the results of your evaluation. Therefore, you should see a healthcare provider who has experience in this area. As a patient, you can typically request a copy of your evaluation results from the professional who completes your assessment.

If you are a Veteran, the Veterans Benefits Administration has section on how to submit a compensation claim for PTSD. You can also call your local VA Medical Center to ask about benefits. Veterans Service Organizations (VSOs) also offer free guidance on completing claims.

Part Five

Child Abuse Preventions, Interventions, and Treatments

Chapter 33

Child Abuse Prevention Strategies

Chapter Contents

Section 33.1

The Need for Prevention and Intervention

This section includes text excerpted from "Acts of Omission: An Overview of Child Neglect," U.S. Department of Health and Human Services (HHS), August 2012. Reviewed May 2016.

Prevention and Intervention

The services and supports that at-risk or neglected children and their families need vary greatly depending on the type of neglect they experienced, the severity of their situation, underlying risks, strengths, and many other factors. Analyzing the information gathered during the investigation and assessment is essential to developing an effective case plan in collaboration with the family, their support network, and related service providers.

Begin Early

Children are more likely to be harmed by neglect the earlier they experience it. Although it can be difficult to prevent neglect and identify it in its early stages, you can have a greater impact on families the earlier you intervene. At this stage, assess the parent's readiness to enhance their parenting abilities and help the family focus on meeting the child's developmental needs. Assume that parents want to improve the quality of their children's care—they just need support to identify and build on their strengths.

Provide Concrete Services First

Most parents cannot focus on interventions like parenting classes when they are still addressing crises in their family. In the early stages of working with a family, be sure basic needs are met before expecting parents to fulfill other aspects of their case plan. Some concrete supports to address include:

• Housing and utilities

• Food and clothing

- Safety for domestic violence victims
- Transportation
- Child care
- Health care and public benefits

Focus on Strengths

You can form better relationships with families when you encourage them to focus on positive parenting strategies and supports they already have in place. The six protective factors described earlier can serve as a framework for assessing families' strengths and helping them identify ways to build upon those strengths to protect their children from harm. The Children's Bureau's Resource Guide for child abuse prevention offers numerous tools and strategies for talking with families about their strengths and incorporating them into service systems.

Offer Customized, Coordinated Services

Be flexible; there is no "one size fits all" solution to addressing neglect. Offer or refer families to a broad array of services and collaborate with other services providers to ensure the family's needs are met. Some of the most common services provided by the Federal child neglect demonstration project grantees included:

- Parent education and support
- Home visits
- Referrals or links to community resources
- Mental health services
- Concrete assistance and crisis intervention

Home visiting programs, which provide in-home services to families with young children, show promise in engaging parents to reduce risks related to child abuse and neglect. Professional or paraprofessional home visitors can build relationships with parents and tailor their visits to address the family's needs and strengths. Some of the topics home visitors may address include:

- The mother's personal health and life choices
- Child health and development

- Environmental concerns such as income, housing, and domestic or community violence

- Family functioning, including adult and child relationships

- Access to services

Supporting Evidence-Based Home Visiting is a Federal initiative to generate knowledge of home visiting practices and models.

Encourage Incremental Change

Most changes don't happen overnight. Especially with families that are stressed by the demands of caring for their child, parents may feel overwhelmed if you expect them to accomplish too many goals too quickly. In collaboration with the family, establish a contract with a timeline for accomplishing specific goals as well as obligations for both you and the parents to meet.

Remember to start with the most basic needs (e.g., food, housing, safety), then address critical underlying issues (e.g., substance abuse, mental health). Once those supports are in place, there will be fewer obstacles to improving higher family functioning. Many programs have found that working with families affected by neglect requires intensive, long-term services to help them achieve changes over time.

Intensive family preservation services provide short-term crisis support to high-risk families to prevent unnecessary child placement in out-of-home care. Children and families experiencing severe neglect may benefit from these kinds of services to address urgent issues, like housing or financial assistance, followed by ongoing family preservation and support to target underlying risk factors.

Address the Social Support Network

Because your time with the family is limited, a strong social support network for the family can reinforce lessons learned and address needs as they arise. Seek out relatives, friends, community members, and other service providers who will help the family practice and build new skills over time. Positive relationships with other caring adults can help support the child's healthy development and serve as a source of respite for parents if they face future crises.

Put Aftercare Services in Place

As the family begins achieving major goals, develop a roadmap for services and supports after more intensive interventions end. An aftercare services plan will ensure opportunities for follow-up and help families maintain improvements over time.

Cultural Competence and Neglect

As with all child protection practice, cultural issues must be taken into consideration both when assessing and intervening with families at risk of neglect. For example, a culture in which shared caregiving is the norm may see no problem with allowing young children to care for their siblings, perhaps in a way that does not conform to cultural norms in the United States.

When working with diverse families, maintain focus on ensuring that children's needs are met and that they are not harmed or endangered. Consult with knowledgeable staff or community members on how best to intervene in a way that is consistent with families' cultural practices.

Section 33.2

Identifying Behaviors in Adults That May Put Children at Risk

This section includes text excerpted from "Recognizing Sexual Abuse," U.S. Department of Justice (DOJ), November 1, 2012. Reviewed May 2016.

Warning Signs That Might Suggest Someone Is Sexually Abusing a Child

The following behaviors could be cause for concern:

- Making others uncomfortable by ignoring social, emotional, or physical boundaries or limits

- Refusing to let a child set any of his or her own limits; using teasing or belittling language to keep a child from setting a limit

- Insisting on hugging, touching, kissing, tickling, wrestling with, or holding a child even when the child does not want this physical contact or attention

- Turning to a child for emotional or physical comfort by sharing personal or private information or activities that are normally shared with adults

- Frequently pointing out sexual images or telling inappropriate or suggestive jokes with children present

- Exposing a child to adult sexual interactions without apparent concern

- Having secret interactions with teens or children (e.g., games, sharing drugs, alcohol, or sexual material) or spending excessive time e-mailing, text-messaging, or calling children or youth

- Being overly interested in the sexuality of a particular child or teen (e.g., talks repeatedly about the child's developing body or interferes with normal teen dating)

- Insisting on or managing to spend unusual amounts of uninterrupted time alone with a child

- Seeming "too good to be true" (e.g., frequently babysits different children for free, takes children on special outings alone, buys children gifts or gives them money for no apparent reason)

- Frequently walking in on children/teens in the bathroom

- Allowing children or teens to consistently get away with inappropriate behaviors

Section 33.3

Preventing Child Sexual Abuse

This section includes text excerpted from "2016 Prevention Resource Guide: Building Community, Building Hope," U.S. Department of Health and Human Services (HHS), 2016.

What You Can Do

To prevent child sexual abuse, it is important to keep the focus on adult responsibility, while teaching children skills to help them protect themselves. Consider the following tips:

- Take an active role in your children's lives. Learn about their activities and people with whom they are involved. Stay alert for possible problems.

- Watch for "grooming" behaviors in adults who spend time with your child. Warning signs may include frequently finding ways to be alone with your child, ignoring your child's need for privacy (e.g., in the bathroom), or giving gifts or money for no particular occasion.

- Ensure that organizations, groups, and teams that your children are involved with minimize one-on-one time between children and adults. Ask how staff and volunteers are screened and supervised.

- Make sure your children know that they can talk to you about anything that bothers or confuses them.

- Teach children accurate names of private body parts and the difference between touches that are "okay" and "not okay."

- Empower children to make decisions about their bodies by allowing them age-appropriate privacy and encouraging them to say "no" when they do not want to touch or be touched by others, even in nonsexual ways.

- Teach children to take care of their own bodies (e.g., bathing or using the bathroom) so they do not have to rely on adults or older children for help.

- Educate children about the difference between good secrets (such as birthday surprises) and bad secrets (those that make the child feel unsafe or uncomfortable)

- Monitor children's use of technology, including cell phones, social networking sites, and messaging. Review contact lists regularly and ask about any people you don't recognize.

- Trust your instincts! If you feel uneasy about leaving your child with someone, don't do it. If you are concerned about possible sexual abuse, ask questions.

- If your child tells you that he or she has been abused, stay calm, listen carefully, and never blame the child. Thank your child for telling you. Report the abuse right away.

Signs of Possible Sexual Abuse

The following may indicate sexual abuse and should not be ignored:

- Unexplained pain, itching, redness, or bleeding in the genital area

- Increased nightmares or bedwetting

- Withdrawn behavior or appearing to be in a trance

- Angry outbursts or sudden mood swings

- Loss of appetite or difficulty swallowing

- Anxiety or depression

- Sudden, unexplained avoidance of certain people or places

- Sexual knowledge, language, or behavior that is unusual for the child's age

Remember: You can help protect your children from sexual abuse by being active in their lives and teaching them safety skills.

Chapter 34

Child Maltreatment Prevention Initiatives

Chapter Contents

Section 34.1

Child Abuse Prevention and Treatment Act (CAPTA)

This section includes text excerpted from "About CAPTA: A Legislative History," U.S. Department of Health and Human Services (HHS), July 2011. Reviewed May 2016.

The key Federal legislation addressing child abuse and neglect is the Child Abuse Prevention and Treatment Act (CAPTA), originally enacted on January 31, 1974 (P.L. 93-247). This Act was amended several times and was most recently amended and reauthorized on December 20, 2010, by the CAPTA Reauthorization Act of 2010 (P.L. 111-320).

CAPTA provides Federal funding to States in support of prevention, assessment, investigation, prosecution, and treatment activities and also provides grants to public agencies and nonprofit organizations, including Indian Tribes and Tribal organizations, for demonstration programs and projects. Additionally, CAPTA identifies the Federal role in supporting research, evaluation, technical assistance, and data collection activities; established the Office on Child Abuse and Neglect; and mandates Child Welfare Information Gateway. CAPTA also sets forth a minimum definition of child abuse and neglect.

The Child Abuse Prevention and Treatment Act (CAPTA) was originally enacted in P.L. 93-247. The act was later amended by the Child Abuse Prevention and Treatment and Adoption Reform Act of 1978 (P.L. 95-266, 4/24/78). The law was completely rewritten in the Child Abuse Prevention, Adoption and Family Services Act of 1988 (P.L. 100-294, 4/25/88). It was further amended by the Child Abuse Prevention Challenge Grants Reauthorization Act of 1989 (P.L. 101-126, 10/25/89) and the Drug Free School Amendments of 1989 (P.L. 101-226, 12/12/89).

The Community-Based Child Abuse and Neglect Prevention Grants program was originally authorized by sections 402 through 409 of the Continuing Appropriations Act for FY 1985 (P.L. 98-473, 10/12/84). The Child Abuse Prevention Challenge Grants Reauthorization Act of 1989 (P.L. 101-126) transferred this program to the Child Abuse Prevention and Treatment Act, as amended.

A new title III, Certain Preventive Services Regarding Children of Homeless Families or Families at Risk of Homelessness, was added to the Child Abuse and Neglect Prevention and Treatment Act by the Stewart B. McKinney Homeless Assistance Act Amendments of 1990 (P.L. 101-645, 11/29/90).

The Child Abuse Prevention and Treatment Act was amended and reauthorized by the Child Abuse, Domestic Violence, Adoption, and Family Services Act of 1992 (P.L. 102-295, 5/28/92) and amended by the Juvenile Justice and Delinquency Prevention Act Amendments of 1992 (P.L. 102-586, 11/4/92).

CAPTA was amended by the Older American Act Technical Amendments of 1993 (P.L. 103-171, 12/2/93) and the Human Services Amendments of 1994 (P.L. 103-252, 5/19/94).

CAPTA was further amended by the Child Abuse Prevention and Treatment Act Amendments of 1996 (P.L. 104-235, 10/3/96), which amended title I, replaced the Title II Community-Based Family Resource Centers program with a new Community-Based Family Resource and Support Program, and repealed Title III, Certain Preventive Services Regarding Children of Homeless Families or Families at Risk of Homelessness.

CAPTA was further amended by the Keeping Children and Families Safe Act of 2003 (P.L. 108-36, 6/25/03), which amended title I and replaced Title II Community-Based Family Resource and Support Program with Community-Based Grants for the Prevention of Child Abuse and Neglect.

CAPTA most recently was amended by the CAPTA Reauthorization Act of 2010 (P.L. 111-320, 12/20/10), which amended both titles I and II.

Section 34.2

Child Welfare System

This section includes text excerpted from "How the Child Welfare System Works," U.S. Department of Health and Human Services (HHS), February 2013.

Overview

The child welfare system is a group of services designed to promote the well-being of children by ensuring safety, achieving permanency, and strengthening families to care for their children successfully. While the primary responsibility for child welfare services rests with the States, the Federal Government plays a major role in supporting States in the delivery of services through funding of programs and legislative initiatives.

The primary responsibility for implementing Federal child and family legislation rests with the Children's Bureau, within the Administration on Children, Youth and Families, Administration for Children and Families, U.S. Department of Health and Human Services (HHS). The Children's Bureau works with State and local agencies to develop programs that focus on preventing child abuse and neglect by strengthening families, protecting children from further maltreatment, reuniting children safely with their families, or finding permanent families for children who cannot safely return home.

Most families first become involved with their local child welfare system because of a report of suspected child abuse or neglect (sometimes called "child maltreatment"). Child maltreatment is defined by CAPTA as serious harm (neglect, physical abuse, sexual abuse, and emotional abuse or neglect) caused to children by parents or primary caregivers, such as extended family members or babysitters. Child maltreatment also can include harm that a caregiver allows to happen or does not prevent from happening to a child. In general, child welfare agencies do not intervene in cases of harm to children caused by acquaintances or strangers. These cases are the responsibility of law enforcement.

The child welfare system is not a single entity. Many organizations in each community work together to strengthen families and keep children safe. Public agencies, such as departments of social services or child and family services, often contract and collaborate with private child welfare agencies and community-based organizations to provide services to families, such as in-home family preservation services, foster care, residential treatment, mental health care, substance abuse treatment, parenting skills classes, domestic violence services, employment assistance, and financial or housing assistance.

Child welfare systems are complex, and their specific procedures vary widely by State. The purpose of this section is to give a brief overview of the purposes and functions of child welfare from a national perspective. Child welfare systems typically:

- Receive and investigate reports of possible child abuse and neglect

- Provide services to families that need assistance in the protection and care of their children

- Arrange for children to live with kin or with foster families when they are not safe at home

- Arrange for reunification, adoption, or other permanent family connections for children leaving foster care

What Happens When Possible Abuse or Neglect Is Reported

Any concerned person can report suspicions of child abuse or neglect. Most reports are made by "mandatory reporters"—people who are required by State law to report suspicions of child abuse and neglect. As of August 2012, statutes in approximately 18 States and Puerto Rico require any person who suspects child abuse or neglect to report it. These reports are generally received by child protective services (CPS) workers and are either "screened in" or "screened out." A report is screened in when there is sufficient information to suggest an investigation is warranted. A report may be screened out if there is not enough information on which to follow up or if the situation reported does not meet the State's legal definition of abuse or neglect. In these instances, the worker may refer the person reporting the incident to other community services or law enforcement for additional help.

What Happens After a Report Is "Screened In"

CPS caseworkers, often called investigators or assessment workers, respond within a particular time period, which may be anywhere from a few hours to a few days, depending on the type of maltreatment alleged, the potential severity of the situation, and requirements under State law. They may speak with the parents and other people in contact with the child, such as doctors, teachers, or child care providers. They also may speak with the child, alone or in the presence of caregivers, depending on the child's age and level of risk. Children who are believed to be in immediate danger may be moved to a shelter, a foster home, or a relative's home during the investigation and while court proceedings are pending. An investigator also engages the family, assessing strengths and needs and initiating connections to community resources and services.

Some jurisdictions now employ an alternative, or differential, response system. In these jurisdictions, when the risk to the children involved is considered low, the CPS caseworker focuses on assessing family strengths, resources, and difficulties and on identifying supports and services needed, rather than on gathering evidence to confirm the occurrence of abuse or neglect.

At the end of an investigation, CPS caseworkers typically make one of two findings—unsubstantiated (unfounded) or substantiated (founded). These terms vary from State to State. Typically, a finding of unsubstantiated means there is insufficient evidence for the worker to conclude that a child was abused or neglected, or what happened does not meet the legal definition of child abuse or neglect. A finding of substantiated typically means that an incident of child abuse or neglect, as defined by State law, is believed to have occurred. Some States have additional categories, such as "unable to determine," that suggest there was not enough evidence to either confirm or refute that abuse or neglect occurred.

The agency will initiate a court action if it determines that the authority of the juvenile court (through a child protection or dependency proceeding) is necessary to keep the child safe. To protect the child, the court can issue temporary orders placing the child in shelter care during the investigation, ordering services, or ordering certain individuals to have no contact with the child. At an adjudicatory hearing, the court hears evidence and decides whether maltreatment occurred and whether the child should be under the continuing jurisdiction of the court. The court then enters a disposition, either at that hearing or at a separate hearing, which may result in the court ordering a parent to comply with services necessary to alleviate the abuse or neglect. Orders can also contain provisions regarding visitation between the parent and the child, agency obligations to provide the parent with services, and services needed by the child.

What Happens in Substantiated (Founded) Cases

If a child has been abused or neglected, the course of action depends on State policy, the severity of the maltreatment, an assessment of the child's immediate safety, the risk of continued or future maltreatment, the services available to address the family's needs, and whether the child was removed from the home and a court action to protect the child was initiated. The following general options are available:

- **No or low risk**—The family's case may be closed with no services if the maltreatment was a one-time incident, the child is considered to be safe, there is no or low risk of future incidents, and any services the family needs will not be provided through the child welfare agency but through other community based resources and service systems.

- **Low to moderate risk**—Referrals may be made to community-based or voluntary in-home child welfare services if the CPS worker believes the family would benefit from these services and the child's present and future safety would be enhanced. This may happen even when no abuse or neglect is found, if the family needs and is willing to participate in services.

- **Moderate to high risk**—The family may again be offered voluntary in-home services to address safety concerns and help reduce the risks. If these are refused, the agency may seek intervention by the juvenile dependency court. Once there is a judicial determination that abuse or neglect occurred, juvenile dependency court may require the family to cooperate with in-home services if it is believed that the child can remain safely at home while the family addresses the issues contributing to the risk of future maltreatment. If the child has been seriously harmed, is considered to be at high risk of serious harm, or the child's safety is threatened, the court may order the child's removal from the home or affirm the agency's prior removal of the child. The child may be placed with a relative or in foster care.

What Happens to Parents

Caregivers who are found to have abused or neglected a child are generally offered support and treatment services or are required by a juvenile dependency court to participate in services that will help keep their children safe. In cases of low risk, in-home services and supports may be provided, including parent education, child care, counseling, safety planning, and more.

In more severe cases or fatalities, police are called on to investigate and may file charges in criminal court against the perpetrators of child maltreatment. In many States, certain types of abuse, such as sexual abuse and serious physical abuse, are routinely referred to law enforcement.

Whether or not criminal charges are filed, the name of the person committing the abuse or neglect may be placed on a State child maltreatment registry if abuse or neglect is confirmed. A registry is a central database that collects information about maltreated children and individuals who are found to have abused or neglected those children. These registries are usually confidential and used for internal child protective purposes only. However, they may be used in background checks for certain professions that involve working with children to protect children from contact with individuals who may mistreat them.

What Happens to Children

Depending on the severity of the case, children may remain at home or be removed into foster care.

In-Home. In low-risk cases, children may remain in their own homes with their families, and the families may receive in-home services and supports. These may include parent education, safety planning, counseling, and more. Families may also be connected with community services that provide concrete help (e.g., housing, food) as well as services such as therapy, parent training, and support groups.

Out-of-Home. Most children in foster care are placed with relatives or foster families, but some may be placed in a group or residential setting. While a child is in foster care, he or she attends school and should receive medical care and other services as needed. The child's family also receives services to support their efforts to reduce the risk of future maltreatment and to help them, in most cases, be reunited with their child. Visits between parents and their children and between siblings are encouraged and supported, following a set plan.

Every child in foster care should have a permanency plan. Families typically participate in developing a permanency plan for the child and a service plan for the family, and these plans guide the agency's work. Family reunification, except in unusual and extreme circumstances, is the permanency plan for most children. In some cases, when prospects for reunification appear less likely, a concurrent permanency plan is developed. If the efforts toward reunification are not successful, the plan may be changed to another permanent arrangement, such as adoption or transfer of custody to a relative.

Federal law requires the court to hold a permanency hearing, which determines the permanent plan for the child, within 12 months after the child enters foster care and every 12 months thereafter. Many courts review each case more frequently to ensure that the agency is actively pursuing permanency for the child.

Whether or not they are adopted, older youth in foster care should receive support in developing some form of permanent family connection, in addition to transitional or Independent Living services, to assist them in being self-sufficient when they leave foster care between the ages of 18 and 21.

Chapter 35

Infant Safe Haven Laws

Safe Haven Laws across the United States

Many State legislatures have enacted legislation to address infant abandonment and infanticide in response to a reported increase in the abandonment of infants. Beginning in Texas in 1999, "Baby Moses laws" or infant safe haven laws have been enacted as an incentive for mothers in crisis to safely relinquish their babies to designated locations where the babies are protected and provided with medical care until a permanent home is found. Safe haven laws generally allow the parent, or an agent of the parent, to remain anonymous and to be shielded from prosecution for abandonment or neglect in exchange for surrendering the baby to a safe haven.

To date, all 50 States, the District of Columbia, and Puerto Rico have enacted safe haven legislation. The focus of these laws is protecting newborns. In approximately 12 States and Puerto Rico, infants who are 72 hours old or younger may be relinquished to a designated safe haven. Approximately 19 States accept infants up to 1 month old. Other States specify varying age limits in their statutes.

Who May Leave a Baby at a Safe Haven

In most States with safe haven laws, either parent may surrender his or her baby to a safe haven. In 4 States and Puerto Rico, only the

This chapter includes text excerpted from "Infant Safe Haven Laws," U.S. Department of Health and Human Services (HHS), February 2013.

mother may relinquish her infant. Idaho specifies that only a custodial parent may surrender an infant. In the District of Columbia, an infant may be relinquished only by a custodial parent who is a resident of the District. In approximately 11 States, an agent of the parent (someone who has the parent's approval) may take a baby to a safe haven for a parent. In California, Kansas, and New York, if the person relinquishing the infant is someone other than a parent, he or she must have legal custody of the child. Eight States do not specify the person who may relinquish an infant.

Safe Haven Providers

The purpose of safe haven laws is to ensure that relinquished infants are left with persons who can provide the immediate care needed for their safety and well-being. To that end, approximately 16 States and Puerto Rico require parents to relinquish their infants only to a hospital, emergency medical services provider, or health-care facility. In 27 States, fire stations also are designated as safe haven providers. Personnel at police stations or other law enforcement agencies may accept infants in 25 States. In 5 States, emergency medical personnel responding to 911 calls may accept an infant. In addition, 4 States allow churches to act as safe havens, but the relinquishing parent must first determine that church personnel are present at the time the infant is left.

Responsibilities of Safe Haven Providers

The safe haven provider is required to accept emergency protective custody of the infant and to provide any immediate medical care that the infant may require. In 13 States and the District of Columbia, when the safe haven receiving the baby is not a hospital, the baby must be transferred to a hospital as soon as possible. The provider is also required to notify the local child welfare department that an infant has been relinquished.

In 24 States and the District of Columbia, the provider is required to ask the parent for family and medical history information. In 16 States and the District of Columbia, the provider is required to attempt to give the parent or parents, information about the legal repercussions of leaving the infant and information about referral services. In 4 States, a copy of the infant's numbered identification bracelet may be offered to the parent as an aid to linking the parent to the child if reunification is sought at a later date.

Immunity from Liability for Providers

In 44 States and the District of Columbia, safe haven laws protect providers who accept custody of relinquished infants from liability for anything that might happen to the infant while in their care, unless there is evidence of major negligence on the part of the provider.

Protections for Parents

In approximately 13 States and the District of Columbia, anonymity for the parent or agent of the parent is expressly guaranteed in statute. In 26 States and Puerto Rico, the safe haven provider cannot compel the parent or agent of the parent to provide identifying information. In addition, 14 States provide an assurance of confidentiality for any information that is voluntarily provided by the parent.

In addition to the guarantee of anonymity, most States provide protection from criminal liability for parents who safely relinquish their infants. Approximately 34 States, the District of Columbia, and Puerto Rico do not prosecute a parent for child abandonment when a baby is relinquished to a safe haven. In 16 States, safe relinquishment of the infant is an affirmative defense in any prosecution of the parent or his/her agent for any crime against the child, such as abandonment, neglect, or child endangerment.

The privileges of anonymity and immunity are forfeited in most States if there is evidence of child abuse or neglect.

Consequences of Relinquishment

Once the safe haven provider has notified the local child welfare department that an infant has been relinquished, the department assumes custody of the infant as an abandoned child. The department has responsibility for placing the infant, usually in a preadoptive home, and for petitioning the court for termination of the birth parents' parental rights. Before the baby is placed in a preadoptive home, 14 States and the District of Columbia require the department to request the local law enforcement agency to determine whether the baby has been reported as a missing child. In addition, 5 States require the department to check the putative father registry before a termination of parental rights petition can be filed.

Approximately 20 States and the District of Columbia have procedures in place for a parent to reclaim the infant, usually within a specified time period and before any petition to terminate parental rights has been granted. Five States also have provisions for a

271

nonrelinquishing father to petition for custody of the child. In 17 States and Puerto Rico, the act of surrendering an infant to a safe haven is presumed to be a relinquishment of parental rights to the child, and no further parental consent is required for the child's adoption.

Chapter 36

Sex Offender Registries and Community Notice Programs

Chapter Contents

Section 36.1

The Dru Sjodin *National Sex Offender Public Website (NSOPW)*

This section includes text excerpted from "About NSOPW," U.S. Department of Justice (DOJ), December 2012. Reviewed May 2016.

The *Dru Sjodin* National Sex Offender Public Website (NSOPW), www.nsopw.gov, is an unprecedented public safety resource that provides the public with access to sex offender data nationwide. NSOPW is a partnership between the U.S. Department of Justice and state, territorial, and tribal governments, working together for the safety of adults and children.

First established in 2005 as the National Sex Offender Public Registry (NSOPR), NSOPW was renamed by the Adam Walsh Child Protection and Safety Act of 2006 in honor of 22-year-old college student Dru Sjodin of Grand Forks, North Dakota, a young woman who was kidnapped and murdered by a sex offender who was registered in Minnesota.

NSOPW is the only U.S. government Website that links public state, territorial, and tribal sex offender registries from one national search site. Parents, employers, and other concerned residents can utilize the Website's search tool to identify location information on sex offenders residing, working, and attending school not only in their own neighborhoods but in other nearby states and communities. In addition, the Website provides visitors with information about sexual abuse and how to protect themselves and loved ones from potential victimization.

NSOPW's advanced search tool provides information about sex offenders through a number of search options:

- Search by name nationally or with an individual Jurisdiction

- Search by address (if provided by Jurisdiction)

- Search by zip code

- Search by county (if provided by Jurisdiction)

- Search by city/town (if provided by Jurisdiction)

NSOPW presents the most up-to-date information as provided by each Jurisdiction. Information is hosted by each Jurisdiction, not by NSOPW or the federal government. The search criteria available for searches are limited to what each individual Jurisdiction may provide. Search results should be verified by visiting the providing Jurisdiction's Public Registry Website for further information and/or guidance.

Section 36.2

Sex Offender Registries and Community Notice Programs

This section includes text excerpted from "Sex Offender Registration and Notification Act (SORNA)," U.S. Department of Justice (DOJ), June 3, 2015.

Purposes of the Sex Offender Registration and Notification Act (SORNA)

Sex offender registration and notification programs are important for public safety purposes. Sex offender registration is a system for monitoring and tracking sex offenders following their release into the community. The registration provides important information about convicted sex offenders to local and federal authorities and the public, such as offender's name, current location and past offenses. Currently, the means of public notification includes sex offender websites in all states, the District of Columbia, and some territories. Some states involve other forms of notice.

Within a specified timeframe, each jurisdiction is required to comply with the federal standards outlined in the Sex Offender Registration and Notification Act (SORNA). Jurisdictions include all 50 states, the District of Columbia, the principal U.S. territories, and federally recognized Indian tribes.

Failure to Register

It is a federal crime for an individual to knowingly fail to register or update his or her registration as required pursuant to the Sex

Offender Registration and Notification Act (SORNA). For example, a sex offender is required to update their registration in each jurisdiction they reside, are employed, or attend school. Offenders convicted of this crime face statutory penalties.

CEOS's Role

CEOS works with the High Technology Investigative Unit (HTIU), the Federal Bureau of Investigation (FBI) and United States Attorney's Offices around the country to investigate and prosecute sex offenders who fail to register pursuant to the Sex Offender Registration and Notification Act (SORNA).

In addition, CEOS attorneys conduct trainings to educate law enforcement officials, investigators, prosecutors, and others about the national sex offender registration system. Moreover, CEOS designs, implements, and supports strategies, legislative proposals, and policy initiatives relating to the enforcement of SORNA.

Chapter 37

Reporting Child Abuse

Child Custody and Visitation

- With the exception of international parental kidnapping, child custody and visitation matters are generally handled by local and state authorities, and not by the federal government.

- To report a child custody or visitation issue, contact your local or state law enforcement agency.

Child Pornography

- To report an incident involving the possession, distribution, receipt, or production of child pornography, file a report on the National Center for Missing and Exploited Children (NCMEC)'s website at www.cybertipline.com, or call 1-800-843-5678. Your report will be forwarded to a law enforcement agency for investigation and action.

- You may also wish to report the incident to federal, state, or local law enforcement personnel.

This chapter contains text excerpted from the following sources: Text under the heading "Child Custody and Visitation" is excerpted from "Child Exploitation and Obscenity Section (CEOS)," U.S. Department of Justice (DOJ), June 3, 2015; Text under the heading "Penalties for Failure to Report and False Reporting of Child Abuse and Neglect" is excerpted from "Penalties for Failure to Report and False Reporting of Child Abuse and Neglect," Child Welfare Information Gateway, August 2015.

Child Sexual Abuse

- Child sexual abuse matters are generally handled by local and state authorities, and not by the federal government.

- To report a child sexual abuse issue, contact your local or state law enforcement agency.

Child Support Enforcement

- Child support enforcement matters are generally handled by local and state authorities, and not by the federal government. To report a child support enforcement issue, contact your local or state law enforcement agency.

- You may also wish to contact your local "Title IV-D" agency, which is required by federal law to provide child support enforcement services to anyone who requests such services. To locate your local "Title IV-D" agency visit the U.S Department of Health and Human Services, Office of Child Support Enforcement's website at www.acf.hhs.gov/programs/cse.

Extraterritorial Sexual Exploitation of Children

- To report an incident or suspicious situation that may involve the extraterritorial sexual exploitation of children, call the National Human Trafficking Resource Center (NHTRC) at 1-888-3737-888, or file a confidential online report at www.polarisproject.org/what-we-do/national-human-trafficking-hotline/report-a-tip. Your report will be forwarded to a law enforcement agency for investigation and action.

- You can also report an incident or suspicious situation to Immigration and Customs Enforcement / Homeland Security Investigations (ICE) by calling the ICE hotline at 1-866-347-2423, or emailing ICE at predator@DHS.gov

International Parental Kidnapping

- To report an international parental kidnapping situation, contact the U.S. Department of State, Office of Children's Issues. This office coordinates efforts to seek the return of children abducted by their parents to foreign countries. Call the office at 1-202-312-9700, or visit their website at travel.state.gov/abduction/country/country_3781.html.

- You can also file a missing child report with the National Center for Missing and Exploited Children (NCMEC) by calling 1-800-The-Lost (1-800-843-5678).

- You may also wish to report the incident to federal, state, or local law enforcement personnel.

Obscenity

- To report obscene material sent to a child, a misleading domain name or misleading words or images on the Internet, file a report on the National Center for Missing and Exploited Children (NCMEC)'s website at www.cybertipline.com, or call 1-800-843-5678. Your report will be forwarded to a law enforcement agency for investigation and action.

- To report obscene or indecent material broadcast over the radio or television, contact the Federal Communication Commission (FCC), which regulates radio and television broadcasting. You can report a complaint by calling the FCC at 1-888-CALL-FCC (1-888-225-5322), faxing 1-866-418-0232.

- To report obscene material sent through the United States Postal Inspector Service (USPIS), contact your local post office or file a complaint on the U.S Postal Services website at postalinspectors.uspis.gov/contactUs/filecomplaint.aspx.

- To report individuals engaged in fraudulent or unfair trade practices involving unsolicited emails, porn-spam, media violence, or identity theft, contact the Federal Trade Commission (FTC) and file a online consumer complaint form at www.ftccomplaintassistant.gov.

- You may also wish to report the incident to federal, state, or local law enforcement personnel.

Prostitution of Children

- To report an incident or suspicious situation that may involve the prostitution of children, call the National Human Trafficking Resource Center (NHTRC) at 1-888-3737-888, or file a confidential online report at www.polarisproject.org/what-we-do/national-human-trafficking-hotline/report-a-tip. Your report will be forwarded to a law enforcement agency for investigation and action.

- To report an incident involving the sexual exploitation of children, file a report on the National Center for Missing and Exploited Children (NCMEC)'s website at www.cybertipline. com, or call 1-800-843-5678. Your report will be forwarded to a law enforcement agency for investigation and action.

- You may also wish to report the incident to federal, state, or local law enforcement personnel.

Penalties for Failure to Report and False Reporting of Child Abuse and Neglect

Many cases of child abuse and neglect are not reported, even when mandated by law. Therefore, nearly every State and U.S. territory imposes penalties, often in the form of a fine or imprisonment, on mandatory reporters who fail to report suspected child abuse or neglect as required by law. In addition, to prevent malicious or intentional reporting of cases that are not founded, many States and the U.S. Virgin Islands impose penalties against any person who files a report known to be false.

Penalties for Failure to Report

Approximately 48 States, the District of Columbia, American Samoa, Guam, the Northern Mariana Islands, and the Virgin Islands impose penalties on mandatory reporters who knowingly or willfully fail to make a report when they suspect that a child is being abused or neglected.

In Florida, a mandatory reporter who fails to report as required by law can be charged with a felony. Failure to report is classified as a misdemeanor or a similar charge in 40 States and American Samoa, Guam, and the Virgin Islands.

In Arizona and Minnesota, misdemeanors are upgraded to felonies for failure to report more serious situations; while in Connecticut, Illinois, Kentucky, and Guam, second or subsequent violations are classified as felonies.

Twenty States and the District of Columbia, Guam, the Northern Mariana Islands, and the Virgin Islands specify in the reporting laws the penalties for failure to report. Upon conviction, a mandated reporter who fails to report can face jail terms ranging from 30 days to 5 years, fines ranging from $300 to $10,000, or both jail terms and fines. In seven States, harsher penalties may be imposed under certain circumstances.

In 7 States and American Samoa, in addition to any criminal penalties, the reporter may be civilly liable for any damages caused by the failure to report. Florida imposes a fine of up to $1 million on any institution of higher learning, including any State university and non-public college, who fails to report or prevents any person from reporting an instance of abuse committed on the property of the institution or at an event sponsored by the institution.

Obstructing Reports of Abuse or Neglect

Approximately 10 States impose penalties against any employer who discharges, suspends, disciplines, or engages in any action to prevent or prohibit an employee or volunteer from making a report of suspected child maltreatment as required by the reporting laws.

In 6 States, an action to prevent a report is classified as a misdemeanor.

In Connecticut, an employer who interferes with making a report will be charged with a felony. Three States specify the penalties for that action, and in 4 States the employer is civilly liable for damages for any harm caused to the mandatory reporter.

In Pennsylvania, a person commits a felony if he or she uses force, violence, or threat; or offers a bribe to prevent a report; or has a prior conviction for the same or a similar offense. In the Northern Mariana Islands, any person who is convicted of interfering with the good-faith efforts of any person making or attempting to make a report shall be subject to imprisonment for up to 1 year, or a fine of $1,000, or both.

Penalties for False Reporting

Approximately 29 States carry penalties in their civil child protection laws for any person who willfully or intentionally makes a report of child abuse or neglect that the reporter knows to be false. In New York, Ohio, Pennsylvania, and the Virgin Islands, making false reports of child maltreatment is made illegal in criminal sections of State code

Nineteen States and the Virgin Islands classify false reporting as a misdemeanor or similar charge. In Florida, Illinois, Tennessee, and Texas, false reporting is a felony; while in Arkansas, Indiana, Missouri, and Virginia, second or subsequent offenses are upgraded to felonies. In Michigan, false reporting can be either a misdemeanor or a felony, depending on the seriousness of the alleged abuse in the report. No criminal penalties are imposed in California, Maine, Minnesota, Montana, and Nebraska; however, the immunity from civil or criminal action that is provided to reporters of abuse or neglect is not extended to those who make a false report. In South Carolina, in addition to any criminal penalties, the Department of Social Services may bring civil action against the person to recover the costs of investigation and any proceedings related to the investigation.

Eleven States and the Virgin Islands specify the penalties for making a false report. Upon conviction, the reporter can face jail terms ranging from 90 days to 5 years or fines ranging from $500 to $5,000. Florida imposes the most severe penalties: In addition to a court sentence of 5 years and $5,000, the Department of Children and Family Services may fine the reporter up to $10,000. In 6 States, the reporter may be civilly liable for any damages caused by the report.

Chapter 38

Professionals Who Are Required to Report Child Abuse and Neglect

Mandatory Reporters of Child Abuse and Neglect

All States, the District of Columbia, American Samoa, Guam, the Northern Mariana Islands, Puerto Rico, and the U.S. Virgin Islands have statutes identifying persons who are required to report suspected child maltreatment to an appropriate agency, such as child protective services, a law enforcement agency, or a State's toll-free child abuse reporting hotline.

Professionals Required to Report

Approximately 48 States, the District of Columbia, American Samoa, Guam, the Northern Mariana Islands, Puerto Rico, and the Virgin Islands designate professions whose members are mandated

This chapter contains text excerpted from the following sources: Text beginning with the heading "Mandatory Reporters of Child Abuse and Neglect" is excerpted from "Mandatory Reporters of Child Abuse and Neglect," U.S. Department of Health and Human Services (HHS), August 2015; Text under the heading "Clergy as Mandatory Reporters of Child Abuse and Neglect" is excerpted from "Clergy as Mandatory Reporters of Child Abuse and Neglect," U.S. Department of Health and Human Services (HHS), August 2015.

283

by law to report child maltreatment. Individuals designated as mandatory reporters typically have frequent contact with children. Such individuals may include:

- Social workers

- Teachers, principals, and other school personnel

- Physicians, nurses, and other health care workers

- Counselors, therapists, and other mental health professionals

- Child care providers

- Medical examiners or coroners

- Law enforcement officers

Some other professions frequently mandated across the States include commercial film or photograph processors (in 12 States, Guam, and Puerto Rico) and computer technicians (in 6 States). Substance abuse counselors are required to report in 14 States, and probation or parole officers are mandatory reporters in 17 States. Directors, employees, and volunteers at entities that provide organized activities for children, such as camps, day camps, youth centers, and recreation centers, are required to report in 13 States. Six States and the District of Columbia include domestic violence workers on the list of mandated reporters, while six other States and the District of Columbia include animal control or humane officers Illinois includes both domestic violence workers and animal control or humane officers as mandatory reporters. Court-appointed special advocates are mandatory reporters in 11 States. Members of the clergy now are required to report in 27 States and Guam.

Eleven States now have faculty, administrators, athletics staff, and other employees and volunteers at institutions of higher learning, including public and private colleges and universities and vocational and technical schools, designated as mandatory reporters.

Reporting by Other Persons

In approximately 18 States and Puerto Rico, any person who suspects child abuse or neglect is required to report. Of these 18 States, 16 States and Puerto Rico specify certain professionals who must report, but also require all persons to report suspected abuse or neglect, regardless of profession. New Jersey and Wyoming require all persons to report without specifying any professions. In all other States, territories, and the District of Columbia, any person is permitted to report. These voluntary reporters of abuse are often referred to as "permissive reporters."

Institutional Responsibility to Report

The term "institutional reporting" refers to those situations in which the mandated reporter is working (or volunteering) as a staff member of an institution, such as a school or hospital, at the time he or she gains the knowledge that leads him or her to suspect that abuse or neglect has occurred. Many institutions have internal policies and procedures for handling reports of abuse, and these usually require the person who suspects abuse to notify the head of the institution that abuse has been discovered or is suspected and needs to be reported to child protective services or other appropriate authorities.

Statutes in 33 States, the District of Columbia, and the Virgin Islands provide procedures that must be followed in those cases. In 18 States, the District of Columbia, and the Virgin Islands, any staff member who suspects abuse must notify the head of the institution when the staff member feels that abuse or possible abuse should be reported to an appropriate authority. In 9 States, the District of Columbia, and the Virgin Islands, the staff member who suspects abuse notifies the head of the institution first, and then the head or his or her designee is required to make the report. In 9 States, the individual reporter must make the report to the appropriate authority first and then notify the institution that a report has been made.

Laws in 15 States make clear that, regardless of any policies within the organization, the mandatory reporter is not relieved of his or her responsibility to report. In 17 States, an employer is expressly prohibited from taking any action to prevent or discourage an employee from making a report.

Standards for Making a Report

The circumstances under which a mandatory reporter must make a report vary from State to State. Typically, a report must be made when the reporter, in his or her official capacity, suspects or has reason to believe that a child has been abused or neglected. Another standard frequently used is in situations in which the reporter has knowledge of, or observes a child being subjected to, conditions that would reasonably result in harm to the child. In Maine, a mandatory reporter must report when he or she has reasonable cause to suspect that a child is not living with the child's family.

Mandatory reporters are required to report the facts and circumstances that led them to suspect that a child has been abused or neglected. They do not have the burden of providing proof that abuse or neglect has occurred. Permissive reporters follow the same standards when electing to make a report.

Privileged Communications

Mandatory reporting statutes also may specify when a communication is privileged. "Privileged communications" is the statutory recognition of the right to maintain confidential communications between professionals and their clients, patients, or congregants. To enable States to provide protection to maltreated children, the reporting laws in most States and territories restrict this privilege for mandated reporters. All but three States and Puerto Rico currently address the issue of privileged communications within their reporting laws, either affirming the privilege or denying it (i.e., not allowing privilege to be grounds for failing to report)

For instance:

- The physician-patient and husband-wife privileges are the most common to be denied by States.

- The attorney-client privilege is most commonly affirmed.

- The clergy-penitent privilege is also widely affirmed, although that privilege usually is limited to confessional communications and, in some States, denied altogether.

In Louisiana, a mental health or social services practitioner is not required to report if the practitioner is engaged by an attorney to assist in the provision of legal services to a child.

Inclusion of the Reporter's Name in the Report

Most States maintain toll-free telephone numbers for receiving reports of abuse or neglect. Reports may be made anonymously to most of these reporting numbers, but States find it helpful to their investigations to know the identity of reporters. Approximately 19 States, the District of Columbia, American Samoa, Guam, and the Virgin Islands currently require mandatory reporters to provide their names and contact information, either at the time of the initial oral report or as part of a written report. The laws in Connecticut, Delaware, and Washington allow child protection workers to request the name of the reporter. In Wyoming, the reporter does not have to provide his or her identity as part of the written report, but if the person takes and submits photographs or X-rays of the child, his or her name must be provided.

Disclosure of the Reporter's Identity

All jurisdictions have provisions in statute to maintain the confidentiality of abuse and neglect records. The identity of the reporter is specifically protected from disclosure to the alleged perpetrator in 41 States, the District of Columbia, American Samoa, Guam, the Northern Mariana Islands, and Puerto Rico. This protection is maintained even when other information from the report may be disclosed.

Release of the reporter's identity is allowed in some jurisdictions under specific circumstances or to specific departments or officials, for example, when information is needed for conducting an investigation or family assessment or upon a finding that the reporter knowingly made a false report (in Alabama, Arkansas, Connecticut, Kentucky, Louisiana, Minnesota, Nevada, South Dakota, Vermont, and Virginia). In some jurisdictions (California, Florida, Minnesota, Tennessee, Texas, Vermont, the District of Columbia, and Guam), the reporter can waive confidentiality and give consent to the release of his or her name.

Clergy as Mandatory Reporters of Child Abuse and Neglect

Every State, the District of Columbia, American Samoa, Guam, the Northern Mariana Islands, Puerto Rico, and the U.S. Virgin Islands have statutes that identify persons who are required to report child maltreatment under specific circumstances. Approximately 28 States and Guam currently include members of the clergy among those professionals specifically mandated by law to report known or suspected instances of child abuse or neglect. In approximately 18 States and Puerto Rico, any person who suspects child abuse or neglect is required to report it. This inclusive language appears to include clergy but may be interpreted otherwise.

Privileged Communications

As a doctrine of some faiths, clergy must maintain the confidentiality of pastoral communications. This is sometimes referred to as "clergy-penitent privilege," where "penitent" refers to the person consulting the clergy. Mandatory reporting statutes in some States specify the circumstances under which a communication is "privileged" or allowed to remain confidential. Privileged communications may be exempt from the requirement to report suspected abuse or neglect. The privilege of maintaining this confidentiality under State law must be provided by statute. Most States do provide the privilege, typically in rules of evidence or civil procedure. If the issue of privilege is not addressed in the reporting laws, it does not mean that privilege is not granted; it may be granted in other parts of State statutes.

This privilege, however, is not absolute. While clergy penitent privilege is frequently recognized within the reporting laws, it is typically interpreted narrowly in the context of child abuse or neglect. The circumstances under which it is allowed vary from State to State, and in some States it is denied altogether. For example, among the States that list clergy as mandated reporters, Guam, New Hampshire, and West Virginia deny the clergy penitent privilege in cases of child abuse or neglect. Four of the States that enumerate "any person" as a mandated reporter (North Carolina, Oklahoma, Rhode Island, and Texas) also deny clergy-penitent privilege in child abuse cases.

In States where neither clergy members nor "any person" are enumerated as mandated reporters, it is less clear whether clergy are included as mandated reporters within other broad categories of professionals who work with children. For example, in Virginia and Washington, clergy are not enumerated as mandated reporters, but the clergy-penitent privilege is affirmed within the reporting laws.

Many States and territories include Christian Science practitioners or religious healers among professionals who are mandated to report suspected child maltreatment. In most instances, they appear to be regarded as a type of health-care provider. Only 10 States explicitly include Christian Science practitioners among classes of clergy required to report. In those States, the clergy-penitent privilege also is extended to those practitioners by statute.

Chapter 39

Parent Education on Strengthening Family and Reducing Risk of Maltreatment

Parent Education on Strengthening Family and Reducing Risk of Maltreatment

Parent education can promote well-being and strengthen families and communities to prevent child abuse and neglect. The Child Abuse Prevention and Treatment Act (CAPTA), as reauthorized in 2010, identifies parent education as a core prevention service. A significant number of the Federal Children's Bureau's Community-Based Child Abuse and Neglect Prevention (CBCAP) grants fund parent education programs as stand-alone efforts or as part of more comprehensive prevention strategies.

Parent education can be defined as any training, program, or other intervention that helps parents acquire skills to improve their parenting of and communication with their children in order to reduce the risk of child maltreatment and/or reduce children's disruptive

---

This chapter includes text excerpted from "Parent Education to Strengthen Families and Reduce the Risk of Maltreatment," U.S. Department of Health and Human Services (HHS), September 2013.

behaviors. Parent education may be delivered individually or in a group in the home, classroom, or other setting; it may be face-to-face or online; and it may include direct instruction, discussion, videos, modeling, or other formats.

Successful parent education programs help parents acquire and internalize parenting and problem-solving skills necessary to build a healthy family. Research shows that effective parent training and family interventions can change parents' attitudes and behaviors, promote protective factors, and lead to positive outcomes for both parents and children. Protective factors include nurturing and attachment, knowledge of parenting and of child and youth development, parenting competencies, parental resilience, social connections (especially caring adults and positive peers), concrete supports for parents, social and emotional competence of children, involvement in positive activities, and other individual skills such as self-regulation and problem solving and relational skills.

What the Research Shows

Practitioners will want to consider both program characteristics and specific training strategies when selecting a parent education program. Program characteristics refer to broader aspects of a program, such as theoretical grounding or how the program is structured, staffed, and evaluated. Training strategies refer to specific teaching methods that have been found to be effective in working directly with parents.

Key Program Characteristics

The following characteristics have been found to be strong predictors of program effectiveness:

Strength-based focus. A large body of research supports the emphasis on family interventions and education programs that focus on family strengths and resilience instead of family weaknesses and problems. This approach reinforces existing protective factors to prevent the occurrence or recurrence of child abuse and neglect.

Family-centered practice. Family-centered parent training programs focus on family skills training and family activities to help children and parents communicate effectively and take advantage of concrete social supports. Family-centered programs respect the traditions and values of the family and reflect the parents' learning styles, preferences, and cultural beliefs.

Individual and group approaches. A variety of factors—including costs, staffing, and program goals—may determine whether parent education is delivered through a home-based program or in a group setting. Individualized programs have been shown to be more effective than group programs with parents at high risk for child abuse and neglect; however, evidence suggests that a combination of individual and group training may be the most effective approach to changing parents' attitudes about childrearing (e.g., use of corporal punishment, expectations about children's competencies, beliefs about children's responsibilities, etc.)

Qualified staff. Program success is in large part dependent on qualified staff. Program staff should have a sound theoretical grounding as well as hands-on experience in the classroom or working with families and groups in different settings. Staff also should be able to provide culturally competent services consistent with the values of the family and the community.

Targeted service groups. Learning is enhanced when the participants include a clearly defined group of people with common needs or identifying characteristics. Identifying the special needs, traditions, and backgrounds of participants is key to developing and implementing an effective program that uses materials and a format matched to the families being served.

An ecological approach. Programs that consider the multiple influences that impact a family—such as community, school, extended family, work, finances, and more—have been shown to have more success. This approach ties in with targeting the service group to best meet the needs of the family.

Parent partnership. Studies of larger, group-based parent education efforts show the effectiveness of parent partnership and shared leadership in fostering the protective factors. In such programs, parent leaders are active in partnering with parents, modeling relationships and behaviors, and creating opportunities for parents to identify and use the protective factors in their families.

Clear program goals and continuous evaluation. Successful programs maintain individualized and group plans developed in partnership with participants. Progress toward program goals is routinely and effectively evaluated by aggregate analyses using both quantitative and qualitative research methods consistent with the services offered. In addition, these programs have an effective process for gathering consumer feedback and use this information, along with outcome-based evaluation efforts, for continuous quality improvement.

Parent Training Strategies

The following parent training strategies may be employed in a variety of service settings and with multiple target populations. These strategies reinforce protective factors and can be adapted as appropriate to fit program and participant needs.

Promote positive family interaction. Promoting already present positive parent-child interactions and strengthening those interactions—along with decreasing parental directives and commands—have been identified as key components of successful parent education programs.

Involve fathers. Research indicates that father involvement in parent training leads to better outcomes and promotes family cooperation and cohesion. Excluding fathers from parent training programs decreases the likelihood of success.

Use interactive training techniques. Research has consistently shown that active learning approaches have greater success than passive approaches. Interactive methods include activities such as group discussion, role playing, active modeling, homework exercises, and reviewing videos of effective parenting approaches. At least one study has indicated that interactive technology can be an effective way to provide parent education to parents with intellectual disabilities.

Provide opportunities to practice new skills. Offering time for parents to practice new skills with their children during parent training sessions is consistently associated with greater effectiveness of parent education programs. Specific skills associated with larger effects on parent and child behavior include emotional communication skills, the use of time-out, and parenting consistency. These were found to be more effective than other common strategies, such as teaching problem-solving skills or ways to promote children's cognitive, academic, or social skills.

Teach emotional communication skills. Programs that teach parents ways to use relationship-building communication skills, such as active listening or self-reflection for children to recognize their own feelings and emotions, have been found to be more successful than those that do not. Emotional communication skills can improve communication patterns among families by reducing negative comments and allowing children to feel they are included in the communication process.

Encourage peer support. Programs that offer opportunities for parental peer support have a positive impact on children's cognitive outcomes. Peer support also strengthens family bonds and gives parents an opportunity to share their experiences in constructive settings. One recent innovation is the use of Parent Cafés and Community Cafés led by trained parent leaders in parent-friendly environments. The cafés provide a forum for parents, caregivers, and others to engage in conversations about ways to incorporate protective factors into parenting, child development, and self-care.

Considerations for Implementation

Agencies seeking to implement parent education programs have many options. The following are some points to consider when choosing a program:

- Is it evidence-based or evidence-informed?
- Will it fit the agency's target audience, or will it need to be adapted in order to be culturally competent?
- Are there specific program components that are important for what the program needs to achieve?
- What kind of training, staffing qualifications, and skills will be necessary?
- What are the costs involved?
- How will the agency roll out the program?
- How will the agency evaluate the outcomes?

Good implementation practice is crucial to achieving positive outcomes with a parenting program.

Evidence-Based and Evidence Informed Programs

There are many parent education programs that aim to strengthen families and help prevent child abuse and neglect. Many of these programs and their outcomes have been evaluated and rated for their scientific basis. Funding sources often require agencies to use programs that are evidence-based or evidence-informed. However, making that determination can be difficult. The Children's Bureau's Office on Child Abuse and Neglect, in working with its CBCAP grantees, developed definitions for evaluating outcomes by adapting definitions from the California Evidence-Based Clearinghouse for Child Welfare. The four resulting definitions reflect an increasing requirement for scientific evidence:

1. **Emerging and evidence-informed** programs and practices have a strong theoretical foundation and are considered generally accepted practice for preventing abuse or neglect. They may have been evaluated using less rigorous evaluation designs.

2. **Promising** programs and practices have had at least one study using some type of control or comparison group and were found to be effective in promoting positive outcomes to prevent abuse or neglect.

3. **Supported and efficacious** programs or practices are supported by at least two rigorous randomized control trials (or other comparable methodology).

4. **Effective or evidence-based** programs or practices are supported by at least two rigorous randomized control trials (or other comparable methodology) and have been replicated in multiple sites.

This chapter lists selected parent education curricula that have been included on various registries of programs with varying degrees of evidence. Each focuses on specific risk and protective factors. Curriculum availability will vary, and some programs require specific training for group facilitators.

The following list is by no means all-inclusive. It does not constitute an endorsement of any particular program and is provided only as a descriptive tool.

1-2-3 Magic

Program objectives: Help parents learn effective methods of controlling negative behavior, encouraging good behavior, and strengthening the child-parent relationship. The program seeks to encourage gentle but firm discipline without arguing, yelling, or spanking.

Target population: Parents, grandparents, teachers, babysitters, and caretakers working with children.

Delivery setting and format: Conducted in adoptive homes, birth family homes, community agencies, foster homes, hospitals, outpatient clinics, residential care facilities, and schools for groups of 6–25 parents of children approximately 2–12 years of age.

Duration: Recommended for 1.5 hours per session for 4–8 weeks.

Training resources: Training manual available, along with a number of other resources for trainers, parents of young children, parents of teens, and teachers.

Website: www.123magic.com

Registries that cite this program: California Evidence-Based Clearinghouse for Child Welfare

Circle of Security

Program objectives: Enhance attachment security between parents and children through early intervention. Over the course of eight sessions, the focus of the intervention moves from discussing secure attachment and children's needs to the more vulnerable process of parents reflecting on themselves and the defensive behaviors that maintain insecure and disorganized attachment.

Target population: Parents of children birth–5, especially high-risk parents (enrolled in Head Start or Early Head Start).

Delivery setting and format: Eight-session video and discussion protocol led by a trainer.

Duration: 4 weeks.

Training resources: Learn about opportunities for trainers: circleofsecurity.net/seminars

Website: circleofsecurity.net

Registries that cite this program: California Evidence-Based Clearinghouse for Child Welfare

Common Sense Parenting®

Program objectives: Teach practical skills to parents that address issues of communication, discipline, decision-making, relationships, self-control, and school success. The proactive skills and techniques help parents from diverse backgrounds create healthy family relationships that foster safety and well-being at home, in school, and in the community.

Target population: Parents of children ages 6–16, although they also offer resources for parenting younger children.

Delivery setting and format: Parents attend weekly, 2-hour classes led by a certified trainer.

Duration: 6 weeks.

Training resources: Include books and videos for parents: www. parenting.org/common-sense-parenting/resources

Website: www.parenting.org/common-sense-parenting

Registries that cite this program: California Evidence-Based Clearinghouse for Child Welfare

The Incredible Years©

Program objectives: Strengthen parenting competencies (monitoring, positive discipline, confidence) and support parents' involvement in children's school experiences in order to promote children's academic, social, and emotional competencies and reduce conduct problems.

Target population: Parents of children ages birth–12, children 4–8 years old, and teachers of young children (individual curricula may be used separately or in combination).

Delivery setting and format: Conducted in a community agency, outpatient clinic, or school in groups of 12–16 parents. Training includes discussions, problem-solving, skills training, role-play, and DVD vignettes of parent-child interactions.

Duration: Varies from 6 to 20 weeks, depending on the program.

Training resources: Program manual, staff training information, and resources available through the website.

Website: www.incredibleyears.com

Registries that cite this program: Blueprints; California Evidence-Based Clearinghouse for Child Welfare; National Registry of Effective Prevention Programs; Promising Practices Network; What Works, Wisconsin

Nurturing Parenting Programs®

Program objectives: Build nurturing parenting skills as an alternative to abusive and neglectful parenting and child-rearing practices, in order to prevent recidivism in families receiving social services, lower the rate of teenage pregnancies, reduce the rate of juvenile delinquency and alcohol abuse, and stop the intergenerational cycle of child abuse.

Target population: All families at risk for abuse and neglect with children birth to 18 years. The programs have been adapted for special populations, including Hmong families, military families, Hispanic families, African-American families, teen parents, foster and adoptive families, families in alcohol treatment and recovery, parents with special learning needs, and families with children with health challenges. Different programs focus on primary, secondary, or tertiary prevention, or on comprehensive parenting education, depending on the needs of the group.

Delivery setting and format: Conducted in a home- or group-based setting or in a combination of settings. Children meet in a separate group.

Duration: 5–55 sessions, depending on the program.

Training resources: Training manuals, videos, information, and other materials are available at www.nurturingparenting.com/training-workshops.html.

Website: www.nurturingparenting.com

Registries that cite this program: California Evidence-Based Clearinghouse for Child Welfare; National Registry of Effective Prevention Programs; What Works, Wisconsin

Parent-Child Interaction Therapy (PCIT)

Program objectives: Strengthen the parent-child bond, decrease harsh and ineffective discipline and control tactics, improve child social skills and cooperation, and reduce child negative or maladaptive behaviors.

Target population: Parents of children ages 2–7 with behavior problems, including those receiving child welfare services or exposed to violence, those with children on the autism spectrum, adoptive families, foster families, and those from other countries or who speak other languages.

Delivery setting and format: Conducted in an outpatient setting with individual parent-child pairs and live coaching of the parent.

Duration: 14–20 weeks.

Training resources: Mental health professionals with at least a master's degree in psychology, social work, or a related field are eligible for PCIT training. Training involves 40 hours of direct training, with ongoing supervision and consultation for approximately 4–6 months, working with at least two PCIT cases through completion.

Website: www.pcit.org and pcit.ucdavis.edu

Registries that cite this program: Blueprints, California Evidence-Based Clearinghouse for Child Welfare, National Registry of Effective Prevention Programs.

Parent Management Training: The Oregon Model / Parenting through Change

Program objectives: Provide preventive and clinical interventions for families of children with behavioral problems in the externalizing spectrum (e.g., aggression, antisocial behavior, conduct problems, conduct disorder, oppositional defiance, delinquency, and substance use); reduce parental coercion; and improve parenting skills. This program also encourages support from the family or other support system.

Target population: Two parents, single parent, kinship caregivers, and foster parents.

Delivery setting and format: Conducted in home settings or in agency or clinic settings, with 14 group sessions and 20–25 family sessions

Duration: Varies but typically lasts 5–6 months.

Training resources: Training requires 18 workshop days and 12 coaching sessions

Website: www.isii.net

Registries that cite this program: California Evidence-Based Clearinghouse for Child Welfare; Coalition for Evidence-Based Policy; National Registry of Effective Prevention Programs; What Works, Wisconsin

Parents as Teachers

Program objectives: Make regular home visits to families focused on parent-child interaction, development-centered parenting, school readiness, maltreatment prevention, and family well-being. Home visitors support parents throughout pregnancy until their children enter kindergarten, providing medical and developmental screenings and connecting families to groups and to resources as needed.

Target population: At-risk new parents, including teen parents, low-income parents, and single parents.

Delivery setting and format: Conducted in the home.

Duration: 5 years on a weekly, biweekly, or monthly basis, as needed.

Training resources: Parent educators who serve as home visitors receive specific training.

Website: www.parentsasteachers.org

Registries that cite this program: California Evidence-Based Clearinghouse for Child Welfare; National Registry of Effective Prevention Programs; Promising Practices Network; What Works, Wisconsin

Period of Purple Crying

Program objectives: Provide new parents and caregivers with information about normal infant crying in order to prevent infant abuse and educate parents about the dangers of shaking an infant.

Target population: New parents and other caregivers of young infants.

Delivery setting and format: The home and hospital.

Duration: Three 5–10 minute exposures, including in the hospital maternity ward, in prenatal classes or at the first pediatrician visit, and through a media campaign.

Training resources: Online training, as well as a booklet and DVD available at dontshake.org/lms/index.php.

Website: purplecrying.info and dontshake.org

Registries that cite this program: California Evidence-Based Clearinghouse for Child Welfare

SafeCare

Program objectives: Provide in-home skill training to parents in child behavior management, activity planning, home safety, and child health care to prevent child maltreatment.

Target population: Parents with a history or risk of child neglect or abuse.

Delivery setting and format: Conducted in family homes, once per week for approximately 1–2 hours per session.

Duration: 18–20 weeks.

Training resources: Training as a home visitor requires attendance at a 1-week workshop, followed by demonstrated proficiency in delivering SafeCare with a family across four sessions monitored by a SafeCare coach. Typically, it takes 2 months to be fully certified as a SafeCare home visitor.

Website: publichealth.gsu.edu/968.html

Registries that cite this program: California Evidence-Based Clearinghouse for Child Welfare, Promising Practices Network

Supporting Father Involvement

Program objectives: Strengthen fathers' involvement in the family, promote healthy child development, and prevent child abuse.

Target population: Couples or fathers of children aged birth–11 years, especially from low-income families.

Delivery setting and format: Conducted in 2-hour weekly sessions of 4–8 couples or 10–12 fathers in agencies, community centers, or other group settings.

Duration: 16 weeks.

Training resources: Training manuals for the couples group and the fathers group are available through Philip A. Cowan (Email: pcowan@berkeley.edu).

Website: supportingfatherinvolvement.org

Registries that cite this program: California Evidence-Based Clearinghouse for Child Welfare, Promising Practices Network

STEP (Systematic Training for Effective Parenting)

Program objectives: Help parents learn effective ways to relate to their children, how to encourage cooperative behavior in their children, and how not to reinforce unacceptable behaviors. STEP also helps parents change dysfunctional and destructive relationships with their children by offering concrete alternatives to abusive and ineffective methods of discipline and control.

Target population: Parents of children ages birth through teenagers.

Delivery setting and format: Conducted in adoptive homes, birth family homes, community agencies, foster homes, hospitals, outpatient clinics, residential care facilities, and schools in small discussion groups to promote better interaction.

Duration: 7 weeks.

Training resources: Workshops and program manuals available. No special training is required for social workers, counselors, etc., to serve as STEP leaders.

Website: www.steppublishers.com

Registries that cite this program: California Evidence-Based Clearinghouse for Child Welfare, National Registry of Effective Prevention Programs

Triple P-Positive Parenting Program

Program objectives: Prevent severe behavioral, emotional, and developmental problems in children by enhancing the knowledge, skills, and confidence of parents. The Triple P system is a five-level system of interventions that vary by audience, intensity, length, and goal. Level 1 focuses on media messages about parenting to a community population, while Level 5 focuses on offering strategies to parents with specific risk factors (e.g., risk of child abuse) or children with moderate to severe behavior problems.

Target population: Parents and caregivers of children from birth through age 16.

Delivery setting and format: Conducted in adoptive homes, birth family homes, community agencies, foster homes, hospitals, outpatient clinics, residential care facilities, and schools in groups of 10–12 parents of children and adolescents from birth to age 16.

Duration: Varies depending on the type of intervention required.

Training resources: Training information is available at www. triplep-america.com/pages/individual/index.html.

Website: www.triplep-america.com/

Registries that cite this program: Blueprints; California Evidence-Based Clearinghouse for Child Welfare; Coalition for Evidence Based Policy; National Registry of Effective Prevention Programs; Promising Practices Network; What Works, Wisconsin

Chapter 40

Legal Interventions in Suspected Child Abuse Cases

Representation of Children in Child Abuse and Neglect Proceedings

The Federal Child Abuse Prevention and Treatment Act (CAPTA) requires States to document in their State plan provisions for appointing a guardian ad litem (GAL) to represent the child's best interests in every case of abuse or neglect that results in a judicial proceeding. The GAL may be an attorney or a court-appointed special advocate (CASA)—or both—who has received appropriate training.

The GAL represents the child at all judicial proceedings related to the case and has the responsibility to:

- Obtain firsthand a clear understanding of the situation and needs of the child

- Make recommendations to the court concerning the best interests of the child

This chapter includes text excerpted from "Representation of Children in Child Abuse and Neglect Proceedings," U.S. Department of Health and Human Services (HHS), August 2014.

At the State level, statutes specify when the court must appoint a representative for a child who is involved in an abuse and neglect proceeding and whom the court may appoint. As described in the National Council of Juvenile and Family Court Judges' *Resource Guidelines: Improving Court Practice in Child Abuse and Neglect Cases,* there are a number of ways that a child's interests can be represented. In some instances, two or more of these representatives may work on the same case:

- A GAL may be appointed to investigate and represent the child's best interests as described above.

- An attorney may be appointed specifically to represent the child's expressed wishes before the court.

- A CASA may be appointed to assist the court by investigating a child's circumstances and providing recommendations on meeting the child's needs. In some cases, a CASA may serve as the child's GAL as described in CAPTA.

Making the Appointment

All States, the District of Columbia, American Samoa, Guam, the Northern Mariana Islands, Puerto Rico, and the U.S. Virgin Islands provide in their statutes for the appointment of representation for a child involved in a child abuse or neglect proceeding. Approximately 41 States, the District of Columbia, American Samoa, Guam, the Northern Mariana Islands, and the Virgin Islands provide for the appointment of a GAL to represent the best interests of the child. In 15 of these States, the District of Columbia, and the Virgin Islands, the GAL must be an attorney. In other States, volunteers who may or may not be attorneys may serve as GALs.

Seventeen States and Puerto Rico require the appointment of an attorney for the child; seven States require both an attorney and GAL. Oregon requires the appointment of a CASA. In Wisconsin, a child has the right to counsel, and he or she may not be removed from the home unless counsel has been appointed. If the child is under age, the court may appoint a GAL instead of counsel. In 4 States, if the GAL is not an attorney, counsel may be appointed to represent the GAL.

In all cases, the appointment of a GAL, attorney, or CASA is made by the court that has jurisdiction over the child abuse or neglect proceedings. In Louisiana, the attorney may be provided by a Child Advocacy Program. In Maryland, the court appoints an attorney with whom the Department of Human Resources has contracted to provide legal services. In Washington, the court may select a GAL from a rotational registry of qualified GALs.

The Use of Court-Appointed Special Advocates

Approximately 34 States and the Virgin Islands allow for the appointment of a CASA. In 17 of these States, the CASA may serve as the GAL. In 13 States and the U.S. Virgin Islands, the CASA may be appointed in addition to the GAL. A CASA may be appointed in addition to an attorney in five States. In Louisiana and New Mexico, a CASA may be assigned to assist the court, while in Utah a CASA may be selected to assist the court or the child's GAL.

Qualifications and Training

Approximately 46 States, the District of Columbia, and the Virgin Islands address the qualifications and training required for those who can be assigned to represent a child involved in a child abuse or neglect proceeding. While most States that require the appointment of an attorney for the child do not require additional specific training, some States do have certain requirements that must be met. Texas, for example, requires the attorney to have training in child advocacy or experience equivalent to that training, while West Virginia requires 8 hours of continuing legal education per year focusing on the representation of children and child abuse and neglect.

For attorneys serving as GALs, training requirements vary considerably from State to State. In 4 States, additional training is not specified.

In 17 States and the District of Columbia, laws require attorneys to receive training specific to their roles as GALs. For example, Delaware requires GALs to complete training offered by the State Office of the Child Advocate, and Florida requires training to be provided by the Statewide Guardian ad Litem Office. In Georgia, the requirement for training can be satisfied within the State's existing continuing legal education obligations. The statutes in six States provide more specific requirements about the content of training, including knowledge about the needs and protection of children; applicable statutory, regulatory, and case law; and the roles, responsibilities, and duties when representing the best interests of a child.

For nonattorneys acting as GALs and CASAs, the laws in many States provide more detailed training requirements. Typically, an initial training program must be completed before a person may be assigned to a child's case, followed by ongoing in-service training. The training programs are designed to ensure that the child's advocate possesses the knowledge and skills to represent the child's best interests competently. Topics covered in these programs may include:

- Child abuse and neglect

- Child development

- Roles and responsibilities of the child's advocate

- Cultural awareness

- The juvenile court process

- Federal, State, and local laws, regulations, and rules

- Interview techniques and information gathering

- Documentation and report writing

Seven States specify that the training provided to CASAs must comply with standards set by the National Court Appointed Special Advocates Association.

In addition to training requirements, volunteers are screened and interviewed prior to acceptance in a GAL or CASA program. Sixteen States and the Northern Mariana Islands require criminal background checks. Checks of the State's child abuse and neglect registry are required in 10 States. California, Florida, and Idaho require checks of the State's sex offender registry

Specific Duties

The primary responsibility of a GAL is to represent the best interests of a child in child abuse and neglect proceedings. The laws in 41 States, American Samoa, Guam, the Northern Mariana Islands, and the Virgin Islands list specific duties that may be required as part of that responsibility. These duties include, but are not limited to:

- Meeting face-to-face with the child on a regular basis, including before all hearings

- Conducting an independent investigation of the circumstances of the case

- Attending all hearings and staffings related to the case

- Monitoring cases to ensure that court orders for services have been fulfilled

- Submitting written reports to the court

The GAL also is expected to make recommendations to the court about specific actions that would serve the best interests of the child. Sometimes, the GAL's determination of best interests may conflict with the child's expressed wishes. In 25 States, the District of Columbia, Guam, and the Virgin Islands, the GAL is obligated to communicate the child's wishes to the court along with his or her own recommendations. In 14 States, the District of Columbia, and Guam, the court may appoint a separate counsel to represent the child's wishes.

The statutes in 13 States list specific duties for a CASA who is appointed in addition to an attorney or GAL.

- Investigating the case to provide independent, factual information to the court. Typically, these duties may include:

  - Monitoring the case to ensure compliance with court orders

  - Determining whether appropriate services are being offered to the child and family

  - Preparing regular written reports for the court and parties to the case

Chapter 41

Therapy Options for Children Impacted by Abuse

Chapter Contents

Section 41.1

Cognitive Behavioral Therapy for Physical Abuse

This section includes text excerpted from "Alternatives for Families: A Cognitive Behavioral Therapy (AF-CBT)," U.S. Department of Health and Human Services (HHS), January 2013.

Alternatives for Families: A Cognitive Behavioral Therapy (AF-CBT)

Families that experience conflict, coercion, and/or physical abuse create substantial risk to children for the development of significant psychiatric, behavioral, and adjustment difficulties, including aggression, poor interpersonal skills/functioning, and emotional reactivity. Caregivers in such families often report punitive or excessive parenting practices, frequent anger and hyperarousal, and negative child attributions, among other stressful conditions. During the past four decades, research has documented the effectiveness of several behavioral and cognitive behavioral methods, many of which have been incorporated in alternatives for families: a cognitive-behavioral therapy (AF-CBT).

AF-CBT is an evidence-supported intervention that targets (1) diverse individual child and caregiver characteristics related to conflict and intimidation in the home and (2) the family context in which aggression or abuse may occur. This approach emphasizes training in intra- and interpersonal skills designed to enhance self-control and reduce violent behavior. AF-CBT has been found to improve functioning in school-aged children, their parents (caregivers), and their families following a referral for concerns about parenting practices, including child physical abuse.

This section is intended to build a better understanding of the characteristics and benefits of AF-CBT, formerly known as abuse focused cognitive behavioral therapy. It was written primarily to help child welfare caseworkers and other professionals who work with at-risk families make more informed decisions about when to refer children and their parents and caregivers to AF-CBT programs. This information also may help parents, foster parents, and other caregivers understand what they and their children can gain from AF-CBT and what to expect during treatment. In addition, this section may be useful to others with an interest in implementing or participating in effective strategies for the treatment of family conflict, child physical abuse, coercive parenting, and children with externalizing behavior problems.

What Makes AF-CBT Unique?

AF-CBT is designed to intervene with families referred for conflict or coercion, verbal or physical aggression by caregivers (including the use of excessive physical force or threats), behavior problems in children/adolescents, or child physical abuse. The treatment program has been expanded to accommodate children and adolescents with physical abuse or discipline-related trauma symptoms, such as posttraumatic stress disorder (PTSD).

AF-CBT addresses both the risk factors and the consequences of physical, emotional, and verbal aggression in a comprehensive manner. Thus, AF-CBT seeks to address specific clinical targets among caregivers that include heightened anger or hostility, negative perceptions or attributions of their children, and difficulties in the appropriate and effective use of parenting practices, such as ineffective or punitive parenting practices. Likewise, AF-CBT targets children's difficulties with anger or anxiety, trauma-related emotional symptoms, poor social and relationship skills, behavioral problems that include aggression, and dysfunctional attributions. At the family level, AF-CBT addresses coercive family interactions by teaching skills to improve positive family relations and reduce family conflict.

Reflects a Comprehensive Treatment Strategy

The diversity of family circumstances and individual problems associated with family conflict points to the need for a comprehensive treatment strategy that targets both the contributors to caregivers' behavior and children's subsequent behavioral and emotional adjustment. Treatment approaches that focus on several aspects of the problem (for example, a caregiver's parenting skills, a child's anger, family coercion) may have a greater likelihood of reducing re-abuse and more fully remediating mental health problems. Therefore, AF-CBT adopts a comprehensive treatment strategy that addresses the complexity of the issues more completely.

Integrates Several Therapeutic Approaches

AF-CBT combines elements drawn from the following:

- **Cognitive therapy**, which aims to change behavior by addressing a person's thoughts or perceptions, particularly those thinking patterns that create distorted views

- **Behavioral and learning theory,** which focuses on modifying habitual responses (e.g., anger, fear) to identified situations or stimuli

- **Family therapy,** which examines patterns of interactions among family members to identify and alleviate problems, and offers strategies to help reframe how problems are viewed

- **Developmental victimology,** which describes how the specific effects of exposure to traumatic or abusive experiences may vary for children at different developmental stages and across the life span

- **Psychology of aggression**, which describes the processes by which aggression and coercion develop and are maintained, which can help to understand one's history as both a contributor to and victim of aggressive behavior

AF-CBT pulls together many techniques currently used by practitioners, such as behavior and anger management, affect regulation, problem-solving, social skills training, cognitive restructuring, and communication. The advantage of this program is that all of these techniques, relevant handouts, training examples, and outcome measures are integrated in a structured approach that practitioners and supervisors can easily access and use.

Treats Children and Parents Simultaneously

During AF-CBT, school-aged children (5–15) and their caregivers participate in separate but coordinated therapy sessions, often using somewhat parallel treatment materials. In addition, children and parents attend joint sessions together at various times throughout treatment. This approach seeks to address individual and parent-child issues in an integrated fashion.

Discourages Aggressive or Violent Behavior

The AF-CBT approach is designed to promote appropriate and prosocial behavior, while discouraging coercive, aggressive, or violent behavior from caregivers as well as children. Consistent with cognitive-behavioral approaches, AF-CBT includes procedures that target three related ways in which people respond to different circumstances:

- Cognition (thinking)

- Affect (feeling)

- Behavior (doing)

AF-CBT includes training in various psychological skills in each of these response channels that are designed to promote self-control and to enhance interpersonal effectiveness.

Tailors Treatment to Meet Specific Needs and Circumstances

AF-CBT begins with a multisource assessment to identify the nature of the problems the child is experiencing, specific parental and family difficulties that may be contributing to family conflict, and the child's and family's strengths that may help influence change. Tailoring the treatment to the family's specific strengths and challenges is key to efficient outcomes.

Treatment Phases and Key Components

AF-CBT is a short-term treatment typically provided once or twice a week, which may require 18 to 24 hours of service (or longer, based on individual needs) over 4 to 12 months (although treatment may last as long as determined necessary). Treatment includes separate individual sessions with the child and caregiver/parent and joint sessions with at least both of them. Where necessary, family interventions may be applied before, during, or after the individual services. The treatment program for children, caregivers, and families incorporates the use of specific skills, role-playing exercises, performance feedback, and home practice exercises.

Generally, the goals of AF-CBT treatment are to:

- Reduce conflict and increase cohesion in family

- Reduce use of coercion (hostility, anger, verbal aggression, threats) by the caregiver and other family members

- Reduce use of physical force (aggressive behavior) by the caregiver, child, and, as relevant, other family members

- Promote nonaggressive (alternative) discipline and interactions

- Reduce child physical abuse risk or recidivism (prevention of child welfare system involvement or repeated reports/allegations)

- Improve the level of child's safety/welfare and family functioning

Treatment Phases

AF-CBT includes three treatment phases, each with key content that is designed to be relevant for both the caregiver and child. The sequence for conducting the treatment generally proceeds from teaching intrapersonal (e.g., cognitive, affective) skills first, followed by interpersonal skills (e.g., behavioral). Topics/sessions can be flexibly delivered (adapted, abbreviated, or repeated) based on the family's progress and/or treatment needs/goals in each phase. Although AF-CBT has primarily been used in outpatient and home settings, the treatment has been more recently delivered in inpatient and residential settings when there is some ongoing or potential contact between the caregiver and the child.

Phase I : Engagement and Psychoeducation

- Topic 1: Orientation–Caregiver and Child

- Topic 2: Alliance Building and Engagement–Caregiver

- Topic 3: Learning About Feelings and Family Experiences–Child

- Topic 4: Talking About Family Experiences and Psychoeducation–Caregiver

Phase II: Individual Skill-building (Skills Training)

- Topic 5: Emotion Regulation–Caregiver

- Topic 6: Emotion Regulation–Child

- Topic 7: Restructuring Thoughts–Caregiver

- Topic 8: Restructuring Thoughts–Child

- Topic 9: Noticing Positive Behavior–Caregiver

- Topic 10: Assertiveness and Social Skills–Child

- Topic 11: Techniques for Managing Behavior–Caregiver

- Optional Topic12: Imaginal Exposure–Child

* Topic 13: Preparation for Clarification–Caregiver

Phase III: Family Applications

* Topic 14: Verbalizing Healthy Communication–Caregiver and Child
* Topic 15: Enhancing Safety Through Clarification–Caregiver and Child
* Topic 16: Solving Family Problems– Caregiver and Child
* Topic 17: Graduation–Caregiver and Child

Key Components

AB-CBT includes specific therapy elements for children, parents, and families.

Treatment for School-Aged Children. The school-aged child-directed therapy elements include:

* Promoting engagement and treatment motivation by identifying individualized goals
* Identifying the child's exposure to and views of positive experiences and upsetting ones (family hostility, coercion, and violence), including the child's perceptions of the circumstances and consequences of the physical abuse or other conflict
* Educating the child on topics related to child welfare, safety/protection, service participation, and common reactions to abuse and family conflict
* Training in techniques to identify, express, and manage emotions appropriately (e.g., anxiety management, anger control)
* Processing the child's exposure to incidents involving force or family conflict to understand and challenge any dysfunctional thoughts/views that encourage the use of aggression or support self-blame for these situations
* Training in interpersonal skills to enhance social competence and developing social support plans
* For those with significant PTS symptoms, conducting imaginal exposure and helping to articulate the meaning of what happened to the child

Treatment for Parents (or Caregivers)

Parent-directed therapy elements include:

- Education about relevance of the CBT model and physical abuse

- Establishing a commitment to limit physical force

- Encouraging discussion of any incidents involving the use of force within the family

- Reviewing the child's exposure to emotional abuse in the family and providing education about the parameters of abusive experiences (causes, characteristics, and consequences) in order to understand the context in which they occurred

- Teaching affect management skills to help identify and manage reactions to abuse specific triggers, heightened anger, anxiety, and depression to promote self-control

- Identifying and addressing cognitive contributors to abusive behavior in caregivers (i.e., misattributions, high expectations, etc.) and/or their consequences in children (i.e., views supportive of aggression, self-blame, etc.) that could maintain any physically abusive or aggressive behavior

- Teaching parents strategies to support the child and encourage positive behavior using active/listening attention, praise, and rewards

- Training in effective discipline guidelines and strategies (e.g., planned ignoring, withdrawal of privileges, time out,) as alternatives to the use of physical force

- If the caregiver is ready, working on a clarification letter to be read to the child

Treatment for Families (or the Parent and Child)

Parent-child or family therapy elements include:

- Conducting a family assessment using multiple methods and identifying family treatment goals

- Encouraging a commitment to increasing the use of positive behavior as an alternative to the use of force

- Conducting a clarification session in which the caregiver can support the child by providing an apology, taking responsibility

316

for the abuse/conflict, and showing a commitment to safety plans and other rules in order to keep the family safe and intact

- Training in communication skills to encourage constructive interactions

- Training in nonaggressive problem-solving skills with home practice applications

- Involving community and social systems, as needed

Effectiveness of AF-CBT

The effectiveness of AF-CBT is supported by a number of outcome studies, and AF-CBT has been recognized by other experts as a "model" or "promising" treatment program.

Demonstrated Effectiveness in Outcome Studies

During the past four decades, many of the procedures incorporated into AF-CBT have been evaluated by outside investigators as effective in:

- Improving child, parent, and/or family functioning

- Promoting safety and/or reducing abuse risk or re-abuse among various populations of parents, children, and families

These procedures have included the use of stress management and anger-control training, cognitive restructuring, parenting skills training, psychoeducational information regarding the use and impact of physical force and hostility, social skills training, imaginal exposure, and family interventions focusing on reducing conflict.

Foundational studies by Kolko (1996a, 1996b) showed the effectiveness of the individual components of AF-CBT when compared to routine community services with abusive families in terms of improved child, parent, and family outcomes. A more recent study by Kolko, Iselin, and Gully documents the sustainability and clinical benefits of AF-CBT in an existing community clinic serving physically abused children and their families.

Recognition as an Evidence Based Practice

Based on systematic reviews of available research and evaluation studies, several groups of experts and agencies have highlighted AF-CBT as a model program or promising treatment practice:

- AF-CBT is rated a 3, which is a Promising Practice, by the California Evidence-Based Clearinghouse for Child Welfare.

- AF-CBT is featured in the Chadwick Center's (2004) Closing the Quality Chasm in Child Abuse Treatment: Identifying and Disseminating Best Practices

- AB-CBT is featured in Trauma-Informed Interventions: Clinical and Research Evidence and Culture-Specific Information Project, published by the National Child Traumatic Stress Network and the Medical University of South Carolina

- It is approved as an evidence-based treatment (EBT) by the Los Angeles County Office of Mental Health.

- It is included in EBT dissemination efforts being conducted by the Effective Providers for Child Victims of Violence Program of the American Psychological Association

- AF-CBT is included as a promising EBT in the website maintained by the U.S. Office of Justice Programs

- It is included in EBT dissemination activities by the Defending Childhood Initiative sponsored by the Attorney General's Office, U.S. Department of Justice.

- It is currently being disseminated by the National Child Traumatic Stress Network (NCTSN) in a National Learning Collaborative on AF-CBT.

Summary of AF-CBT Outcomes

Parent Outcomes

- Achievement of individual treatment goals related to the use of more effective discipline methods

- Decreased parental reports of overall psychological distress

- Lowered parent-reported child abuse potential (risk)

- Reduction in parent-reported drug use

Child Outcomes

- Reduction in parent-reported severity of children's behavior problems (externalizing behavior), including child-to-parent aggression and likelihood of violating other children's privacy

- Reduction in child anxiety

- Greater child safety from harm

Family Outcomes

- Greater child-reported family cohesion

- Reduced child-reported and parent-reported family conflict

Child Welfare Outcome

- Low rate of abuse recidivism or concerns about the child being harmed

Section 41.2

Parent-Child Interaction Therapy with At- Risk Families

This section includes text excerpted from "Parent-Child Interaction Therapy with At-Risk Families," U.S. Department of Health and Human Services (HHS), January 2013.

Parent-child interaction therapy (PCIT) is a family-centered treatment approach proven effective for abused and at-risk children ages 2 to 8 and their caregivers—birth parents, adoptive parents, or foster or kin caregivers. During PCIT, therapists coach parents while they interact with their children, teaching caregivers strategies that will promote positive behaviors in children who have disruptive or externalizing behavior problems. Research has shown that, as a result of PCIT, parents learn more effective parenting techniques, the behavior problems of children decrease, and the quality of the parent-child relationship improves.

This section is intended to build a better understanding of the characteristics and benefits of PCIT. It was written primarily to help child welfare caseworkers and other professionals who work with at-risk families make more informed decisions about when to refer parents and caregivers, along with their children, to PCIT programs. This information may also help parents, foster parents, and other care-givers understand what they and their children can gain from PCIT and what to expect during treatment. This brief also may be useful to others with an interest in implementing or participating in effective parent-training strategies.

What Makes PCIT Unique?

Introduced in the 1970s as a way to treat young children with seri-ous behavioral problems, PCIT has since been adapted successfully for use with populations who have experienced trauma due to child abuse or neglect. The distinctiveness of this approach lies in the use of live coaching and the treatment of both parent and child together. PCIT is the only evidence-based practice in which the parent and child are treated together throughout the course of all treatment sessions. As a result, it is a more intensive parenting intervention and most applicable for children with serious behavioral problems, parents with significant limitations (e.g., substance abuse, limited intellectual ability, mental health problems), and/or parents at risk for child maltreatment. In randomized testing, including families identified by the child welfare system, PCIT has consistently demonstrated success in improving par-ent-child interactions. Benefits of the model, which have been experi-enced by families along the child welfare continuum, such as at-risk families and those with confirmed reports of maltreatment or neglect, are described below.

Reduces Behavior Problems in Young Children by Improving Parent-Child Interaction

PCIT was originally designed to treat children ages 2 to 8 with disruptive or externalizing behavior problems, including conduct and oppositional defiant disorders. These children are often described as negative, argumentative, disobedient, and aggressive.

PCIT addresses the negative parent-child interaction patterns that contribute to the disruptive behavior of young children. Through PCIT, parents learn to bond with their children and develop more effective parenting styles that better meet their children's needs. For example, parents learn to model and reinforce constructive ways for dealing with emotions, such as frustration. Children, in turn, respond to these healthier relationships and interactions. As a result, children treated using PCIT typically show significant reductions in behavior problems at home and at school.

Treats the Parent and Child Together

While many treatment approaches target either parents or children, PCIT focuses on changing the behaviors of both the parent and child together. Parents learn to model positive behaviors that children can learn from and are trained to act as "agents of change" for their children's behavioral or emotional difficulties. Sitting behind a one-way mirror and coaching the parent through an "ear bug" audio device, therapist's guide parents through strategies that reinforce their children's positive behavior. In addition, PCIT therapists are able to tailor treatment based on observations of parent-child interactions. As such, PCIT can help address specific needs of each parent and child.

Decreases the Risk for Child Physical Abuse and Breaks the Coercive Cycle

PCIT has been found effective for physically abusive parents with children ages 2 to 12. PCIT is appropriate where physical abuse occurs within the context of child discipline, as most physical abuse does. While child behavior problems and child physical abuse often co-occur, PCIT may help change the parental response to challenging child behaviors, regardless of the type of behavior problem.

Foundational research has shown that many complex factors contribute to abusive behaviors, including a coercive relationship between the parent and child. Abusive and at-risk parents often interact in negative ways with their children, use ineffective and inconsistent discipline strategies, and rely too much on punishment. These same parents rarely interact in positive ways with their children (e.g., rewarding good behavior). At the same time, some physically abused and at-risk children learn to be aggressive, defiant, noncompliant, and resistant to parental direction.

The reciprocal negative behaviors of the parent and child create a harmful cycle that often escalates to the point of severe corporal punishment and physical abuse. The negative behaviors of the parent—screaming and threatening—reinforce the negative behaviors of the child—such as unresponsiveness and disobedience, which further aggravates the parent's behavior and may result in violence. PCIT helps break this cycle by encouraging positive interaction between parent and child and training parents in how to implement consistent and nonviolent discipline techniques when children act out.

Parents and caretakers completing PCIT typically:

- Show more positive parenting attitudes and demonstrate improvements in the ways that they listen to, talk to, and interact with their children

- Report less stress

- Use less corporal punishment and physically coercive means to control their children

Offers Support for Caregivers including Foster Parents

PCIT is now recognized as a way to help support foster parents caring for children with behavioral problems by enhancing the relationship between foster parents and foster children and by teaching foster parents behavior management skills. In addition to reporting decreases in child behavior problems, foster parents frequently report less parental stress following PCIT and high levels of satisfaction with the program. One benefit of providing foster parents with PCIT skills is that they can use these same effective parenting skills with future generations of foster children.

Uses Live Coaching

PCIT is a behavioral parent-training model. What makes PCIT different from other parent training programs is the way skills are taught, using live coaching of parents and children together. Live coaching provides immediate prompts to parents while they interact with their children. During the course of this hands-on treatment, parents are guided to demonstrate specific relationship-building and discipline skills.

The benefits of live coaching are significant:

- Parents are provided with opportunities to practice newly taught skills.

- Therapists can correct errors and misunderstandings on the spot.

- Parents receive immediate feedback.

- Parents are offered support, guidance, and encouragement as they learn.

- Treatment gains (e.g., increases in child compliance) are recognized by the parent "in the moment"–which supports continued use of effective parenting skills.

Adaptations for Various Populations

While PCIT was originally applied to Caucasian families, it has been adapted for use with various populations and cultures, including:

322

- Families in which child abuse has occurred
- Trauma victims/survivors
- Children with prenatal exposure to alcohol
- Children aged 18–60 months with externalizing behaviors who were premature births
- Children with developmental delays and/or mental retardation
- Older children
- Foster parents and maltreated children
- African-American families
- Latino and Spanish-speaking families
- Native American families

Limitations of PCIT

While PCIT is very effective in addressing certain types of problems, there are clear limitations to its use. For the following populations, PCIT may not be appropriate, or specific modifications to treatment may be needed:

- Parents who have limited or no ongoing contact with their child
- Parents with serious mental health problems that may include auditory or visual hallucinations or delusions
- Parents who are hearing impaired and would have trouble using the ear bug device, or parents who have significant expressive or receptive language deficits
- Sexually abusive parents, or parents engaging in sadistic physical abuse, or parents with substance abuse issues

Key Components

PCIT is typically provided in 10 to 20 sessions, with an average of 12 to 14 sessions, each lasting about 1 to 1.5 hours. Occasionally, additional treatment sessions are added as needed.

The PCIT curriculum uses a two-phase approach addressing:

1. Relationship enhancement
2. Discipline and compliance

Initially, the therapist discusses the key principles and skills of each phase with the parents. Then, the parents interact with their children and try to implement the particular skills. The therapist typically observes from behind a one-way mirror while communicating with the parent, who wears a small wireless earphone. Although not optimal, clinicians who do not have access to a one-way mirror and ear bug may provide services using in-room coaching. Specific behaviors are tracked on a graph over time to provide parents with feedback about the achievement of new skills and their progress in positive interactions with their child.

Phase 1: Relationship Enhancement (Child-Directed Interaction)

The first phase of treatment focuses on improving the quality of the relationship between the parent and the child. This phase emphasizes building a nurturing relationship and secure bond between parent and child. Phase I sessions are structured so that the child selects a toy or activity, and the parent plays along while being coached by the therapist. Because parents are taught to follow the child's lead, this phase also is referred to as child-directed interaction (CDI).

During Phase I sessions, parents are instructed to use positive reinforcement. In particular, parents are encouraged to use skills represented in the acronym "PRIDE":

- **Praise.** Parents provide praise for a child's appropriate behavior—for example, telling them, "good job cleaning up your crayons"—to help encourage the behavior and make the child feel good about his or her relationship with the parent.

- **Reflection.** Parents repeat and build upon what the child says to show that they are listening and to encourage improved communication.

- **Imitation.** Parents do the same thing that the child is doing, which shows approval and helps teach the child how to play with others.

- **Behavioral Description.** Parents describe the child's activity (e.g., "You're building a tower with blocks") to demonstrate interest and build vocabulary.

- **Enjoyment.** Parents are enthusiastic and show excitement about what the child is doing.

Parents are guided to praise wanted behaviors, like sharing, and to ignore unwanted or annoying behaviors, such as whining (unless the behaviors are destructive or dangerous). In addition, parents are taught to avoid criticisms or negative words—such as "No," "Don't," "Stop," "Quit," or "Not"—and instead concentrate on positive directions.

In addition to the coached sessions, parents are given homework sessions of 5 minutes each day to practice newly acquired skills with their child. Once the parent's skill level meets the program's identified criteria, the second phase of treatment is initiated.

Phase II: Discipline and Compliance (Parent-Directed Interaction)

The second phase of PCIT concentrates on establishing a structured and consistent approach to discipline. During this phase, also known as parent-directed interaction (PDI), the parent takes the lead. Parents are taught to give clear, direct commands to the child and to provide consistent consequences for both compliance and noncompliance. When a child obeys the command, parents are instructed to provide labeled or specific praise (e.g., "Thank you for sitting quietly"). When a child disobeys, however, the parents initiate a timeout procedure. The timeout procedure typically begins with the parent issuing the child a warning and a clear choice of action (e.g., "Put your toys away or go to timeout") and may advance to sending the child to a timeout chair.

Parents are coached in the use of these skills during a play situation where they must issue commands to their child and follow through with the appropriate consequence for compliance/noncompliance. In addition, parents are provided with strategies for managing challenging situations outside of therapy (for example, when a child throws a tantrum in the grocery store or hits another child). Parents also are given homework in this phase to aid in skill acquisition.

Assessments

In addition to clinical interviews, PCIT uses a combination of observational and standardized assessment measures to assess interactions between parent and child, child behaviors, and parental perception of stress related to being a parent, as well as parents' own perceptions of the difficulty of their child's behaviors and their interactions with their child. Assessments are conducted before, during, and after treatment.

Effectiveness of PCIT

The effectiveness of PCIT is supported by a growing body of research and increasingly identified on inventories of model and promising treatment programs.

Demonstrated Effectiveness in Outcome Studies

At least 30 randomized clinical outcome studies and more than 10 true randomized trials have found PCIT to be useful in treating at-risk families and children with behavioral problems. Research findings include the following:

- **Trauma adaptation.** PCIT is now commonly referred to in the cluster of trauma-informed strategies. Trauma adaption to the model was examined in a study of PCIT in meeting the needs of mother-child dyads exposed to Interpersonal Violence (IPV) by reducing children's behavior problems and decreasing mothers' distress

- **Reductions in the risk of child abuse.** In a study of 110 physically abusive parents, only one-fifth (19 percent) of the parents participating in PCIT had re-reports of physically abusing their children after 850 days, compared to half (49 percent) of the parents attending a typical community parenting group. Reductions in the risk of abuse following treatment have been confirmed in other studies among parents who had abused their children

- **Improvements in parenting skills and attitudes.** Research reveals that parents and caretakers completing PCIT typically demonstrate improvements in reflective listening skills, use more prosocial verbalization, direct fewer sarcastic comments and critical statements at their children, improve physical closeness to their children, and show more positive parenting attitudes

- **Improvements in child behavior.** A review of 17 studies that included 628 preschool-aged children identified as exhibiting a disruptive behavior disorder concluded that involvement in PCIT resulted in significant improvements in child behavior functioning. Commonly reported behavioral outcomes of PCIT included both less frequent and less intense behavior problems as reported by parents and teachers, increases in clinic-observed compliance, reductions in inattention and hyperactivity, decreases in observed negative behaviors such as whining or crying, and reductions in the percentage of children who qualified for a diagnosis of disruptive behavior disorder

- **Benefits for parents and other caregivers.** Examining PCIT effectiveness among foster parents participating with their foster children and biological parents referred for treatment because of their children's behavioral problems, researchers found decreases in child behavior problems and caregiver distress for both groups.

- **Lasting effectiveness.** Follow-up studies report that treatment gains are maintained over time

- **Usefulness in treating multiple issues.** Adapted versions of PCIT also have been shown to be effective in treating other issues such as separation anxiety, depression, self-injurious behavior, attention deficit hyperactivity disorder (ADHD), and adjustment following divorce

- **Adaptability for a variety of populations.** Studies support the benefits of PCIT across genders and across a variety of ethnic groups

Recognition as an Evidence Based Practice

Based on systematic reviews of available research and evaluation studies, a number of expert groups have highlighted PCIT as a model program or promising treatment practice, including:

- The California Evidence-Based Clearinghouse for Child Welfare

- The National Child Traumatic Stress Network

- National Crime Victims Research and Treatment Center and The Center for Sexual Assault and Traumatic Stress; Office for Victims of Crime, U.S. Department of Justice

Implementation of PCIT in a Child Welfare Setting

When introducing PCIT as a referral option that child welfare workers may consider for children and families in their caseload, administrators will want to ensure that workers have a clear understanding of how PCIT works, the values that drive it, and its effectiveness. Training for child welfare staff on the basics of PCIT, how to screen at-risk children with behavior problems, and how to make appropriate referrals can expedite families' access to effective treatment options.

A free online training on the fundamentals of PCIT, the "PCIT for Traumatized Children Web Course" can be accessed from the UC Davis PCIT Training Center website (pcit.ucdavis.edu). This is a 10-hour web course with eight separate modules that discuss and show the basics of PCIT treatment and three supplemental modules on cultural considerations of treatment, parent factors affecting PCIT provision, and strategies for engaging parents in treatment. Module 2, "Overview of PCIT," was designed to educate professionals who work with children in the child welfare system. This training may help a child welfare professional decide whether to refer a family to a qualified therapist for PCIT.

Finding a Therapist

Caseworkers should become knowledgeable about commonly used treatments before recommending a treatment provider to families. Caregivers should receive as much information as possible on the treatment options available to them. If PCIT is an appropriate treatment model for a family, seek a provider who has received adequate training, supervision, and consultation in the PCIT model. If feasible, both the caseworker and family should have an opportunity to interview potential PCIT therapists before beginning treatment.

PCIT Training

Mental health professionals with at least a master's degree in psychology, social work, or a related field are eligible for training in PCIT. Training involves 40 hours of direct training, with ongoing supervision and consultation for approximately 4 to 6 months, working with at least two PCIT cases through completion. Fidelity to the model is assessed throughout the supervision and consultation period.

Questions to Ask Treatment Providers

In addition to the appropriate training, it is important to select a treatment provider who is sensitive to the individual and cultural needs of the child, caregiver, and family. Caseworkers recommending a PCIT therapist should ask the treatment provider to explain the course of treatment, the role of each family member, and how the family's cultural background will be addressed. Family members should be involved in this discussion to the extent possible. The child, caregiver, and family should feel comfortable with, and have confidence in, the therapist with whom they will work. Some specific questions to ask a potential therapist regarding PCIT include:

- How will the parent be involved in this process?

- What is the nature of your PCIT training? When were you trained? By whom? How long was the training? Do you have access to follow-up consultation? What resource materials on PCIT are you familiar with? Are you clinically supervised by (or do you participate in a peer supervision group with) others who are PCIT trained?

- Why do you feel that PCIT is the appropriate treatment model for this child? Would the child benefit from other treatment methods after they complete PCIT (i.e., group or individual therapy)?

- What techniques will you use to help the child manage his or her emotions and related behaviors?

- Do you use a standard assessment process to gather baseline information on the functioning of the child and family and to monitor their progress in treatment over time?

- Do you have access to the appropriate equipment for PCIT (one-way mirror, ear bug, video equipment)? If not, how do you plan to structure the sessions to ensure that the PCIT techniques are used according to the model?

- Is there any potential for harm associated with treatment?

Conclusion

PCIT is a parent-training strategy with benefits for many families with child welfare involvement. PCIT's live coaching approach guides parents while they develop needed skills to manage their children's behavior. As parents learn to reinforce positive behaviors, while also setting limits and implementing appropriate discipline techniques, children's behavioral problems decrease. Notably, the risk for re-abuse in these families also declines. PCIT holds much promise to continue helping parents and caregivers build nurturing relationships that strengthen families and provide healthy environments for children to thrive.

Part Six

Parenting Issues and Child Abuse Risks

Chapter 42

Family Matters and Child Abuse Risk

Chapter Contents

Section 42.1

Risk Factors for Potential Abuse by Parents

This section contains text excerpted from the following sources:
Text under the heading "Parental Drug Use as Child Abuse"
is excerpted from "Parental Drug Use as Child Abuse," U.S.
Department of Health and Human Services (HHS), April 2015;
Text under the heading "Child Abuse and Neglect: Risk and
Protective Factors" is excerpted from "Child Abuse and Neglect:
Risk and Protective Factors," Centers for Disease Control
and Prevention (CDC), March 28, 2016.

Abuse of drugs or alcohol by parents and other caregivers can have negative effects on the health, safety, and well-being of children. Approximately 47 States, the District of Columbia, Guam, and the U.S Virgin Islands have laws within their child protection statutes that address the issue of substance abuse by parents. Two areas of concern are the harm caused by prenatal drug exposure and the harm caused to children of any age by exposure to illegal drug activity in their homes or environment.

Prenatal Drug Exposure

The Child Abuse Prevention and Treatment Act (CAPTA) requires States to have policies and procedures in place to notify child protective services (CPS) agencies of substance-exposed newborns (SENs) and to establish a plan of safe care for newborns identified as being affected by illegal substance abuse or having withdrawal symptoms resulting from prenatal drug exposure. Several States currently address this requirement in their statutes. Approximately 19 States and the District of Columbia have specific reporting procedures for infants who show evidence at birth of having been exposed to drugs, alcohol, or other controlled substances; 14 States and the District of Columbia include this type of exposure in their definitions of child abuse or neglect.

Some States specify in their statutes the response the CPS agency must make to reports of SENs. Maine requires the State agency to develop a plan of safe care for the infant. California, Maryland,

Minnesota, Missouri, Nevada, Pennsylvania, and the District of Columbia require the agency to complete an assessment of needs for the infant and for the infant's family and to make a referral to appropriate services. Illinois and Minnesota require mandated reporters to report when they suspect that pregnant women are substance abusers so that the women can be referred for treatment.

Children Exposed to Illegal Drug Activity

There is increasing concern about the negative effects on children when parents or other members of their households abuse alcohol or drugs or engage in other illegal drug-related activity, such as the manufacture of methamphetamines in home-based laboratories. Many States have responded to this problem by expanding the civil definition of child abuse or neglect to include this concern. Specific circumstances that are considered child abuse or neglect in some States include:

- Manufacturing a controlled substance in the presence of a child or on premises occupied by a child

- Exposing a child to, or allowing a child to be present where, chemicals or equipment for the manufacture of controlled substances are used or stored

- Selling, distributing, or giving drugs or alcohol to a child

- Using a controlled substance that impairs the caregiver's ability to adequately care for the child

- Exposing a child to the criminal sale or distribution of drugs

Approximately 34 States and the U.S. Virgin Islands address in their criminal statutes the issue of exposing children to illegal drug activity. For example, in 20 States the manufacture or possession of methamphetamine in the presence of a child is a felony, while in 10 States, the manufacture or possession of any controlled substance in the presence of a child is considered a felony.

Nine States have enacted enhanced penalties for any conviction for the manufacture of methamphetamine when a child was on the premises where the crime occurred. Exposing children to the manufacture, possession, or distribution of illegal drugs is considered child endangerment in 11 States. The exposure of a child to drugs or drug paraphernalia is a crime in eight States and the Virgin Islands. In North Carolina and Wyoming, selling or giving an illegal drug to a child by any person is a felony.

Child Abuse and Neglect: Risk and Protective Factors

A combination of individual, relational, community, and societal factors contribute to the risk of child abuse and neglect. Although children are not responsible for the harm inflicted upon them, certain characteristics have been found to increase their risk of being maltreated. Risk factors are those characteristics associated with child abuse and neglect—they may or may not be direct causes.

Risk Factors for Victimization

Individual Risk Factors

* Children younger than 4 years of age

* Special needs that may increase caregiver burden (e.g., disabilities, mental retardation, mental health issues, and chronic physical illnesses)

Risk Factors for Perpetration

Individual Risk Factors

* Parents' lack of understanding of children's needs, child development and parenting skills

* Parents' history of child maltreatment in family of origin

* Substance abuse and/or mental health issues including depression in the family

* Parental characteristics such as young age, low education, single parenthood, large number of dependent children, and low income

* Nonbiological, transient caregivers in the home (e.g., mother's male partner)

* Parental thoughts and emotions that tend to support or justify maltreatment behaviors

Family Risk Factors

* Social isolation

* Family disorganization, dissolution, and violence, including intimate partner violence

* Parenting stress, poor parent-child relationships, and negative interactions

Community Risk Factors

• Community violence

• Concentrated neighborhood disadvantage (e.g., high poverty and residential instability, high unemployment rates, and high density of alcohol outlets), and poor social connections.

Protective Factors for Child Maltreatment

Protective factors buffer children from being abused or neglected. These factors exist at various levels. Protective factors have not been studied as extensively or rigorously as risk factors. However, identifying and understanding protective factors are equally as important as researching risk factors.

There is scientific evidence to support the following protective factor:

Family Protective Factors

• Supportive family environment and social networks

Several other potential protective factors have been identified. Research is ongoing to determine whether the following factors do indeed buffer children from maltreatment.

Family Protective Factors

• Nurturing parenting skills

• Stable family relationships

• Household rules and child monitoring

• Parental employment

• Adequate housing

• Access to health care and social services

• Caring adults outside the family who can serve as role models or mentors

Community Protective Factors

• Communities that support parents and take responsibility for preventing abuse

Section 42.2

Domestic Violence and Child Abuse

This section includes text excerpted from "Domestic Violence and the Child Welfare System," U.S. Department of Health and Human Services (HHS), October 2014.

Domestic Violence

Domestic violence is a devastating social problem that affects every segment of the population. It is critical for child welfare professionals and other providers who work with children who have experienced abuse to understand the relationship between domestic violence and child maltreatment, as many families experiencing domestic violence also come to the attention of the child welfare system.

Increasingly, child welfare professionals, domestic violence victim advocates, courts, and other community stakeholders are working together to address the impact of domestic violence on children. This bulletin discusses the extent of the overlap between domestic violence and child welfare, some of the effects of domestic violence on child witnesses, and the trend toward a more collaborative, community wide response to the issue. It also features promising practices from States and local communities.

Scope of the Problem

Estimates of the number of children who have been exposed to domestic violence each year vary. Research suggests that nearly 30 million children in the United States will be exposed to some type of family violence before the age of 17, and there is a 30 to 60 percent overlap of child maltreatment and domestic violence. The most comprehensive data collected on this issue were gathered by the National Survey of Children's Exposure to Violence (NATSCEV), sponsored by the Office of Juvenile Justice and Delinquency Prevention (OJJDP) and the CDC. Researchers surveyed 4,549 children and youth ages 17 and younger between January and May 2008. Findings show that more than 11 percent of children and youth were exposed to some form of family violence within the past year, and 26 percent were exposed to at least one form of family violence during their lifetimes. Extrapolating these findings to the general population yields an estimate of more than 8 million children and youth who were exposed to family violence in the past year and more than 18 million exposed to family violence during their lifetime.

Large numbers of children come in contact with domestic violence service providers each year. Every year, the National Network to End Domestic Violence (NNEDV) conducts a 1-day, unduplicated count of adults and children seeking domestic violence services in the United States. On September 12, 2012, the NNEDV census found that "18,968 children and 16,355 adults found safety in emergency shelters and transitional housing, while 5,815 children and 23,186 adults received advocacy and support through nonresidential services" (National Network to End Domestic Violence, 2013).

Exposure to both domestic violence and child maltreatment can have immediate and, often, long-term impact on children and youth.

Impact of Domestic Violence on Children

Children who have been exposed to domestic violence are more likely than their peers to experience a wide range of difficulties, and the potential effects vary by age and developmental stage. The challenges faced by children and youth exposed to domestic violence generally fall into three categories:

- **Behavioral, social, and emotional problems.** Children in families experiencing domestic violence are more likely than other children to exhibit signs of depression and anxiety; higher levels of anger and/or disobedience; fear and withdrawal; poor peer, sibling, and social relationships; and low self-esteem.

- **Cognitive and attitudinal problems.** Children exposed to domestic violence are more likely than their peers to experience difficulties in school and with concentration and task completion; score lower on assessments of verbal, motor, and cognitive skills; lack conflict resolution skills; and possess limited problem solving skills. Children exposed to domestic violence also are more likely to exhibit pro-violence attitudes.

- **Long-term problems.** In addition to higher rates of delinquency and substance use, exposure to domestic violence is also one of several adverse childhood experiences (ACEs) that have been shown be risk factors for many of the most common causes of death in the United States, including alcohol abuse, drug abuse, smoking, obesity, and more.

Additional factors that influence the impact of domestic violence on children include:

- **Nature of the violence.** Children who witness frequent and severe forms of violence or fail to observe their caretakers resolving conflict may undergo more distress than children who witness fewer incidences of physical violence and experience positive interactions between their caregivers.

- **Age of the child.** Younger children appear to exhibit higher levels of emotional and psychological distress than older children. Children ages 5 and younger may experience developmental regression—the loss of acquired skills—or disruptions in eating or sleeping habits. Adolescents may exhibit impulsive and/or reckless behavior, such as substance use or running away (National Child Traumatic Stress Network, n.d.). Age-related differences can result from older children's more fully developed cognitive abilities, which help them to better understand the violence and select various coping strategies to alleviate upsetting symptoms. Additionally, because very young children are more likely to have closer physical proximity to and stronger emotional dependence on their mothers (often the victims of domestic violence), they may be more susceptible to and exhibit enhanced trauma symptoms

- **Elapsed time since exposure.** Children often have heightened levels of anxiety and fear immediately after a violent event. Fewer observable effects are seen in children as time passes after the violent event.

- **Gender.** In general, boys exhibit more externalized behaviors (e.g., aggression and acting out), while girls exhibit more internalized behaviors (e.g., withdrawal and depression).

- **Presence of child physical or sexual abuse.** Children who witness domestic violence and are physically or sexually abused are at higher risk for emotional and psychological maladjustment than children who witness violence and are not abused.

Despite these findings, not all children exposed to domestic violence will experience negative effects. Children's risk levels and reactions to domestic violence exist on a continuum; some children demonstrate enormous resiliency, while others show signs of significant maladaptive adjustment. Protective factors such as social competence, intelligence, high self-esteem, and a supportive relationship with an adult (especially a nonabusive parent) can help protect children from the adverse effects of exposure to domestic violence. It's important for domestic violence, child welfare, and other child-serving professionals to understand the impact of trauma on child development and how to minimize its effects without causing additional trauma.

Responding to Domestic Violence

Often families impacted by domestic violence may be involved with child welfare and child-serving community agencies. It is important to work with State domestic violence coalitions and local domestic violence programs to ensure an understanding of the dynamics of domestic violence, how abusive parents affect children, and how to support the safety of both children and nonabusive parents. Promising practices for building and sustaining community partnerships include:

- Building and sustaining relationships and partnerships with employees of other agencies and systems that affect family safety

- Establishing a shared vision for practice based on safety for all family members

- Understanding various perspectives and work processes and acknowledging the experience and skills of staffs in other agencies

- Developing joint protocols and policies to guide practice

Investing in meaningful training and technical assistance partnerships is critical to supporting victims of domestic violence and their children. Domestic violence coalitions, local domestic violence shelter programs, Tribal domestic violence programs, and culturally specific community-based organizations are all an integral part of any coordinated healthcare and social service response to domestic violence.

Each State, the District of Columbia, Puerto Rico, the U.S. Virgin Islands, Guam, the Commonwealth of the Northern Mariana Islands, and American Samoa have a Domestic Violence Coalition. These coalitions are connected to more than 2,000 local domestic violence programs receiving funding from FYSB's Family Violence Prevention and Services Program (FVPSA).

Addressing the issue of domestic violence requires a community wide response. While there are some challenges to responding to this serious social problem, the emergence of trauma-informed care and differential response are fostering cross-system collaboration to protect children and strengthen families.

Challenges

Although adult and child victims often are found in the same families, child welfare and domestic violence programs have traditionally responded separately to victims. This focus on the safety and protection of only one victim can lead to unintended consequences. For example, removing children from their homes and placing them in out-of-home care can cause additional trauma. Individual therapies focused on parents may not help rebuild family relationships or strengthen protective factors to prevent future violence or abuse. In recent years, however, enhanced collaboration among child and family-serving organizations and domestic violence programs has led to more comprehensive services to better meet the needs of both children and adults affected by domestic violence.

One example of enhanced collaboration efforts is the groundbreaking Greenbook Initiative, which was composed of six demonstration sites working on issues related to the intersection of domestic violence and child maltreatment. The projects implemented guidelines and policies outlined in the 1999 publication *Domestic Violence and Child Maltreatment Cases: Guidelines for Policy and Practice* (the Greenbook). The demonstration sites were funded from 2000 to 2007, and many service providers, agencies, and the courts continue to implement guidelines put forth by the Greenbook.

Still, challenges in responding to the issue of domestic violence and child maltreatment continue. Domestic violence is not always reported to authorities or identified by caseworkers. Of the data gathered through NATSCEV, authorities knew about approximately one-half (49 percent) of the incidents of children witnessing domestic violence. While a majority of children with reports of abuse or neglect remain at home after an investigation, they may remain in a home where they experience domestic violence.

The National Survey of Child and Adolescent Well-Being II found that one-quarter of the caregivers for children with reports of maltreatment—and who remained in the home following investigation—indicated having experienced domestic violence within the previous 12 months. Caseworkers for those families identified active domestic violence in 1 out of 10, highlighting the possibility that domestic violence is under identified in some child welfare cases.

A Trauma-Informed Approach

Trauma-informed practice—the services and programs specifically designed to address and respond to the impact of traumatic stress—help children and families build resiliency and prevent further trauma. The importance of this approach has become especially evident in child welfare, since the majority of children and families involved with child welfare have experienced some form of past trauma (Wilson, 2013). A trauma-informed approach means that all service providers share values and goals, focus on promoting healing and preventing further trauma, and work to identify and eliminate the abuse or violence that caused the trauma. One helpful resource has been made available by the Children's Bureau's National Resource Center for Child Protective Services (NRC CPS), which sponsored a webinar series focused on domestic violence and child protection.

The National Center on Domestic Violence, Trauma and Mental Health (NCDVTMH) offers the Creating Trauma-Informed Services: Tipsheet Series, which includes *Tips for Supporting Children and Youth Exposed to Domestic Violence: What You Might See and What You Can Do.* This tip sheet for child advocates outlines ways to support children who have been exposed to violence at home and tips for supporting parents as they help their children heal from trauma. Divided by age group—infants, toddlers, preschoolers; school-age children; and adolescents—the tip sheet lists signs and symptoms of violence exposure and corresponding tips for offering support.

Collaborative Approaches

Despite their differences, child welfare advocates and domestic violence service providers share significant goals that can help bridge the gap between them. These include:

- Ending violence against adults and children

- Ensuring children's safety

- Protecting adult victims so their children are not harmed by violence

- Promoting parents' strengths

- Deferring CPS intervention—as long as child safety is preserved—and referring adult and child victims to community-based services

The National Resource Center for Permanency and Family Connections, formerly the National Resource Center for Family-Centered Practice and Permanency Planning (Toussaint, 2006), suggests the following policies to align efforts of child abuse and domestic violence practitioners:

- Identify and assess domestic violence in all child welfare cases

- Provide services to families where domestic violence has been identified (even if child abuse had not been substantiated), including helping abused women protect themselves and their children using noncoercive, supporting and empowering interventions whenever possible.

- Hold perpetrators of domestic violence accountable for stopping the violent behavior in order to protect children.

To help judges hold perpetrators accountable, the NCJFCJ developed the *Checklist to Promote Perpetrator Accountability in Dependency Cases Involving Domestic Violence.*

In recent years, increased awareness of the co-occurrence of domestic violence and child abuse has compelled both child welfare systems and domestic violence programs to reevaluate their interventions with families experiencing both forms of violence. Many professionals now acknowledge that communities can serve families better by allocating resources to build partnerships among domestic violence service providers, child protective service providers, and an array of informal and formal systems within the community. National, State, and local initiatives are demonstrating that a collective ownership and intolerance for abuse against adults and children alike can form the foundation of a coordinated and comprehensive approach to ending child abuse and domestic violence. Additionally, the 2010 reauthorization of the Child Abuse Prevention and Treatment Act authorized grants to develop or expand effective collaborations between child protective service and domestic violence service entities.

Institutional and societal changes can begin to eliminate domestic violence only when service providers integrate their expertise, resources, and services into an expansive network. New practices are enhancing cross-system understanding and interactions between agencies and communities. New protocols are institutionalizing change and ensuring that child welfare workers and domestic violence advocates benefit from the lessons learned by their predecessors and colleagues.

A collaborative approach to working with families that experience the co-occurrence of domestic violence and child maltreatment has a number of potential benefits: families receive more comprehensive and coordinated services, while avoiding redundant interviews and program requirements; agencies can effectively identify and provide appropriate services; and caseworkers can minimize blaming of the adult victim, hold batterers accountable, and advocate on behalf of all family members. To improve collaboration within and among systems and to engage new community partners in keeping families safe, organizations must have certain strategies. While some of these are described in more detail later in this section, examples of strategies to improve collaboration include:

- Collaborative learning and practice as a prelude to new policies

- New strategies to address issues of race, culture, and gender

- Greater participation by survivor mothers and children

- Greater investment in community

- Differential responses for families based on risk

- Therapeutic and other services and supports for mothers and children

- Greater accountability for men who batter and greater attention to the roles they continue to play as fathers and providers

- Broad, meaningful engagement of men as allies in protecting children

FYSB's Family Violence Prevention and Services Program (FVPSA) funds a network of culturally specific resource centers that work to address the impact of domestic violence and provide culturally specific programming and culturally relevant responses for the African-American, Asian and Pacific Islander, and Hispanic and Latina communities.

The Asian and Pacific Islander Institute on Domestic Violence produced a publication that aims to share the voices of immigrant, refugee, and indigenous women who are survivors of intimate partner violence and who have been involved with child protective services. By gathering and sharing the experiences of these women, the project hoped the information would help with the development of policies, practices, and interventions that more effectively address the issue of family violence. *Battered Mothers Involved With Child Protective Services: Learning from Immigrant, Refugee and Indigenous Women's Experiences.*

Responding Early: Teens and Dating Violence

Children and youth learn about healthy relationships by watching and modeling the relationships they witness. Children who are exposed to domestic violence may later repeat the abuse they see, thinking that it is a normal part of relationships. This can be especially concerning with young adults forging their first romantic relationships. Child welfare professionals, domestic violence victim advocates, and related professionals can work together to help youth understand that healthy relationships are nonviolent relationships, and they can help young people who have experienced dating violence develop resilience and heal.

In addition to a web section on teen dating violence, the CDC offers a 1-hour training for youth-serving organizations to help young people understand the risk factors of dating violence. *Dating Matters: Understanding Teen Dating Violence Prevention*

Other resources with information and materials on teen dating violence include the following:

- Child Welfare Information Gateway's web section on teen dating violence prevention that offers links to prevention programs and other materials on the subject.

- The National Online Resource Center on Violence against Women's resource collection on collaborative and multilevel approaches to the prevention of and response to teen dating violence.

- The National Center for Victims of Crime's bulletins for teens that define teen dating violence and the signs and symptoms of abuse.

- Break the Cycle: Empowering Youth to End Domestic Violence, which provides comprehensive dating abuse prevention programs exclusively to young people, including tools for action, training, and a Dating Violence 101 section.

Section 42.3

Postpartum Depression

This section includes text excerpted from "Postpartum Depression Facts," National Institutes of Health (NIH), December 13, 2013.

What Is Postpartum Depression?

Postpartum depression is a mood disorder that can affect women after childbirth. Mothers with postpartum depression experience feelings of extreme sadness, anxiety, and exhaustion that may make it difficult for them to complete daily care activities for themselves or for others.

What Causes Postpartum Depression?

Postpartum depression does not have a single cause, but likely results from a combination of physical and emotional factors. Postpartum depression does not occur because of something a mother does or does not do.

After childbirth, the levels of hormones (estrogen and progesterone) in a woman's body quickly drop. This leads to chemical changes in her brain that may trigger mood swings. In addition, many mothers are unable to get the rest they need to fully recover from giving birth. Constant sleep deprivation can lead to physical discomfort and exhaustion, which can contribute to the symptoms of postpartum depression.

What Are the Symptoms of Postpartum Depression?

Some of the more common symptoms a woman may experience include:

- Feeling sad, hopeless, empty, or overwhelmed

- Crying more often than usual or for no apparent reason

- Worrying or feeling overly anxious

- Feeling moody, irritable, or restless

347

- Oversleeping, or being unable to sleep even when her baby is asleep

- Having trouble concentrating, remembering details, and making decisions

- Experiencing anger or rage

- Losing interest in activities that are usually enjoyable

- Suffering from physical aches and pains, including frequent headaches, stomach problems, and muscle pain

- Eating too little or too much

- Withdrawing from or avoiding friends and family

- Having trouble bonding or forming an emotional attachment with her baby

- Persistently doubting her ability to care for her baby

- Thinking about harming herself or her baby.

How Can a Woman Tell If She Has Postpartum Depression?

Only a health care provider can diagnose a woman with postpartum depression. Because symptoms of this condition are broad and may vary between women, a healthcare provider can help a woman figure out whether the symptoms she is feeling are due to postpartum depression or something else. A woman who experiences any of these symptoms should see a healthcare provider right away.

How Is Postpartum Depression Different from the "Baby Blues"?

The "baby blues" is a term used to describe the feelings of worry, unhappiness, and fatigue that many women experience after having a baby. Babies require a lot of care, so it's normal for mothers to be worried about, or tired from, providing that care. Baby blues, which affects up to 80 percent of mothers, includes feelings that are somewhat mild, last a week or two, and go away on their own.

With postpartum depression, feelings of sadness and anxiety can be extreme and might interfere with a woman's ability to care for herself or her family. Because of the severity of the symptoms, postpartum depression usually requires treatment. The condition, which occurs in nearly 15 percent of births, may begin shortly before or any time after childbirth, but commonly begins between a week and a month after delivery.

Are Some Women More Likely to Experience Postpartum Depression?

Some women are at greater risk for developing postpartum depression because they have one or more risk factors, such as:

* Symptoms of depression during or after a previous pregnancy

* Previous experience with depression or bipolar disorder at another time in her life

* A family member who has been diagnosed with depression or other mental illness

* A stressful life event during pregnancy or shortly after giving birth, such as job loss, death of a loved one, domestic violence, or personal illness

* Medical complications during childbirth, including premature delivery or having a baby with medical problems

* Mixed feelings about the pregnancy, whether it was planned or unplanned

* A lack of strong emotional support from her spouse, partner, family, or friends

* Alcohol or other drug abuse problems. Postpartum depression can affect any woman regardless of age, race, ethnicity, or economic status

Postpartum depression can affect any woman regardless of age, race, ethnicity, or economic status.

How Is Postpartum Depression Treated?

There are effective treatments for postpartum depression. A woman's health care provider can help her choose the best treatment, which may include:

* **Counseling/Talk Therapy:** This treatment involves talking one-on-one with a mental health professional (a counselor, therapist, psychologist, psychiatrist, or social worker). Two types of

counseling shown to be particularly effective in treating postpartum depression are:

1. Cognitive behavioral therapy (CBT), which helps people recognize and change their negative thoughts and behaviors; and

2. Interpersonal therapy (IPT), which helps people understand and work through problematic personal relationships.

- **Medication:** Antidepressant medications act on the brain chemicals that are involved in mood regulation. Many antidepressants take a few weeks to be most effective. While these medications are generally considered safe to use during breastfeeding, a woman should talk to her healthcare provider about the risks and benefits to both herself and her baby.

These treatment methods can be used alone or together.

What Can Happen If Postpartum Depression Is Left Untreated?

Without treatment, postpartum depression can last for months or years. In addition to affecting the mother's health, it can interfere with her ability to connect with and care for her baby and may cause the baby to have problems with sleeping, eating, and behavior as he or she grows.

How Can Family and Friends Help?

Family members and friends may be the first to recognize symptoms of postpartum depression in a new mother. They can encourage her to talk with a health care provider, offer emotional support, and assist with daily tasks such as caring for the baby or the home.

Section 42.4

Military Deployment and Child Abuse Risk

This section contains text excerpted from the following sources: Text under the heading "Children Coping with Deployment" is excerpted from "Children Coping with Deployment," U.S. Department of Veterans Affairs (VA), August 13, 2015; Text under the heading "How Deployment Stress Affects Children and Families: Research Findings" is excerpted from "How Deployment Stress Affects Children and Families: Research Findings," U.S. Department of Veterans Affairs (VA), February 23, 2016.

Children Coping with Deployment

The children of military personnel face many challenges because of deployment to war. Kids need to understand why their parent has to leave, where they are going, and how long they will be away. If you are being deployed, take time to talk to your children about your feelings, what you do on your military job, and what you think of your job. Help them know where you will be and plan ahead to keep in touch regularly and often.

Children also need to understand what will happen when the deployed person returns home. The amount kids can understand and how they cope depends on age and how mature they are.

Protecting Children from Fear

We cannot protect our children from all that is bad. Yet we can learn to talk to our children about war. Use language that is easy to understand and does not hide the truth. Protect children from needless worries and concerns. Provide them with a sense of security and safety. Children should be assured that everything is being done to bring their loved one home safely and to protect families at home.

It is important to take the time to discuss and share our own concerns and fears. Do this with other adults, loved ones, friends or counselors, and this will help make it easier on children. Seeking social support from adults outside of the family is one way to manage our own stress. Researchers have found that parents who are able to handle upsetting, traumatic, or conflicting issues can serve as a buffer for the child.

Non-Military Kids

Civilian children may be concerned and feel afraid too. They may be learning about war from TV, radio, online, or from other sources like friends and school. Children may know someone who has a parent or loved one who went to war. They may be concerned for that person's safety. Parents will need to respond to these concerns. The everyday security of family life may be challenged.

Listen and Watch

All parents need to take the time to listen, observe, and talk to their children about what is happening around them. This can teach children good listening and communication skills, respect and support for differing opinions, and ways to manage fears and anxieties.

Even if you prepare and talk to a child, he or she will still be affected. Look for signs of stress. If children have been through trauma in their lives or have difficulties in school or with friends, they may be particularly open to feeling any changes in their sense of safety.

The Effects of Deployment on Children

Talk to Help Children Deal with War

Take the time to talk about war and deployment. Remember that talking can only make your family stronger. Don't ignore the subject. Do not minimize your child's concerns or stressors. Many parents would like to ignore the situation because thinking about war makes them feel vulnerable and powerless to protect their children.

Children need a real message about what is happening around them. Children are very good at knowing when things are being hidden from them. Be truthful and honest regardless of the age of your child, without overburdening him or her.

Children in different age groups will understand differently:

- Very young children are concerned with present everyday life. They need to feel safe. They are affected by the presence or absence of loved ones.

- Younger children may be confused by names of people and places that mean little to them. They may need help in forming basic ideas and understanding.

- Preteens and adolescents will be developing more abstract thinking about ideas and issues and concern for world events. They will be forming strong opinions they want recognized as their own. They may hear ideas from their peers. These ideas and feelings may be in agreement with their families' opinions or not. Yet their ideas and thoughts need to be heard and respected.

Talk about Feelings

Encourage your children to freely talk about their concerns and feelings. All children want to be included in family matters. They want to be listened to and understood. They have ideas and feelings but may not know how to express them, or how to handle them. "If war is bad, why is mommy going to war?" "If war is bad, why are we doing it?" "Is killing other people ok?"

Don't be afraid to talk about your feelings, even if you are conflicted or confused. If children know adults are being honest and respectful to them, they will feel safer. Do the best you can, even when you don't know all the answers.

Make Your Child Feel as Secure as Possible

Make your child feel as secure as possible without changing the facts. For example, you might say to a very young child, "War is happening in another country, far away. But you are safe here and we will take care of you." Or, "Your (dad, mom) will be serving with men and women who will do the best job possible to protect (him, her) and bring (him, her) home safely."

Provide reassurance about the future. Be hopeful about the future. "Yes these are hard times, but we are hopeful that people will be able to overcome their differences and live more peacefully in the future."

Accept Different Opinions

Try to look at and explain the points of view from all sides of a conflict. Teach the importance of respect and give and take. Be sure that children understand that violence is not always the best solution. Whether you are for or against war, take the time to explain how democracy works. Explain how to respect all points of view, just as in your family, each person wants their opinion to be respected and heard.

Explain why you agree or disagree with war in terms your child can understand. For example: "I don't like war, but it seems this is the best way to keep us safe," or "I understand why some people want to fight, but I believe that the only way to peace is negotiation, not violence."

Things to Do to Help Children Cope with War

- Provide extra attention, care, and physical closeness.

- Understand that they may be angry (and perhaps rightly so).

- Limit exposure to news, especially when news repeats and is violent. Younger children should be shielded from this kind of news as much as possible. It will needlessly increase their worry of events they don't understand.

- Respect your child's timing and ways of coping. Very young children may want to close their eyes or just go out and play. Don't confront children or force them to talk about things when they don't want to.

- Keep an open door for the absent parent or loved one. Talk with him or her as often as possible, and for important dates like birthdays, holidays, etc. Talk about what it will be like when that person returns and what it would be like if they were here now. This is really important for younger children who may not understand why their loved one is not here.

- Help your children develop and enjoy fun activities. Distraction can make time go by faster.

- Stick to routines and plan for upcoming events.

- Suggest positive and creative ways of coping for older children and adolescents (create scrapbooks and videos, write letters, take photos).

- Discuss things. Let kids know they can talk about how they feel. Accept how they feel and don't tell them they should not feel that way.

- Tell kids their feelings are normal. Be prepared to tell them many times.

If stress becomes out of hand, seek support from Military Family Assistance Centers available in each state. They will understand and may direct you to support groups that can help as well. It may be helpful for children to talk in groups with other children whose parents are deployed.

How Deployment Stress Affects Children and Families: Research Findings

How Many Families Are Affected by Deployment?

By the end of 2008, 1.7 million American Service Members had served in Operation Enduring Freedom and Operation Iraqi Freedom (OEF/OIF). Military personnel serving in Iraq and Afghanistan run the risk of developing problems such as depression, posttraumatic stress disorder (PTSD), anxiety, and traumatic brain injury due to their deployment. Studies of these returning service members and Veterans have found rates of 4% to 14% for depression, 12% to 25% for PTSD, 11% to 19% for traumatic brain injury, and 18% to 35% for any mental health risk or concern.

Forty-three percent of active duty service members have children. These children face the challenges inherent in having a parent deployed. Many of them must also cope with living with a parent who returns profoundly changed by war. Most families will be able to overcome these adversities through the support of family, friends, and community. Others, however, will need additional help from service providers to strengthen their resilience, access needed services, and readjust to life post-deployment. Veterans themselves recognize the need for such services. In a recent study of Veterans receiving treatment for PTSD, nearly 80% were interested in greater family involvement in their care.

What Are the Effects of Deployment on Children and Families?

While frequent moves, absence of the military parent, and other stresses are common for military families, the deployment of a parent to a combat zone represents a challenge of a different magnitude. For the parent who stays behind (usually the mother) increased family responsibilities, financial issues, isolation, and fear for their spouse's safety can cause anxiety, loneliness, sadness, and a feeling of being overwhelmed.

Children's reactions to a parent's deployment vary by child, and more broadly, by a child's developmental stage, age, and presence of any preexisting psychological or behavioral problems. Very young children may exhibit separation anxiety, temper tantrums, and changes in eating habits. School-age children may experience a decline in academic performance, and have mood changes or physical complaints. Adolescents may become angry and act out, or withdraw and show signs of apathy.

Especially for young children, the mental health of the at-home parent is often a key factor affecting the child's distress level. Parents reporting clinically significant stress are more likely to have children identified as "high risk" for psychological and behavioral problems.

What Are the Effects of Returning from Deployment on Children and Families?

Older studies of Vietnam Veterans demonstrate the negative impact on families of war-related PTSD. These Veterans have higher levels of marital problems, family violence, and partner distress. Their children present more behavioral problems than do those of Veterans without PTSD. Veterans with the highest levels of symptomology had families with the worst functioning. The numbing and avoidance experienced by Veterans with PTSD is associated with lower parenting satisfaction. The difficulty these Veterans have experiencing emotions and their sense of detachment may make it difficult for them in their personal relationships, and may even lead to behavioral problems on the part of their children.

More recent studies of personnel deployed to Afghanistan and Iraq have looked at family functioning in the near-term post-deployment period. In one study, soldiers' dissociative symptoms, sexual problems, and sleep disturbances had the greatest impact on relationships. The total number of traumatic events experienced, either during the war or in other contexts, did not significantly affect relationship satisfaction. In a sample referred for mental health evaluation, 75% of Veterans with partners reported at least one family adjustment issue. Fifty-four percent of these Veterans reported shouting with, shoving, or pushing current or former partners. Symptoms of depression were associated with family problems generally and domestic abuse in particular. Among Veterans with children, those with more severe PTSD and depression were more likely to report that their children were afraid of them or lacked warmth towards them.

Summary

Information from previous conflicts and from the ongoing conflicts in Iraq and Afghanistan indicates that the effects of war go far beyond the deployed service member. Children and families struggle both with changes resulting from an absent parent or spouse as well as changes when the absent service member returns.

The mental health of the at-home parent plays a crucial role in children's adjustment during deployment. The mental health of the returning service member also affects the children as well as family functioning and relationship satisfaction. Therefore, it is important that the needs of the entire family are considered. Pilot programs both within and outside VA are currently underway to address this important issue.

Chapter 43

Parental Substance Abuse and Child Abuse Risks

Chapter Contents

Section 43.1

Connection between Substance Abuse and Child Abuse

This section includes text excerpted from "Parental Substance Use and the Child Welfare System," U.S. Department of Health and Human Services (HHS), October 2014.

Parental Substance Use and the Child Welfare System

Many families receiving child welfare services are affected by parental substance use. Identifying substance abuse and meeting the complex needs of parents with substance use disorders and those of their children can be challenging. Over the past two decades, innovative approaches coupled with new research and program evaluation have helped point to new directions for more effective, collaborative, and holistic service delivery to support both parents and children. This bulletin provides child welfare workers and related professionals with information on the intersection of substance use disorders and child maltreatment and describes strategies for prevention, intervention, and treatment, including examples of effective programs and practices.

The Relationship between Substance Use Disorders and Child Maltreatment

It is difficult to provide precise, current statistics on the number of families in child welfare affected by parental substance use or dependency since there is no ongoing, standardized, national data collection on the topic. In a 1999 report to Congress, the U.S. Department of Health and Human Services (HHS) reported that studies showed that between one-third and two-thirds of child maltreatment cases were affected by substance use to some degree. More recent research reviews suggest that the range may be even wider. The variation in estimates may be attributable, in part, to differences in the populations studied and the type of child welfare involvement (e.g., reports, substantiation, out-of-home placement); differences in how substance use (or substance abuse or substance use disorder) is defined and measured;

and variations in State and local child welfare policies and practices for case documentation of substance abuse.

Children of Parents with Substance Use Disorders

An estimated 12 percent of children in this country live with a parent who is dependent on or abuses alcohol or other drugs. Based on data from the period 2002 to 2007, the National Survey on Drug Use and Health (NSDUH) reported that 8.3 million children under 18 years of age lived with at least one substance dependent or substance-abusing parent. Of these children, approximately 7.3 million lived with a parent who was dependent on or abused alcohol, and about 2.2 million lived with a parent who was dependent on or abused illicit drugs. While many of these children will not experience abuse or neglect, they are at increased risk for maltreatment and entering the child welfare system.

For more than 400,000 infants each year (about 10 percent of all births), substance exposure begins prenatally. State and local surveys have documented prenatal substance use as high as 30 percent in some populations. Based on NSDUH data from 2011 and 2012, approximately 5.9 percent of pregnant women aged 15 to 44 were current illicit drug users. Younger pregnant women generally reported the greatest substance use, with rates approaching 18.3 percent among 15- to 17-year-olds. Among pregnant women aged 15 to 44 years old, about 8.5 percent reported current alcohol use, 2.7 percent reported binge drinking, and 3 percent reported heavy drinking.

Parental Substance Abuse as a Risk Factor for Maltreatment and Child Welfare Involvement

Parental substance abuse is recognized as a risk factor for child maltreatment and child welfare involvement. Research shows that children with parents who abuse alcohol or drugs are more likely to experience abuse or neglect than children in other households. One longitudinal study identified parental substance abuse (specifically, maternal drug use) as one of five key factors that predicted a report to child protective services (CPS) for abuse or neglect. Once a report is substantiated, children of parents with substance use issues are more likely to be placed in out-of-home care and more likely to stay in care longer than other children. The National Survey of Child and Adolescent Well-Being (NSCAW) estimates that 61 percent of infants and 41 percent of older children in out-of-home care are from families with active alcohol or drug abuse.

According to data in the Adoption and Foster Care Analysis and Reporting System (AFCARS), parental substance abuse is frequently reported as a reason for removal, particularly in combination with neglect. For almost 31 percent of all children placed in foster care in 2012, parental alcohol or drug use was the documented reason for removal, and in several States that percentage surpassed 60 percent (National Data Archive on Child Abuse and Neglect, 2012). Nevertheless, many caregivers whose children remain at home after an investigation also have substance abuse issues. NSCAW found that the need for substance abuse services among in-home caregivers receiving child welfare services was substantially higher than that of adults nationwide (29 percent as compared with 20 percent, respectively, for parents ages 18 to 25, and 29 percent versus 7 percent for parents over age 26).

Role of Co-Occurring Issues

While the link between substance abuse and child maltreatment is well documented, it is not clear how much is a direct causal connection and how much can be attributed to other co-occurring issues. National data reveal that slightly more than one-third of adults with substance use disorders have a co-occurring mental illness. Research on women with substance abuse problems shows high rates of post-traumatic stress disorder (PTSD), most commonly stemming from a history of childhood physical and/or sexual assault. Many parents with substance abuse problems also experience social isolation, poverty, unstable housing, and domestic violence. These co-occurring issues may contribute to both the substance use and the child maltreatment. Evidence increasingly points to a critical role of stress and reactions within the brain to stress, which can lead to both drug-seeking activity and inappropriate caregiving.

Impact of Parental Substance Use on Children

The way parents with substance use disorders behave and interact with their children can have a multifaceted impact on the children. The effects can be both indirect (e.g., through a chaotic living environment) and direct (e.g., physical or sexual abuse). Parental substance use can affect parenting, prenatal development, and early childhood and adolescent development. It is important to recognize, however, that not all children of parents with substance use issues will suffer abuse, neglect, or other negative outcomes.

Parenting

A parent's substance use disorder may affect his or her ability to function effectively in a parental role. Ineffective or inconsistent parenting can be due to the following:

- Physical or mental impairments caused by alcohol or other drugs

- Reduced capacity to respond to a child's cues and needs

- Difficulties regulating emotions and controlling anger and impulsivity

- Disruptions in healthy parent-child attachment

- Spending limited funds on alcohol and drugs rather than food or other household needs

- Spending time seeking out, manufacturing, or using alcohol or other drugs

- Incarceration, which can result in inadequate or inappropriate supervision for children

- Estrangement from family and other social supports

Family life for children with one or both parents that abuse drugs or alcohol often can be chaotic and unpredictable. Children's basic needs—including nutrition, supervision, and nurturing—may go unmet, which can result in neglect. These families often experience a number of other problems—such as mental illness, domestic violence, unemployment, and housing instability—that also affect parenting and contribute to high levels of stress. A parent with a substance abuse disorder may be unable to regulate stress and other emotions, which can lead to impulsive and reactive behavior that may escalate to physical abuse.

Different substances may have different effects on parenting and safety. For example, the threats to a child of a parent who becomes sedated and inattentive after drinking excessively differ from the threats posed by a parent who exhibits aggressive side effects from methamphetamine use. Dangers may be posed not only from use of illegal drugs, but also, and increasingly, from abuse of prescription drugs (pain relievers, anti-anxiety medicines, and sleeping pills). Polysubstance use (multiple drugs) may make it difficult to determine the specific and compounded effects on any individual. Further, risks for the child's safety may differ depending upon the level and severity of parental substance use and associated adverse effects.

Prenatal and Infant Development

The effects of parental substance use disorders on a child can begin before the child is born. Maternal drug and alcohol use during pregnancy have been associated with premature birth, low birth weight, slowed growth, and a variety of physical, emotional, behavioral, and cognitive problems. Research suggests powerful effects of legal drugs, such as tobacco, as well as illegal drugs on prenatal and early childhood development.

Fetal alcohol spectrum disorders (FASD) are a set of conditions that affect an estimated 40,000 infants born each year to mothers who drank alcohol during pregnancy (Prevention First, n.d.). Children with FASD may experience mild to severe physical, mental, behavioral, and/ or learning disabilities, some of which may have lifelong implications (e.g., brain damage, physical defects, attention deficits). In addition, increasing numbers of newborns—approximately 3 per 1,000 hospital births each year—are affected by neonatal abstinence syndrome (NAS), a group of problems that occur in a newborn who was exposed prenatally to addictive illegal or prescription drugs.

The full impact of prenatal substance exposure depends on a number of factors. These include the frequency, timing, and type of substances used by pregnant women; co-occurring environmental deficiencies; and the extent of prenatal care. Research suggests that some of the negative outcomes of prenatal exposure can be improved by supportive home environments and positive parenting practices.

Child and Adolescent Development

Children and youth of parents who use or abuse substances and have parenting difficulties have an increased chance of experiencing a variety of negative outcomes:

- Poor cognitive, social, and emotional development
- Depression, anxiety, and other trauma and mental health symptoms
- Physical and health issues
- Substance use problems

Parental substance use can affect the well-being of children and youth in complex ways. For example, an infant who receives inconsistent care and nurturing from a parent engaged in addiction-related behaviors may suffer from attachment difficulties that can then interfere with the growing child's emotional development. Adolescent children of parents with substance use disorders, particularly those who have experienced child maltreatment and foster care, may turn to substances themselves as a coping mechanism. In addition, children of parents with substance use issues are more likely to experience trauma and its effects, which include difficulties with concentration and learning, controlling physical and emotional responses to stress, and forming trusting relationships.

Child Welfare Laws Related to Parental Substance Use

In response to concerns over the potential negative impact on children of parental substance abuse and illegal drug-related activities, approximately 47 States and the District of Columbia have child protection laws that address some aspect of parental substance use. Some States have expanded their civil definitions of child abuse and neglect to include a caregiver's use of a controlled substance that impairs the ability to adequately care for a child and/or exposure of a child to illegal drug activity (e.g., sale or distribution of drugs, home-based meth labs). Exposure of children to illegal drug activity is also addressed in 33 States' criminal statutes.

Federal and State laws also address prenatal drug exposure. The Child Abuse Prevention and Treatment Act (CAPTA) requires States receiving CAPTA funds to have policies and procedures for health-care personnel to notify CPS of substance-exposed newborns and to develop procedures for safe care of affected infants. As yet, there are no national data on CAPTA-related reports for substance-exposed newborns. In some State statutes, substance abuse during pregnancy is considered child abuse and/or grounds for termination of parental rights. State statutes and State and local policies vary widely in their requirements for reporting suspected prenatal drug abuse, testing for drug exposure, CPS response, forced admission to treatment of pregnant women who use drugs, and priority access for pregnant women to State funded treatment programs.

Service Delivery Challenges

Despite the fact that a large percentage of parents who are investigated in child protection cases require treatment for alcohol or drug dependence, the percentage of parents who actually receive services is limited, compared to the need. Also, many parents who begin treatment do not complete it. Historically, insufficient collaboration has hindered the ability of child welfare, substance abuse treatment, and family/dependency court systems to support these families.

Child welfare agencies face a number of difficulties in serving children and families affected by parental substance use disorders, including:

- **Insufficient service availability** or scope of services to meet existing needs

- **Inadequate funds** for services and/or dependence on client insurance coverage

- **Difficulties in engaging** and retaining parents in treatment

- **Knowledge gaps** among child welfare workers to meet the comprehensive needs of families with substance use issues

- **Lack of coordination** between the child welfare system and other services and systems, including hospitals that may screen for drug exposure, treatment agencies, mental health services, criminal justice system, and family/dependency courts

- **Differences in perspectives and timeframes,** reflecting different guiding policies, philosophies, and goals in child welfare and substance abuse treatment systems (for example, a focus on the safety and wellbeing of the child without sufficient focus on parents' recovery)

A critical challenge for child welfare professionals is meeting legislative requirements regarding child permanency while allowing for sufficient progress in substance abuse recovery and development of parenting capacity. The Adoption and Safe Families Act (ASFA) requires that a child welfare agency file a petition for termination of parental rights if a child has been in foster care for 15 of the past 22 months, unless it is not in the best interest of the child. Many agencies struggle with adhering to this timeframe due to problems with accessing substance abuse services in a timely manner. In addition, treatment may take many months (often longer than the ASFA timeline allows), and achieving sufficient stability to care for children may take even longer. Addressing addiction can require extended recovery periods, and relapses can occur.

Innovative Prevention and Treatment Approaches

While parental substance abuse continues to be a major challenge in child welfare, the past two decades have witnessed some new and more effective approaches and innovative programs to address child protection for families where substance abuse is an issue. Some examples of promising and innovative prevention and treatment approaches include the following:

- **Promotion of protective factors**, such as social connections, concrete supports, and parenting knowledge, to support families and buffer risks

- **Early identification of at-risk families** in substance abuse treatment programs and through expanded prenatal screening initiatives so that prevention services can be provided to promote child safety and well-being in the home

- **Priority and timely access** to substance abuse treatment slots for mothers involved in the child welfare system

- **Gender-sensitive treatment** and support services that respond to the specific needs, characteristics, and co-occurring issues of women who have substance use disorders

- **Family-centered treatment services,** including inpatient treatment for mothers in facilities where they can have their children with them and programs that provide services to each family member

- **Recovery coaches or mentoring** of parents to support treatment, recovery, and parenting

- **Shared family care** in which a family experiencing parental substance use and child maltreatment is placed with a host family for support and mentoring.

Promising Child Welfare Casework Practices

In working with families affected by substance abuse, child welfare workers can use a variety of strategies to help meet parents' needs while also promoting safety, permanency, and well-being of their children. To begin, workers need to build their understanding of parental substance use issues, its signs, the effects on parenting and child safety, and what to expect during a parent's treatment and recovery. Specific casework practice strategies reflect:

Family engagement. Engagement strategies that help motivate parents to enter and remain in substance abuse services are critical to enhancing treatment outcomes. An essential part of this process is partnering with parents to develop plans that address individual needs, such as a woman's own trauma history, as well as needs for support services like child care and transportation. Child welfare workers can help create supportive environments, build nonjudgmental relationships, and implement evidence based motivational approaches, such as motivational interviewing.

Routine screening and assessment. Screening family members for possible substance use disorders with the use of brief, validated, and culturally appropriate tools should be a routine part of child welfare investigation and case monitoring. Once a substance use issue has been identified through screening, alcohol and drug treatment providers can conduct more in depth assessments of its nature and extent, the impact on the child, and recommended treatment. Find more information on screening tools and collaborative strategies:

- Screening and Assessment for Family Engagement, Retention and Recovery

- Protecting Children in Families Affected by Substance Use Disorders

Individualized treatment and case plans. Caseworkers can help match parents with evidence-based treatment programs and support services that meet their specific needs. Working collaboratively with families, alcohol and drug treatment professionals, and the courts, caseworkers can help develop and coordinate case and treatment plans.

Support of parents in treatment and recovery. Child welfare workers can support parents in their efforts to build coping and parenting skills, help them pay attention to triggers for substance-using behaviors, and work collaboratively on safety plans to protect children during a potential relapse. Workers also can help coordinate services, make formal and informal connections, and encourage parents in looking forward to their role as caregivers.

Providing services for children of parents with substance use issues. Given the developmental and emotional effects of parental substance abuse on children and youth in child welfare, it is important that child welfare workers collaborate with behavioral/mental health professionals to conduct screenings and assessments and link children and youth to appropriate, evidence-based services that promote wellness. Individualized services should address the child or youth's strengths and needs, trauma symptoms, effects associated with prenatal or postnatal exposure to parental substance use, and risk for developing substance use disorders themselves.

Permanency planning. ASFA and treatment timeframes become significant considerations in permanency plans and reunification goals in families affected by substance abuse. Concurrent planning, in which an alternative permanency plan is pursued at the same time as the reunification plan, can play an important part in ensuring that children achieve permanency in a timely manner. For instance, guardianship by a relative or adoption by foster parents might be the concurrent goal if family reunification is not viable.

Systems Change and Collaboration

Since the late 1990s, systems-level collaboration and service integration strategies have been increasingly implemented to coordinate services from child welfare, treatment, dependency courts, and other service systems for families affected by substance use. Communication and active collaboration across systems help ensure that parents in need of substance abuse treatment are identified and receive appropriate treatment in a timely manner, while children's intervention needs are also addressed. To meet complex needs, collaborative practice provides access to a wider array of resources than is traditionally available from an individual system. Collaborative and integrated strategies have shown promising results— women remain in treatment longer, are more likely to reduce substance use, and are more likely to remain or reunite with their children.

Family treatment drug courts (also known as family drug courts and dependency drug courts) represent a cross-system approach with demonstrated success. These courts use judicial system authority and collaborative partnerships to support timely substance abuse treatment for parents, provision of a wide range of services for families, and monitoring of recovery components. Evaluations have linked these courts with improvements in treatment enrollment, treatment completion, and family reunification.

Examples of other cross-systems changes to overcome traditional "siloed" approaches include:

- **Cross-training** of child welfare and substance abuse treatment professionals to build an understanding of each other's systems, legal requirements (e.g., ASFA), goals, approaches, and shared interests

- **Collocation of substance abuse specialists** in child welfare offices to assess and engage parents, provide services to families, and offer training and consultation services to child welfare workers

- **Cross-system partnerships**, based on shared principles that ensure coordinated services through formal linkages (such as interagency agreements) between child welfare, treatment, and other community agencies

- **Cross-system information sharing** related to screening and assessment results, case plans, treatment plans, and progress toward goals, which can support professionals in each system to make informed decisions, while still adhering to confidentiality parameters

- **Joint planning and case management** to help safeguard against parents becoming overwhelmed by multiple and potentially conflicting requirements of different systems

- **Wraparound and comprehensive community services** that address multiple service needs of parents and children, including those related to parenting skills, mental health, health, domestic violence, housing, employment, income support, education, and child care

- **Flexible financing strategies** that leverage or combine various funding streams to address the needs of substance abuse treatment for families involved in child welfare

- **Linked data systems** that track progress toward shared system objectives and achievement of desired outcomes while also promoting shared accountability

Conclusion

As new demonstration and innovation projects continue to be implemented, expanded, and evaluated, the field continues to learn more about promising and effective approaches to holistically address the complex needs of families with substance use issues. In particular, there is a continuing call for and movement toward enhanced collaboration among child welfare, substance abuse treatment, courts, and other systems to provide coordinated and comprehensive services to both children and their parents. Further, the use of enhanced and linked information systems will improve the collective ability to track and share the results of collaborative efforts to achieve better outcomes for these families and children.

Section 43.2

Substance Abuse during Pregnancy

This section includes text excerpted from "Substance Use While Pregnant and Breastfeeding," National Institute on Drug Abuse (NIDA), July 2015.

Substance Use While Pregnant and Breastfeeding

Research shows that use of tobacco, alcohol, or illicit drugs or abuse of prescription drugs by pregnant women can have severe health consequences for infants. This is because many substances pass easily through the placenta, so substances that a pregnant woman takes also, to some degree, reach the baby. Recent research shows that smoking tobacco or marijuana, taking prescription pain relievers, or using illegal drugs during pregnancy is associated with double or even triple the risk of stillbirth.

Regular drug use can produce dependence in the newborn, and the baby may go through withdrawal upon birth. Most research in this area has focused on the effects of opioid misuse (prescription pain relievers or heroin). However, more recent data has shown that use of alcohol, barbiturates, benzodiazepines, and caffeine during pregnancy may also cause the infant to show withdrawal symptoms at birth. The type and severity of an infant's withdrawal symptoms depend on the drug(s) used, how long and how often the birth mother used, how her body breaks the drug down, and whether the infant was born full term or prematurely.

Symptoms of drug withdrawal in a newborn can develop immediately or up to 14 days after birth and can include:

- blotchy skin coloring
- diarrhea
- excessive or high-pitched crying

- abnormal sucking reflex
- fever
- hyperactive reflexes

- increased muscle tone
- irritability
- poor feeding
- rapid breathing
- increased heart rate
- seizures

- sleep problems
- slow weight gain
- stuffy nose and sneezing
- sweating
- trembling
- vomiting

Effects of using some drugs could be long-term and possibly fatal to the baby

- low birth weight
- birth defects
- small head circumference
- premature birth
- sudden infant death syndrome (SIDS)

Risks of Stillbirth from Substance Use in Pregnancy

- Tobacco use—1.8 to 2.8 times greater risk of stillbirth, with the highest risk found among the heaviest smokers
- Marijuana use—2.3 times greater risk of stillbirth
- Evidence of any stimulant, marijuana, or prescription pain reliever use—2.2 times greater risk of stillbirth
- Passive exposure to tobacco—2.1 times greater risk of stillbirth

Illegal Drugs

Marijuana

More research needs to be done on how marijuana use during pregnancy could impact the health and development of infants, given changing policies about access to marijuana, as well as significant increases over the last decade in the number of pregnant women seeking substance use disorder treatment for marijuana use.

There is no human research connecting marijuana use to the chance of miscarriage, although animal studies indicate that the risk for miscarriage increases if marijuana is used early in pregnancy. Some associations have been found between marijuana use during pregnancy and future developmental and hyperactivity disorders in children. Evidence is mixed as to whether marijuana use by pregnant women is associated with low birth rate or premature birth, although long-term use may elevate these risks. Pregnant women are strongly discouraged from using marijuana, given its potential to negatively impact the developing brain.

Some women report using marijuana to treat severe nausea associated with their pregnancy; however, there is no research confirming that this is a safe practice, and it is generally not recommended. Women considering using medical marijuana while pregnant should not do so without checking with their healthcare providers. Animal studies have shown that moderate concentrations of delta-9-tetrahydrocannabinol (or THC, the main psychoactive ingredient in marijuana), when administered to mothers while pregnant or nursing, could have long-lasting effects on the child, including increasing stress responsivity and abnormal patterns of social interactions. Animal studies also show learning deficits in prenatally exposed individuals.

Human research has shown that some babies born to women who used marijuana during their pregnancies display altered responses to visual stimuli, increased trembling, and a high-pitched cry, which could indicate problems with neurological development. In school, marijuana-exposed children are more likely to show gaps in problem-solving skills, memory, and the ability to remain attentive. More research is needed, however, to disentangle marijuana-specific effects from those of other environmental factors that could be associated with a mother's marijuana use, such as an impoverished home environment or the mother's use of other drugs. Prenatal marijuana exposure is also associated with an increased likelihood of a person using marijuana as a young adult, even when other factors that influence drug use are considered.

Very little is known about marijuana use and breastfeeding. One study suggests that moderate amounts of THC find their way into breast milk when a nursing mother uses marijuana. Some evidence shows that exposure to THC through breast milk in the first month of life could result in decreased motor development at 1 year of age. There have been no studies to determine if exposure to THC during nursing is linked to effects later in the child's life. With regular use, THC can accumulate in human breast milk to high concentrations. Because a baby's brain is still forming, THC consumed in breast milk could affect brain development. Given all these uncertainties, nursing mothers are discouraged from using marijuana. New mothers using medical marijuana should be vigilant about coordinating care between the doctor recommending their marijuana use and the pediatrician caring for their baby.

Stimulants (Cocaine and Methamphetamine)

Some may recall news items about "crack babies," a term coined in the 1980s to describe babies born to mothers who smoked cocaine while pregnant. These babies were initially predicted to suffer from severe, irreversible cognitive and behavioral consequences, including reduced intelligence and social skills. These purported effects turned out to be somewhat exaggerated. However, it is not completely known how a pregnant woman's cocaine use affects her child, since cocaine-using women are more likely to also use other drugs such as alcohol, to have poor nutrition, or to not seek prenatal care. All of these factors can affect a developing fetus, making it difficult to isolate the effects of cocaine.

Research does show, however, that pregnant women who use cocaine are at higher risk for maternal migraines and seizures, premature membrane rupture, and placental abruption (separation of the placental lining from the uterus). Pregnancy is accompanied by normal cardiovascular changes, and cocaine abuse exacerbates these changes—sometimes leading to serious problems with high blood pressure (hypertensive crises), spontaneous miscarriage, preterm labor, and difficult delivery. Babies born to mothers who use cocaine during pregnancy may also have low birth weight and smaller head circumferences, and are shorter in length than babies born to mothers who do not use cocaine. They also show symptoms of irritability, hyperactivity, tremors, high-pitched cry, and excessive sucking at birth. These symptoms may be due to the effects of cocaine itself, rather than withdrawal, since cocaine and its metabolites are still present in the baby's body up to 5 to 7 days after delivery.

Pregnant women who use methamphetamine have a greater risk of preeclampsia (high blood pressure and possible organ damage), premature delivery, and placental abruption. Their babies are more likely to be smaller and to have low birth weight. In a large, longitudinal study of children prenatally exposed to methamphetamine, exposed children had increased emotional reactivity and anxiety/depression, were more withdrawn, had problems with attention, and showed cognitive problems that could lead to poorer academic outcomes.

MDMA (Ecstasy, Molly)

What little research exists on the effects of MDMA use in pregnancy suggests that prenatal MDMA exposure may cause learning, memory, and motor problems in the baby.

Heroin

Heroin use during pregnancy can result in neonatal abstinence syndrome (NAS). NAS occurs when heroin passes through the placenta to the fetus during pregnancy, causing the baby to become dependent on opioids. Symptoms include excessive crying, high-pitched cry, irritability, seizures, and gastrointestinal problems, among others. NAS requires hospitalization of the affected infant and possibly treatment with morphine or methadone to relieve symptoms; researchers have also studied buprenorphine for this purpose. The medication is gradually tapered off until the baby adjusts to being opioid-free.

Medications

Prescription and Over-the-Counter (OTC) Drugs

Pregnancy can be a confusing time for pregnant women facing many choices about legal drugs, like tobacco and alcohol, as well as prescription and over-the-counter (OTC) drugs that may affect their baby. These are difficult issues for researchers to study because scientists cannot give potentially dangerous drugs to pregnant women. Here are some of the known facts about popular medications and pregnancy:

There are more than 6 million pregnancies in the United States every year, and pregnant women take an average of three to five prescription drugs while pregnant. The U.S. Food and Drug Administration (FDA) recently issued new rules on drug labeling to provide clearer instructions for pregnant and nursing women, including a summary of the risks of use during pregnancy and breastfeeding, a discussion of the data supporting the summary, and other information to help prescribers make safe decisions.

Even so, we know little about the effects of taking most medications during pregnancy. This is because pregnant women are often not included in studies to determine safety of new medications before they come on the market. A recent study shows that use of short-acting prescription opioids such as oxycodone during pregnancy, especially when combined with tobacco and/or certain antidepressant medications, is associated with an increased likelihood of neonatal abstinence syndrome (NAS) in the infant.

Although some prescription and OTC medications are safe to take during pregnancy, a pregnant woman should tell her doctor about all prescription medications, OTC cold and pain medicines, and herbal or dietary supplements she is taking or planning to take. This will allow her doctor to weigh the risks and benefits of a medication during pregnancy. In some cases, the doctor may recommend the continued use of specific medications, even though they could have some impact on the fetus. Suddenly stopping the use of a medication may be more risky for both the mother and baby than continuing to use the medication while under a doctor's care.

Some prescription and OTC medications are generally compatible with breastfeeding, and the American Academy of Pediatrics maintains a list of such substances. Others, such as some anti-anxiety and antidepressant medications, have unknown effects (AAP Committee on Drugs, 2001), so mothers who are using these medications should consult with their doctor before breastfeeding. Nursing mothers should contact their infant's health care provider if their infants show any of these reactions to the breast milk: diarrhea, excessive crying, vomiting, skin rashes, loss of appetite, or sleepiness.

Other Substances

Alcohol

Alcohol use while pregnant can result in Fetal Alcohol Spectrum Disorders (FASD), a general term that includes Fetal Alcohol Syndrome, partial Fetal Alcohol Syndrome, alcohol-related disorders of brain development, and alcohol-related birth defects. These effects can last throughout life, causing difficulties with motor coordination, emotional control, schoolwork, socialization, and holding a job.

There is currently little research into how a nursing mother's alcohol use might affect her breastfed baby. What science suggests is that, contrary to folklore, alcohol does not increase a nursing mother's milk production, and it may disrupt the breastfed child's sleep cycle. The American Academy of Pediatrics (AAP) recommends that alcohol drinking should be minimized during the months a woman nurses and daily intake limited to no more than 2 ounces of liquor, 8 ounces of wine, or two average beers for a 130-pound woman. In this case, nursing should take place at least 2 hours after drinking to allow the alcohol to be reduced or eliminated from the mother's body and milk. This will minimize the amount of alcohol passed to the baby.

Nicotine (Tobacco Products and e-Cigarettes)

Almost 16 percent of pregnant women in the United States have smoked in the past month. Carbon monoxide and nicotine from tobacco smoke may interfere with the oxygen supply to the fetus. Nicotine also readily crosses the placenta, and concentrations of this drug in the blood of the fetus can be as much as 15 percent higher than in the mother. Smoking during pregnancy increases the risk for certain birth defects, premature birth, miscarriage, and low birth weight and is estimated to have caused 1,015 infant deaths annually from 2005 through 2009. Newborns of smoking mothers also show signs of stress and drug withdrawal consistent with what has been reported in infants exposed to other drugs. In some cases, smoking during pregnancy may be associated with sudden infant death syndrome (SIDS), as well as learning and behavioral problems and an increased risk of obesity in children. In addition, smoking more than one pack a day during pregnancy nearly doubles the risk that the affected child will become addicted to tobacco if that child starts smoking. Even a mother's secondhand exposure to cigarette smoke can cause problems; such exposure is associated with premature birth and low birth weight.

Recent research provides strong support that nicotine is a gateway drug, making the brain more sensitive to the effects of other drugs such as cocaine. This shows that pregnant women who use nicotine may be affecting their baby's brain in ways they may not anticipate. Because e-cigarettes typically also contain nicotine, those products may also pose a risk to the baby's health. More research is needed.

Similar to pregnant women, nursing mothers are also advised against using tobacco. New mothers who smoke should be aware that nicotine is passed through breast milk, so tobacco use can impact the infant's brain and body development—even if the mother never smokes near the baby. There is also evidence that the milk of mothers who smoke smells and may taste like cigarettes. It is unclear whether this will make it more likely that exposed children may find tobacco flavors/smells more appealing later in life.

Secondhand Smoke

Newborns exposed to secondhand smoke are at greater risk for SIDS, respiratory illnesses (asthma, respiratory infections, and bronchitis), ear infections, cavities, and increased medical visits and hospitalizations. If a woman smokes and is planning a pregnancy, the ideal time to seek smoking cessation help is before she becomes pregnant.

Chapter 44

Disciplining Your Child

Chapter Contents

Section 44.1

Setting Structure and Rules

This section includes text excerpted from "Essentials for Parenting Toddlers and Preschoolers," Centers for Disease Control and Prevention (CDC), May 17, 2014.

Creating Structure and Rules

Does your child have meltdowns when you change from one activity to another? Do you have trouble getting your child to follow a regular schedule? Consistent routines and rules help create order and structure your day. Things go more smoothly when you and your child know what to expect.

Keys to Creating Structure

1. Consistency, predictability, and follow-through are important for creating structure in the home.

2. Respond to your child's behavior the same way every time. When you are consistent, the behaviors you like will happen more often and problem behaviors are less likely to happen.

3. Routines and daily schedules help you and your child. You both know what to expect each day. Routines can also improve your child's behavior and your relationship with your child.

4. A family rule is a clear statement about behaviors that are never okay, such as hitting and running in the house. You can change your child's behavior when there are clear consequences for breaking the rule.

5. Keep things positive! Reward and praise your child for following routines and rules. This makes it more likely that your child will follow the routines and rules in the future.

Building Blocks of Structure

It's normal for young children to test the limits. That's how they learn what is right and wrong. But, it can be frustrating and really test our patience as parents! One way to keep control and help children learn is to create structure. Structure is created by consistent routines and rules. Rules teach children what behaviors are okay and not okay. Routines teach children what to expect throughout the day. Structure helps children learn responsibility and self-control.

There are three key ingredients to building structure in the home:

1. **Consistency**—*doing the same thing every time*

2. **Predictability**—*expecting or knowing what is going to happen*

3. **Follow-through**—*enforcing the consequence*

What Are These Things? How Can You Use Them in Your Family?

Consistency means that you respond to your child's behavior the same way every time. You respond the same no matter what is going on or how you're feeling. Misbehaviors are less likely to occur again if you always use the same consequence, like ignoring or time-out. Good behaviors are likely to be repeated if you let your child know you like them. This doesn't mean that you need to give **consistent** attention to ALL of your child's behaviors. Think about something you want your child to do more often. This could be sharing, cleaning up, or following directions. To increase those behaviors, praise them each time you see them occur. Your consistent response will help those behaviors happen more often.

Following through means that you do what you say you will do in response to your child's behaviors. This is often called the "say what you mean and mean what you say." If you tell your child a behavior will be punished, you punish it every time it happens. If you tell your child he will be rewarded for a behavior, you give him the reward after he has done what you asked. To be **consistent** and **predictable,** we need to **follow through**. Follow-through is important for ALL behaviors. This includes behaviors we like and don't like.

How Do Consistency, Predictability, and Follow-Through Help Create Structure?

A structure that helps your child learn to behave has routines and rules that are consistent, predictable, and have follow through. There is a basic routine you follow and rules you live by on most days of the week. You set appropriate expectations and limits for your child's behaviors. Your child learns how you are going to respond to behaviors that are okay or not okay.

Structure helps parents and their kids. Kids feel safe and secure because they know what to expect. Parents feel confident because they know how to respond, and they respond the same way each time. Routines and rules help structure the home and make life more predictable.

When Can You Start Creating Structure with Routines and Rules?

Creating structure at any age can help your child and you. Children can begin learning routines and rules at a very young age. You can begin with routines for important activities of the day, like meals, bedtime, or in the morning. Or you can use routines to help your child learn important behaviors, like getting dressed.

Section 44.2

Importance of Giving Directions

This section includes text excerpted from "Essentials for Parenting Toddlers and Preschoolers," Centers for Disease Control and Prevention (CDC), May 17, 2014.

Giving Directions

Do you sometimes feel like your child doesn't listen? Do you get into power struggles when you want your child to do something? A positive relationship is your most important tool for getting your child to listen and follow directions. It is also important to give clear directions that fit your child's age. Good directions can help reduce the chance that your child will forget or misunderstand what you've said. Good directions can help you have positive daily interactions with your child.

Keys to Giving Good Directions

1. Make sure you have your child's attention when you give a direction.

2. Be clear about what you want your child to do and when she needs to do it.

3. Ask your child to repeat the direction back to you to make sure he understands.

4. Avoid asking questions when you want your child to do something. Asking a question gives your child the chance to say, "No!"

5. Give one direction at a time.

6. Model good listening skills during special playtime and give your child positive attention for good listening.

Why Are Good Directions Important?

Toddlers and preschoolers are exploring and discovering their world. They are also learning about what is right and wrong. Good directions are useful in many situations.

Good directions set limits on your child's behavior and let him know how he is expected to behave or what he should do.
Our job as parents is to teach our children how to behave. Sometimes it may feel like you spend more time correcting misbehaviors than you spend teaching good behaviors. But, when you give good directions, you tell your child exactly what behaviors you expect. This means that instead of saying, "Stop it!", "Quit!", or "Don't do that!" you tell your child exactly what you want him to do. For example, you might say, "Please walk instead of running in the house" or "Please sit so that I can put on your shoes."

When you give your child choices with your directions, you also encourage his independence. For example, if you want your child to get dressed but it does not matter what he wears, you can give him two choices. You can say, "Please put on the gray pants or the blue ones." Of course, your direction should be at a level your child can understand or it won't work. If your child does not know his colors, this would not be a good direction.

Good directions are helpful when you need your child to do something specific or to stop your child from doing something harmful or dangerous.
If your child is doing something harmful or dangerous, a good direction can stop the misbehavior. For example, if your child is standing in a chair, you can say, "Please sit with your bottom on the chair." If your child is dangerously tipping the chair back, you can say, "Please keep the chair on the floor."

Good directions prevent misbehaviors. If your child is doing what you told him to do, he can't misbehave at the same time. Good directions can prevent misbehaviors. For example, if you see that your child is about to throw a toy, you can give him a direction to redirect his behavior. You might say, "Please put the toy on the floor gently." The direction lets your child know what behavior you expect from him.

Use Consequences for Not Following Directions. Anytime you give a direction, use consequences if your child does not listen. When you are first learning to give good directions, it is helpful to ask yourself if you have the time and energy to follow through with a consequence. For consequences to work, you need to follow through with the consequences each time. If you do not have time, it is probably best not to give a direction. Instead, you can assist your child with the task. For example, if you are running late in the morning and your child has not put on his clothes, you may decide to help him put his clothes on instead of giving a direction.

Practice, Practice, Practice. Giving good directions is a skill that is not always easy so practice will help. Practice and follow-through for not listening will also help your child learn that he needs to listen to your direction. Practice when you have time to follow through if your child does not listen. Over time, your child will learn that when you give directions, you expect him to listen to you. But it will take some time for your child to learn that you mean what you say. It is perfectly normal for children not to follow directions some of the time. However, it is important to be prepared for that and have a plan for immediately following through with a consequence.

At other times, your child may test you to see how much he can get away with before you use a consequence. Remember that no excuse gets him out of the consequence if he has been given enough time to follow directions. When your child does what you tell him to do, praise him for listening and following directions.

Steps in Giving Directions

Giving good directions takes practice. Here are a few things to keep in mind.

Step 1: Get Your Child's Attention

Make sure your child hears and pays attention to your direction. This means that you will need to be close to your child and make eye contact. You may need to say your child's name. It is sometimes helpful to bend over, squat, or sit next to your child so you are on the same level and face-to-face.

Step 2: Give the Direction

Tell your child exactly what you want him to do. Here are some tips for giving good directions.

Be sure the direction fits your child's age. Make sure your child is able to do what you have told him to do. For example, a 2-year-old can take your hand before crossing the street, but he can't mop the floor. Remember that inability is not the same as disobeying.

Tell your child exactly what behavior you want to see. Your words are important. A good direction will clearly tell your child what you expect. The direction is specific and not stated as a question. While using the words "No", "Don't," "Quit," or "Stop" are an everyday part of parenting a toddler and preschooler, the direction only tells the child what not to do. This may stop the misbehavior momentarily, but it does not tell the child what behaviors are expected now and in the future. To give good directions:

- **Be specific.** Tell your child exactly what you want him to do. Avoid unclear directions like "be good," "straighten up," and "clean up" because they can mean different things to different people. For example, when you say "straighten up," you may want your child to stop spitting water, but she may hear "stand up straight." A specific direction is "Swallow the water." Sometimes parents will just say the child's name when giving a direction. For example, if your son, John, is banging a toy on the table, you might say, "John!" and expect him to stop banging and play with his toys nicely. To make this a good, specific direction, you might say, "Stop banging the table. Play nicely with your toy."

- **Make it a statement.** Tell your child what to do rather than asking if he wants to do the activity. For instance, it is better to say "Put your toys away in the closet" than "Would you put your toys away in the closet?" Sometimes when we give directions, we accidentally make them into questions by using agreement words like "OK". For example, "Get dressed now, OK?" is a question. Questions give your child the option to say "yes" or "no". If you want your direction followed avoid questions.

Tell your child the behavior you want to see.

Let your child know exactly what behavior to do. If you are unsure what to say to stop a misbehavior, it may be helpful to think of the opposite of the misbehavior. For example, saying, "Don't throw that toy!" may stop your child from throwing a toy momentarily but it may not result in what you really want. Instead, you might say, "Please put the toy on the table" or "Please play nicely with the toy."

Give one direction at a time.

Toddlers and preschoolers have a very short attention span. If you tell your child to do more than one thing, he may not be able to remember all of the instructions. By giving one direction at a time, you can make sure the direction is clear, your child is more likely to remember and follow the direction, and you can praise your child more often.

Give the direction in a neutral tone.

If a child does not follow a direction immediately, parents will sometimes raise their voice and repeat the direction. Sometimes, parents end up yelling. This can send the message that the child does not need to follow the direction until the parent is yelling. To avoid the yelling trap, provide directions in a neutral, firm voice with no yelling or pleading. If you consistently use a neutral tone and follow through with consequences when your child does not obey, your child will learn that you are serious the first time a direction is given.

Be polite and respectful.

Most parents want their children to use good manners. One way to help your child learn good manners is for you to model good behaviors like being polite and respectful when giving directions. For example, you can start directions with the word "please." When used consistently, the word please can serve as a signal to your child that an important direction is about to come. Eye contact and using a calm voice to give the direction are other ways to model good manners.

Use gestures.

For toddlers and preschoolers, it is a good idea to use gestures along with directions so your child has a visual cue of what is expected. For example, if you state, "Please put the toys on the floor in your toy box," you can point to the toys you want him to put away and then point to the toy box. You could walk from where the toys are on the floor to the toy box while giving the direction.

Choose your words carefully.

How parents word directions can affect who your child thinks needs to act. For instance, only use the word "let's" in your direction if you plan to help your child. If you say, "Let's put your toys away," you should plan to help your child put the toys away. If you want your child to do as you directed, you can just say, "Please put your toys away."

Give your child choices when possible.

Choices are a great way to develop your child's independence and teach them important decision-making skills. Directions with limited choices, like only two options, are best for young children. For example, if you want your daughter to get ready for school, you can give her a choice by saying "It is time to get ready for school. You can wear the yellow dress or the jogging suit. Please make a choice and put on your clothes now." By offering choices, you are giving your daughter the chance to make a decision about what she wants to wear, but you are still communicating that it is time to get dressed. Make sure you are comfortable with whichever choice your child makes.

Provide carefully timed explanations.

Some children may want to know "why" they have to do something. Your child may ask "why" out of simple curiosity or because they want to delay having to listen. One way to avoid this problem is to provide an explanation before giving the direction. For example, "It's time for us to go to the store. Please put on your shoes." If your child still asks why, he is probably trying to delay doing what you have told him to do. You should ignore his question and follow through with the consequence if he does not put on his shoes.

Step 3: Check Compliance

In this step, you will be checking to see whether your child complied or did what you told him to do. Most children will respond within 5-10 seconds or within a short amount of time after you give the direction. The time frame will vary a little with each child and family. If your child does what you told him to do, follow through with a positive consequence, like praise. If your child does not follow your direction within a short amount of time, remain calm and follow through with a negative consequence. Determining if your child has followed your direction may not always be easy, even when directions are clear and fit the child's age. Some examples are:

Doing something slightly different.

- Sometimes children respond to directions in a slightly different way than was expected by the parent. For example, a parent might tell a child to put his crayons in the closet, but the child puts his blocks in the closet instead. This is considered not following directions as long as you are sure that your child knows the difference between the crayons and the blocks.

Dawdling or stalling.

- Sometimes children do not immediately do what they are told. Instead they may say, "In a minute," or they may tell you they are going to finish something else before following the direction. This type of behavior is referred to as dawdling and is an example of not following directions.

Pretending not to hear.

- Many children ignore a parent's directions in an attempt to delay or avoid having to do what the parent has said. As long as you get your child's attention and are sure that your child heard your instructions, the direction should not be repeated. If your child does not respond within a short amount of time, the behavior should be considered not following directions.

Following part of the direction.

- Children sometimes follow through with part of a direction but not the entire direction. For example, you tell your child to put her toys away, and she puts her dolls away but leaves other toys out. This is an example of not following the entire direction. If your child does only part of a direction, it is possible she needs to be taught what "put your toys away" means. In this example, you could say, "Good job of putting your dolls away. Now put the other toys away. Please put your blocks in the toy box." Continue in this way until the child understands that all of these things are toys.

Following directions with a bad attitude.

- Children may sometimes follow the direction but with a bad attitude. For example, you tell your daughter to put her toys away. She was enjoying playing with her toys, so she stomps across the room, picks up her toys, throws them in the toy box, and whines "I don't want to put my toys away." Even though she is following directions with a bad attitude, she is still doing what you told her to do. In this case, you can ignore the bad attitude and let her know you like that she followed your direction. If having a good attitude is important to you, you can include that as part of the direction. For example, you could say, "Please put the toys away as quiet as a mouse." Remember that all of us, including adults, have to do things we do not want to do sometimes, and sometimes we also do it with an "attitude."

Undoing.

- Children sometimes test the limits by initially doing what the parent tells them to do and then undoing it. For example, you tell your son to put his toys in the toy box. Your son puts the toys away but then decides to pull two trucks back out of the box. In this case, your child followed your direction because he put the toys away and the direction didn't include anything about leaving the toys in the toy box. If you have a child who will test the limits by undoing, provide really specific directions. You might tell your son, "Put all of the toys in the toy box and leave them in the box."

Step 4: Add a Consequence

Consequences can be positive or negative. Positive consequences let your child know you are happy with his behavior. Labeled praises, hugs, or high fives are examples of positive consequences and let your child know you are happy he followed your directions. If you praise your child, you might say, "Great job putting on your shirt all by yourself!" This praise tells your child exactly what you liked about his behavior.

Negative consequences are things you do after your child's behavior to show you are not happy with the behavior. Examples of negative consequences include delay of a privilege and time-out. If your child does not follow your direction, you can give him one warning and tell him what to expect for not following your direction. For example, you might say, "Pick up your toys or you will go to time-out." If he still does not follow your direction, follow through with the consequence immediately. As your directions get better and your child learns to follow your directions, use warnings less often. Also, try to avoid repeating a direction over and over. Warnings and repeating directions teach your child he does not have to listen the first time you give a direction.

He will learn it is only important to listen after you have given a warning or repeated the direction. Always follow through with consequences if your child does not follow directions.

Even if your child receives a consequence, he still has to follow the direction. After the consequence, you should give your child the direction again. If your child follows the direction, you can praise him for following the direction. If your child fails to follow directions again, you should repeat the same negative consequence so that he learns he has to follow your direction to avoid the consequence. This is why you need to make sure you have plenty of time to follow through with consequences. It may take several attempts to get your child to follow your directions.

Once your child follows your direction and the consequence is over, go back to positive interactions with him.

Section 44.3

Using Discipline and Consequences on Your Child

This section includes text excerpted from "Essentials for Parenting Toddlers and Preschoolers," Centers for Disease Control and Prevention (CDC), May 27, 2014.

Using Discipline and Consequences

Did you know that what you do right after any of your child's behavior makes a difference? This may be why your child has good behavior some days and not others. Learning how to use discipline and consequences can help you have more good days with your child. It can also help you get behaviors you like to happen more.

Keys to Using Discipline and Consequences

1.   Use social rewards (like hugs and kisses) more than material rewards (like toys or candy). Social rewards can be given often and are more powerful!

2. Sticker charts or similar reward programs can help change your child's behavior.

3. Ignoring misbehavior means taking away your attention. It helps stop misbehaviors like tantrums, whining, and interrupting.

4. Want to reduce misbehavior?

5. Distracting your child can help stop misbehaviors. It works by getting your child to think and do something else so he doesn't continue to misbehave.

6. Toddlers and preschoolers have short attention spans. Give consequences right after a misbehavior so they can remember what they did that you do not like.

7. Use consequences that match your child's age and stage of development.

Why Are Discipline and Consequences Important?

From time to time, your child is going to do things you don't like. He'll do things that are dangerous. He'll do things you don't want him to do again. He'll also do a lot of things you like. The consequence or what happens right after your child's behaviors makes the behavior more or less likely to happen again. Consequences can be both positive and negative.

Positive and Negative Consequences

Positive consequences show your child she has done something you like. Your child is more likely to repeat the behavior when you use positive consequences. Positive consequences include things like rewards, praise, and attention. Use positive consequences as much as possible for behaviors you would like your child to do again.

Negative consequences. let your child know you do not like what she has done. Your child is less likely to repeat the behavior when you use negative consequences. Negative consequences are also called discipline. Negative consequences include things like ignoring, distraction, loss of a privilege, and time-out. Use negative consequences for behaviors you would like your child to stop. It's a good idea to start with ignoring and distraction, especially for young children. Other consequences may be needed if ignoring and distraction don't work or are not possible. Natural consequences, delay or removal of privileges, and time-out can be used to stop misbehavior. More information about these consequences is provided below.

Ignoring. Children sometimes throw tantrums, whine, and interrupt just to get your attention. When you take away your attention from your child and these misbehaviors, the behaviors often stop. When ignoring, do not make eye contact with your child or talk to him. Ignore anything your child does to get your attention.

Distraction. When you distract your child, you get him to focus on something else. By doing this, he stops the misbehavior. You can use distraction anywhere. You just have to be prepared. Crayons and paper, toys, and small games are things you can keep with you to distract your child. You can also make up games. For example, if your child is whining in the grocery store, you could play the "show me" game. Ask your child to name or point to everything on the aisle that is the color blue or in the shape of a square.

Natural consequences. Natural consequences are things that happen because of what we do or how we act. If you tell your child to play carefully with a toy but she continues to bang it, the toy may break. In this case, your child has experienced the natural consequence of playing roughly with the toy. Although it is good for your child to learn from his mistakes, natural consequences should never put the child at risk. Do not allow your child to do anything that could hurt him or others, such as playing with matches or running into the street.

Delay of a privilege and logical (or common sense) consequences Delaying a privilege means that your child has to wait to get something she really wants. You might tell your child, "After you pick up your toys, you can go out and play". Or, "When you take three more bites of your dinner, you can have dessert." Removal of privileges means taking away the items or activities your child enjoys most. For young children, removing privileges is often called logical (or common sense) consequences. The consequences are logically related to the misbehavior. You might take away toys or crayons that are not handled carefully. You might turn off the TV if your children are arguing about the channel. If your child spills something on purpose, a logical consequence is having your child clean-up the mess.

Time-out. Time-out removes the child from where he is misbehaving. Time-out puts the child in a place that is free of anything or anyone that might provide attention. If your child hits his brother, you can give him time-out. Time-outs, when used the right way, really work at reducing a child's misbehaviors.

Tips on Discipline and Negative Consequences

The negative consequences used to decrease misbehavior should relate to the misbehavior and the seriousness of the misbehavior when possible. If your child is not playing nicely at the park, you can simply take her home. In this case, the negative consequence of going home fits the misbehavior at the park. Negative consequences should never deprive the child of basic essentials, such as food, a bath, or school.

After any consequence your child does not like, go back to being positive with your child. Remember that consequences should be directed at the behavior and not at the person. Avoid saying things like, "You never do anything right." These comments can be damaging to your child's self-esteem and to the parent-child relationship. It was the behavior that was the problem, not the child.

Use of Rewards

The way you respond right after your child's behaviors makes the behavior more or less likely to happen again. Behaviors are more likely to happen again when followed by a positive consequence like a reward. This is true for all behaviors, even those you don't want to happen again. Rewards are things like attention, going to the park, small toys, or other things your child likes such as hugs and kisses.

Rewards can be used to encourage your child's good behaviors. They also help get your child to do more of the things you want her to do. Rewards that happen right after a behavior are best. Sometimes rewards can't be given right away but should be given as soon as possible. Rewards don't work as well when they are given long after a behavior. This is true especially for toddlers and preschoolers. Their memory is not as good as it is for older children.

When you first start using rewards, reward the behavior you like every time it occurs. Tell your child exactly what she did that you liked and why she is getting the reward. If you don't tell her what you liked, she will not know what to do next time to be rewarded. You could say, "I am so happy you put your toys away without being asked. Now we get to read two extra books before sleepy time!"

Why are Rewards Important?

Rewards are important for many reasons. First, rewards can be used to increase self-esteem. Toddlers and preschoolers hear the words "no," "don't," "stop," and "quit" many times during the day. This is normal and one of the ways they learn right from wrong. But when children hear these things over and over, their self-esteem can begin to suffer. They may begin to believe they cannot do anything correctly. Rewards can be used to increase self-esteem. When a child earns a reward, he knows he has done something good and something you like.

Rewards can also help improve your relationship with your child. When you give a reward to your child, you and your child are both happy. You are happy because your child has done something you like. Your child is also happy because she is getting something she likes.

Types of Rewards

There are several types of rewards. Most people think of toys, candy, or other things that cost money as rewards. These are called material rewards. Another type of reward is a social reward. Social rewards are cheap or free and can be even more powerful than material rewards. They also can be given more often and immediately after behaviors you like. Affection, praise, or attention from you are examples of social rewards.

Examples of Social Rewards

1. *Affection*–Rewarding your child with your affection lets her know you approve of what she did. This includes hugs, kisses, a high five, a smile, a pat on the back, or an arm around the shoulder.

2. *Praise*–Praise happens when parents say things like "Great job," "Way to go," or "Good boy/girl." These words show approval, but they do not tell children exactly what behavior you liked. Specific (or labeled) praise tells a child exactly what behavior you liked.

   Examples of labeled praise are:

   "Great job playing quietly while I was on the telephone!"

   "You were a great helper when you put all your toys in the closet today!"

   "Thank you for using your inside voice."

3. *Attention and Activities*–Extra time with you or a special activity can be a powerful reward for young children. Some examples include playing a favorite game, reading a story, going to the park, and helping with dinner. Other activities such as going to the movies, the zoo, or skating can also be used, but these activities may not always be available or affordable.

Tips for Using Rewards

Using social and material rewards together may increase how quickly your child's behavior changes. You can decrease the use of rewards after your child is doing what you want regularly and consistently.

When using material rewards, the rewards must be items your child likes or really enjoys. If your child doesn't like or enjoy the reward, he will not be interested in earning it. Praise and attention should always be used with material rewards. Praise and attention play an important role in making the parent-child relationship positive.

When picking rewards be creative and come up with a variety of rewards to use with each of your children. Remember that all children are different and like different things. What may be rewarding for one child may not be for another. Children will also get bored easily. If they receive the same rewards each time, that reward will be less powerful over time.

When children are younger, small rewards go a long way. A sticker or smiley face and parental attention are usually all that is required to encourage good behaviors. This changes as children get older and other rewards become more important.

Reward Programs

A rewards program is a way to keep track of how often your child does what you like. For young children, a chart is often used. Social and material rewards can be used as part of the reward program. You watch your child's behavior and when you catch him doing what you like, you provide a reward. Rewards could be a sticker, a smiley face, a check mark, or an ink stamp. Praise and attention from you can also be used as the reward. The rewards need to be specific to your child's age, ability level, and preferences.

Chapter 45

Improving Parenting Skills

Chapter Contents

Section 45.1

Parenting Tips

This section includes text excerpted from "Child
Development," Centers for Disease Control and
Prevention (CDC), March 15, 2016.

Positive Parenting Tips

As a parent you give your children a good start in life—you nurture,
protect and guide them. Parenting is a process that prepares your child
for independence. As your child grows and develops, there are many
things you can do to help your child. These links will help you learn
more about your child's development, positive parenting, safety, and
health at each stage of your child's life.

Infants (0-1 year of age)

Developmental Milestones

Skills such as taking a first step, smiling for the first time, and
waving "bye-bye" are called developmental milestones. Developmental
milestones are things most children can do by a certain age. Children
reach milestones in how they play, learn, speak, behave, and move
(like crawling, walking, or jumping).

In the first year, babies learn to focus their vision, reach out, explore,
and learn about the things that are around them. Cognitive, or brain
development means the learning process of memory, language, thinking, and reasoning. Learning language is more than making sounds
("babble"), or saying "ma-ma" and "da-da." Listening, understanding,
and knowing the names of people and things are all a part of language
development. During this stage, babies also are developing bonds of
love and trust with their parents and others as part of social and emotional development. The way parents cuddle, hold, and play with their
baby will set the basis for how they will interact with them and others.

In the first year, babies learn to focus their vision, reach out,
explore, and learn about the things that are around them. Cognitive,
or brain development means the learning process of memory, language,

thinking, and reasoning. Learning language is more than making sounds ("babble"), or saying "ma-ma" and "da-da." Listening, understanding, and knowing the names of people and things are all a part of language development. During this stage, babies also are developing bonds of love and trust with their parents and others as part of social and emotional development. The way parents cuddle, hold, and play with their baby will set the basis for how they will interact with them and others.

Positive Parenting Tips

Following are some things you, as a parent, can do to help your baby during this time:

- Talk to your baby. She will find your voice calming.

- Answer when your baby makes sounds by repeating the sounds and adding words. This will help him learn to use language.

- Read to your baby. This will help her develop and understand language and sounds.

- Sing to your baby and play music. This will help your baby develop a love for music and will help his brain development.

- Praise your baby and give her lots of loving attention.

- Spend time cuddling and holding your baby. This will help him feel cared for and secure.

- Play with your baby when she's alert and relaxed. Watch your baby closely for signs of being tired or fussy so that she can take a break from playing.

- Distract your baby with toys and move him to safe areas when he starts moving and touching things that he shouldn't touch.

- Take care of yourself physically, mentally, and emotionally. Parenting can be hard work! It is easier to enjoy your new baby and be a positive, loving parent when you are feeling good yourself.

Toddlers (1-2 years of age)

Developmental Milestones

Skills such as taking a first step, smiling for the first time, and waving "bye-bye" are called developmental milestones. Developmental milestones are things most children can do by a certain age. Children reach milestones in how they play, learn, speak, behave, and move (like crawling, walking, or jumping).

During the second year, toddlers are moving around more, and are aware of themselves and their surroundings. Their desire to explore new objects and people also is increasing. During this stage, toddlers will show greater independence; begin to show defiant behavior; recognize themselves in pictures or a mirror; and imitate the behavior of others, especially adults and older children. Toddlers also should be able to recognize the names of familiar people and objects, form simple phrases and sentences, and follow simple instructions and directions.

Positive Parenting Tips

Following are some of the things you, as a parent, can do to help your toddler during this time:

• Read to your toddler daily.

• Ask her to find objects for you or name body parts and objects.

• Play matching games with your toddler, like shape sorting and simple puzzles.

• Encourage him to explore and try new things.

• Help to develop your toddler's language by talking with her and adding to words she starts. For example, if your toddler says "baba", you can respond, "Yes, you are right? that is a bottle."

• Encourage your child's growing independence by letting him help with dressing himself and feeding himself.

• Respond to wanted behaviors more than you punish unwanted behaviors (use only very brief time outs). Always tell or show your child what she should do instead.

• Encourage your toddler's curiosity and ability to recognize common objects by taking field trips together to the park or going on a bus ride.

Toddlers (2-3 years of age)

Developmental Milestones

Skills such as taking turns, playing make believe, and kicking a ball, are called developmental milestones. Developmental milestones are things most children can do by a certain age. Children reach milestones in how they play, learn, speak, behave, and move (like jumping, running, or balancing).

Because of children's growing desire to be independent, this stage is often called the "terrible twos." However, this can be an exciting time for parents and toddlers. Toddlers will experience huge thinking, learning, social, and emotional changes that will help them to explore their new world, and make sense of it. During this stage, toddlers should be able to follow two- or three-step directions, sort objects by shape and color, imitate the actions of adults and playmates, and express a wide range of emotions.

Positive Parenting Tips

Following are some of the things you, as a parent, can do to help your toddler during this time:

- Set up a special time to read books with your toddler.
- Encourage your child to take part in pretend play.
- Play parade or follow the leader with your toddler.
- Help your child to explore things around her by taking her on a walk or wagon ride.
- Encourage your child to tell you his name and age.
- Teach your child simple songs like Itsy Bitsy Spider, or other cultural childhood rhymes.
- Give your child attention and praise when she follows instructions and shows positive behavior and limit attention for defiant behavior like tantrums. Teach your child acceptable ways to show that she's upset.

Preschoolers (3-5 years of age)

Developmental Milestones

Skills such as naming colors, showing affection, and hopping on one foot are called developmental milestones. Developmental milestones are things most children can do by a certain age. Children reach milestones in how they play, learn, speak, behave, and move (like crawling, walking, or jumping).

As children grow into early childhood, their world will begin to open up. They will become more independent and begin to focus more on adults and children outside of the family. They will want to explore and ask about the things around them even more. Their interactions with family and those around them will help to shape their personality and their own ways of thinking and moving. During this stage, children should be able to ride a tricycle, use safety scissors, notice a difference between girls and boys, help to dress and undress themselves, play with other children, recall part of a story, and sing a song.

Positive Parenting Tips

Following are some of the things you, as a parent, can do to help your preschooler during this time:

- Continue to read to your child. Nurture her love for books by taking her to the library or bookstore.

- Let your child help with simple chores.

- Encourage your child to play with other children. This helps him to learn the value of sharing and friendship.

- Be clear and consistent when disciplining your child. Explain and show the behavior that you expect from her. Whenever you tell her no, follow up with what he should be doing instead.

- Help your child develop good language skills by speaking to him in complete sentences and using "grown up" words. Help him to use the correct words and phrases.

- Help your child through the steps to solve problems when she is upset.

- Give your child a limited number of simple choices (for example, deciding what to wear, when to play, and what to eat for snack).

Middle Childhood (6-8 years of age)

Developmental Milestones

Middle childhood brings many changes in a child's life. By this time, children can dress themselves, catch a ball more easily using only their hands, and tie their shoes. Having independence from family becomes more important now. Events such as starting school bring children this age into regular contact with the larger world. Friendships become more and more important. Physical, social, and mental skills develop quickly at this time. This is a critical time for children to develop confidence in all areas of life, such as through friends, schoolwork, and sports.

Here is some information on how children develop during middle childhood:

Emotional/Social Changes. Children in this age group might:

- Show more independence from parents and family.
- Start to think about the future.
- Understand more about his or her place in the world.
- Pay more attention to friendships and teamwork.
- Want to be liked and accepted by friends.

Thinking and Learning. Children in this age group might:

- Show rapid development of mental skills.
- Learn better ways to describe experiences and talk about thoughts and feelings.
- Have less focus on one's self and more concern for others.

Positive Parenting Tips

Following are some things you, as a parent, can do to help your child during this time:

- Show affection for your child. Recognize her accomplishments.
- Help your child develop a sense of responsibility—ask him to help with household tasks, such as setting the table.
- Talk with your child about school, friends, and things she looks forward to in the future.
- Talk with your child about respecting others. Encourage him to help people in need.
- Help your child set her own achievable goals—she'll learn to take pride in herself and rely less on approval or reward from others.
- Help your child learn patience by letting others go first or by finishing a task before going out to play. Encourage him to think about possible consequences before acting.
- Make clear rules and stick to them, such as how long your child can watch TV or when she has to go to bed. Be clear about what behavior is okay and what is not okay.

- Do fun things together as a family, such as playing games, reading, and going to events in your community.

- Get involved with your child's school. Meet the teachers and staff and get to understand their learning goals and how you and the school can work together to help your child do well.

- Continue reading to your child. As your child learns to read, take turns reading to each other.

- Use discipline to guide and protect your child, rather than punishment to make him feel bad about himself. Follow up any discussion about what not to do with a discussion of what to do instead.

- Praise your child for good behavior. It's best to focus praise more on what your child does ("you worked hard to figure this out") than on traits she can't change ("you are smart").

- Support your child in taking on new challenges. Encourage her to solve problems, such as a disagreement with another child, on her own.

- Encourage your child to join school and community groups, such as a team sports, or to take advantage of volunteer opportunities.

Middle Childhood (9-11 years of age)

Developmental Milestones

Your child's growing independence from the family and interest in friends might be obvious by now. Healthy friendships are very important to your child's development, but peer pressure can become strong during this time. Children who feel good about themselves are more able to resist negative peer pressure and make better choices for themselves. This is an important time for children to gain a sense of responsibility along with their growing independence. Also, physical changes of puberty might be showing by now, especially for girls. Another big change children need to prepare for during this time is starting middle or junior high school.

Here is some information on how children develop during middle childhood:

Emotional/Social Changes. Children in this age group might:

- Start to form stronger, more complex friendships and peer relationships. It becomes more emotionally important to have friends, especially of the same sex.

- Experience more peer pressure.

- Become more aware of his or her body as puberty approaches. Body image and eating problems sometimes start around this age.

Thinking and Learning. Children in this age group might:

- Face more academic challenges at school.

- Become more independent from the family.

- Begin to see the point of view of others more clearly.

- Have an increased attention span.

Positive Parenting Tips

Following are some things you, as a parent, can do to help your child during this time:

- Spend time with your child. Talk with her about her friends, her accomplishments, and what challenges she will face.

- Be involved with your child's school. Go to school events; meet your child's teachers.

- Encourage your child to join school and community groups, such as a sports team, or to be a volunteer for a charity.

- Help your child develop his own sense of right and wrong. Talk with him about risky things friends might pressure him to do, like smoking or dangerous physical dares.

- Help your child develop a sense of responsibility—involve your child in household tasks like cleaning and cooking. Talk with your child about saving and spending money wisely.

- Meet the families of your child's friends.

- Talk with your child about respecting others. Encourage her to help people in need. Talk with her about what to do when others are not kind or are disrespectful.

- Help your child set his own goals. Encourage him to think about skills and abilities he would like to have and about how to develop them.

- Make clear rules and stick to them. Talk with your child about what you expect from her (behavior) when no adults are present.

If you provide reasons for rules, it will help her to know what to do in most situations.

• Use discipline to guide and protect your child, instead of punishment to make him feel badly about himself.

• When using praise, help your child think about her own accomplishments. Saying "you must be proud of yourself" rather than simply "I'm proud of you" can encourage your child to make good choices when nobody is around to praise her.

• Talk with your child about the normal physical and emotional changes of puberty.

• Encourage your child to read every day. Talk with him about his homework.

• Be affectionate and honest with your child, and do things together as a family.

Young Teens (12-14 years of age)

Developmental Milestones

This is a time of many physical, mental, emotional, and social changes. Hormones change as puberty begins. Most boys grow facial and pubic hair and their voices deepen. Most girls grow pubic hair and breasts, and start their period. They might be worried about these changes and how they are looked at by others. This also will be a time when your teen might face peer pressure to use alcohol, tobacco products, and drugs, and to have sex. Other challenges can be eating disorders, depression, and family problems. At this age, teens make more of their own choices about friends, sports, studying, and school. They become more independent, with their own personality and interests, although parents are still very important.

Here is some information on how young teens develop:

Emotional/Social Changes. Children in this age group might:

• Show more concern about body image, looks, and clothes.

• Focus on themselves; going back and forth between high expectations and lack of confidence.

• Experience more moodiness.

• Show more interest in and influence by peer group.

- Express less affection toward parents; sometimes might seem rude or short-tempered.

- Feel stress from more challenging school work.

- Develop eating problems.

- Feel a lot of sadness or depression, which can lead to poor grades at school, alcohol or drug use, unsafe sex, and other problems.

   Thinking and Learning. Children in this age group might:

- Have more ability for complex thought.

- Be better able to express feelings through talking.

- Develop a stronger sense of right and wrong.

Positive Parenting Tips

Following are some things you, as a parent, can do to help your child during this time:

- Be honest and direct with your teen when talking about sensitive subjects such as drugs, drinking, smoking, and sex.

- Meet and get to know your teen's friends.

- Show an interest in your teen's school life.

- Help your teen make healthy choices while encouraging him to make his own decisions.

- Respect your teen's opinions and take into account her thoughts and feelings. It is important that she knows you are listening to her.

- When there is a conflict, be clear about goals and expectations (like getting good grades, keeping things clean, and showing respect), but allow your teen input on how to reach those goals (like when and how to study or clean).

Teenagers (15-17 years of age)

Developmental Milestones

This is a time of changes for how teenagers think, feel, and interact with others, and how their bodies grow. Most girls will be physically mature by now, and most will have completed puberty. Boys might still be maturing physically during this time. Your teen might have

407

concerns about her body size, shape, or weight. Eating disorders also can be common, especially among girls. During this time, your teen is developing his unique personality and opinions. Relationships with friends are still important, yet your teen will have other interests as he develops a more clear sense of who he is. This is also an important time to prepare for more independence and responsibility; many teenagers start working, and many will be leaving home soon after high school.

Here is some information on how teens develop:

Emotional/Social Changes. Children in this age group might:

- Have more interest in the opposite sex.

- Go through less conflict with parents.

- Show more independence from parents.

- Have a deeper capacity for caring and sharing and for developing more intimate relationships.

- Spend less time with parents and more time with friends.

- Feel a lot of sadness or depression, which can lead to poor grades at school, alcohol or drug use, unsafe sex, and other problems.

Thinking and Learning. Children in this age group might:

- Learn more defined work habits.

- Show more concern about future school and work plans.

- Be better able to give reasons for their own choices, including about what is right or wrong.

Positive Parenting Tips

Following are some things you, as a parent, can do to help your teen during this time:

- Talk with your teen about her concerns and pay attention to any changes in her behavior. Ask her if she has had suicidal thoughts, particularly if she seems sad or depressed. Asking about suicidal thoughts will not cause her to have these thoughts, but it will let her know that you care about how she feels. Seek professional help if necessary.

- Show interest in your teen's school and extracurricular interests and activities and encourage him to become involved in activities such as sports, music, theater, and art.

- Encourage your teen to volunteer and become involved in civic activities in her community.

- Compliment your teen and celebrate his efforts and accomplishments.

- Show affection for your teen. Spend time together doing things you enjoy.

- Respect your teen's opinion. Listen to her without playing down her concerns.

- Encourage your teen to develop solutions to problems or conflicts. Help your teenager learn to make good decisions. Create opportunities for him to use his own judgment, and be available for advice and support.

- If your teen engages in interactive Internet media such as games, chat rooms, and instant messaging, encourage her to make good decisions about what she posts and the amount of time she spends on these activities.

- If your teen works, use the opportunity to talk about expectations, responsibilities, and other ways of behaving respectfully in a public setting.

- Talk with your teen and help him plan ahead for difficult or uncomfortable situations. Discuss what he can do if he is in a group and someone is using drugs or under pressure to have sex, or is offered a ride by someone who has been drinking.

- Respect your teen's need for privacy.

- Encourage your teen to get enough sleep and exercise, and to eat healthy, balanced meals.

Section 45.2

Coping with Infant Crying

This section includes text excerpted from "Communication and Your Newborn," © 1995–2016. The Nemours Foundation KidsHealth®. Reprinted with permission.

Do you remember your baby's very first cry? From the moment of birth, babies begin to communicate.

At first, your newborn's cries may seem like a foreign language. But before you know it, you'll learn your baby's "language" and be able to answer your little one's needs.

How Babies Communicate

Babies are born with the ability to cry, which is how they communicate for a while. Your baby's cries generally tell you that something is wrong: an empty belly, a wet bottom, cold feet, being tired, or a need to be held and cuddled, etc.

Sometimes what a baby needs can be identified by the type of cry— for example, the "I'm hungry" cry may be short and low-pitched, while "I'm upset" may sound choppy. Before you know it, you'll probably be able to recognize which need your baby is expressing and respond accordingly.

But babies also can cry when feeling overwhelmed by all of the sights and sounds of the world—or for no clear reason at all. So if your baby cries and you aren't able to console him or her immediately, remember that crying is one way babies shut out stimuli when they're overloaded.

While crying is the main way that babies communicate, they also use other, more subtle forms. Learning to recognize them is rewarding and can strengthen your bond with your baby.

A newborn can tell the difference between a human voice and other sounds. Try to pay attention to how your little one responds to your voice, which is already associated with care: food, warmth, touch.

If your baby is crying in the bassinet, see how quickly your approaching voice quiets him or her. See how closely your baby listens when you talk in loving tones. Your baby may not yet coordinate looking and listening, but even when staring into the distance, will be paying close attention to your voice as you speak. Your baby may subtly adjust body position or facial expression, or even move the arms and legs in time with your speech.

Sometime during your newborn's first month, you may get a glimpse of a first smile—a welcome addition to your baby's communication skills!

What Should I Do?

As soon as you hold your baby after birth, you'll begin to communicate with each other by exchanging your first glances, sounds, and touches. Babies quickly learn about the world through their senses.

As the days after birth pass, your newborn will become accustomed to seeing you and will begin to focus on your face. The senses of touch and hearing are especially important, though.

Your baby will be curious about noises, but none more so than the spoken voice. Talk to your baby whenever you have the chance. Even though your baby doesn't understand what you're saying, your calm, reassuring voice conveys safety. Your newborn is learning about life with almost every touch, so provide lots of tender kisses and your little one will find the world a soothing place.

Communicating with newborns is a matter of meeting their needs. Always respond to your newborn's cries—babies cannot be spoiled with too much attention. Indeed, quick responses to babies' cries lets them know that they're important and worthy of attention.

There will probably be times when you have met all needs, yet your baby continues to cry. Don't despair—your little one might be overstimulated, have too much energy, or just need a good cry for no apparent reason.

It's common for babies to have a fussy period about the same time every day, generally between early evening and midnight. Though all newborns cry and show some fussiness, when an infant who is otherwise healthy cries for more than 3 hours per day, more than 3 days per week for at least 3 weeks, it is a condition known as colic. This can be upsetting, but the good news is that it's short-lived—most babies outgrow it at around 3 or 4 months of age.

Try to soothe your baby. Some are comforted by motion, such as rocking or being walked back and forth across the room, while others respond to sounds, like soft music or the hum of a vacuum cleaner. It may take some time to find out what best comforts your baby during these stressful periods.

Should I Be Concerned?

Talk to your doctor if your baby seems to cry for an unusual length of time, if the cries sound odd to you, or if the crying is associated with decreased activity, poor feeding, or unusual breathing or movements. Your doctor will be able to reassure you or look for a medical reason for your baby's distress. Chances are there is nothing wrong, and knowing this can help you relax and stay calm when your baby is upset.

Here are some other reasons for prolonged crying:

- The baby is ill. A baby who cries more when being held or rocked may be sick. Call your doctor, especially if the baby has a temperature of 100.4°F (38°C) or more.

- The baby has an eye irritation. A scratched cornea or "foreign body" in a baby's eye can cause redness and tearing. Call your doctor.

- The baby is in pain. An open diaper pin or other object could be hurting the baby's skin. Take a close look everywhere, even each finger and toe (sometimes hair can get wrapped around a baby's tiny digits and cause pain; this is known as a hair tourniquet).

If you have any questions about your newborn's ability to see or hear, contact your doctor immediately. Even newborns can be tested using sophisticated equipment, if necessary. The sooner a potential problem is caught, the better it can be treated.

Section 45.3

Taming Tempers

This section includes text excerpted from "Taming Tempers," © 1995–2016. The Nemours Foundation/KidsHealth®. Reprinted with permission.

Parents expect temper tantrums from 2- and 3-year-olds. But angry outbursts don't necessarily stop after the toddler years. Older kids sometimes have trouble handling anger and frustration, too.

Some kids only lose their cool once in a while, but others seem to have a harder time when things don't go their way. Kids who tend to have strong reactions by nature will need more help from parents to manage their tempers.

Controlling outbursts can be difficult for kids—and helping them learn to do so is a tough job for the parents who love them. Try to be patient and positive, and know that these skills take time to develop and that just about every child can improve with the right coaching.

A Parent's Role

Managing kids can be a challenge. Some days keeping the peace while keeping your cool seems impossible. But whether you're reacting to an occasional temper flare-up or a pattern of outbursts, managing your own anger when things get heated will make it easier to teach kids to do the same.

To help tame a temper, try to be your child's ally—you're both rooting for your child to triumph over the temper that keeps leading to trouble.

While your own patience may be frayed by angry outbursts, opposition, defiance, arguing, and talking back, it's during these episodes that you need your patience most. Of course you feel angry, but what counts is how you handle that.

Reacting to kids' meltdowns with yelling and outbursts of your own will only teach them to do the same (and actually is associated with an increase in children's negative behaviors). But keeping your cool and calmly working through a frustrating situation lets you show—and teach—appropriate ways to handle anger and frustration.

Let's say you hear your kids fighting over a toy in the other room. You have ignored it, hoping that they would work it out themselves. But the arguing turns into screaming and soon you hear doors slamming, the thump of hitting, and crying. You decide to get involved before someone gets really hurt.

By the time you arrive at the scene of the fight, you may be at the end of your own rope. After all, the sound of screaming is upsetting, and you may be frustrated that your kids aren't sharing or trying to get along. (And you know that this toy they're fighting over is going to be lost, broken, or ignored before long anyway!)

So what's the best way for you to react? With your own self-control intact. Teaching by example is your most powerful tool. Speak calmly, clearly, and firmly—not with anger, blame, harsh criticisms, threats, or putdowns.

Of course, that's easier said than done. But remember that you're trying to teach your kids how to handle anger. If you yell or threaten, you'll model and ingrain the exact kinds of behavior you want to discourage. Your kids will see that you're so angry and unable to control your own temper that you can't help but scream—and that won't help them learn not to scream.

What You Can Do

Regulating emotions and managing behavior are skills that develop slowly over time during childhood. Just like any other skills, your kids will need to learn and practice them, with your help.

If it's unusual for your child to have a tantrum, when one does happen, clearly but calmly review the rules. Saying something like "I know you're upset, but no yelling and no name-calling, please" might be all your child needs to hear to regain composure. Then patiently give an instruction, like "tell me what you're upset about" or "please apologize to your brother for calling him that name." In this way, you're guiding your child back to acceptable behavior and encouraging self-control.

Also, tell your child what will happen if he or she doesn't calm down—for example, "If you don't calm down, you need to go to your room until you're able to stop screaming."

Kids whose temper outbursts are routine might lack the self-control necessary to deal with frustration and anger and need more help managing those emotions. These steps can help:

Help kids put it into words. If your child is in the middle of an outburst, find out what's wrong. If necessary, use a time-out to get your child to settle down or remind him or her about house rules and expectations—"There's no yelling or throwing stuff; please stop that right now and cool it." Remind your child to talk to you without whining, sulking, or yelling. Once your child calms down, ask what got him or her so upset. You might say, "Use your words to tell me what's wrong and what you're mad about." This helps your child put emotions into words and figure out what, if anything, needs to be done to solve the problem. However, don't push too hard for your child to talk right then. He or she may need some time to reflect before being ready to talk.

Listen and respond. Once your child puts the feelings into words, it's up to you to listen and say that you understand. If your child is struggling for words, offer some help: "so that made you angry," "you must have felt frustrated," or "that must have hurt your feelings." Offer to help find an answer if there's a problem to be solved, a conflict to be mended, or an apology to be made. Many times, feeling listened to and understood is all kids need to calm down. But while acknowledging your child's feelings, make it clear that strong emotions aren't an excuse for bad behavior. "I know you're mad, but it's still not OK to hit." Then tell your child some things to try instead. Some kids really just need to be "heard" first.

Create clear ground rules and stick to them. Talk about house rules regularly so your kids know what you expect of them. Be clear about what is and what is not acceptable without using threats, accusations, or putdowns. Your kids will get the message if you make clear, simple statements about what's off limits and explain what you do want them to do. You might say: "There's no yelling in this house. Use your words to tell me what's upsetting you."

Here are some other good-behavior rules to try:

- In this family, we don't hit, push, or shove.
- There's no screaming allowed.
- There's no door-slamming in our house.
- There's no name calling.
- We don't say mean things in this family.
- You may not throw things or break things on purpose.

Coping Strategies for Kids

Kids who've learned that it's not OK to yell, hit, and throw stuff when they're upset need other strategies for calming down when they're angry. Offer some ideas to help them learn safe ways to get the anger out or to find other activities that can create a better mood.

Take a Break from the Situation.

Tell your kids that it's OK to walk away from a conflict to avoid an angry outburst. By moving to another part of the house or the backyard, a child can get some space and work on calming down.

Find a Way to (Safely) Get the Anger Out.

There may be no punching walls, but you can suggest some good ways for a child to vent. Doing a bunch of jumping jacks, dancing around the bedroom, or going outside and doing cartwheels are all good choices. Or your child can choose to write about or draw a picture of what is so upsetting.

Learn to Shift.

This one is tough for kids—and adults, too. Explain that part of calming down is moving from a really angry mood to a more in-control mood. Instead of thinking of the person or situation that caused the anger, encourage kids to think of something else to do that might bring about a better mood—like a walk around the block, a bike ride, playing a game, reading a favorite book, digging in the garden, or listening to a favorite song. Try one of these things together so you both see how doing something different can change the way a person feels.

Building a Strong Foundation

Fortunately, really angry episodes don't happen too often for most kids. Those with temper troubles often have an active, strong-willed style and extra energy that needs to be discharged.

Try these steps during the calm times—they can prevent problems before they start by helping kids learn and practice skills needed to manage the heat of the moment:

Make sure kids get enough sleep. Sleep is very important to their well-being. The link between a lack of sleep and a child's behavior isn't always obvious. When adults are tired, they can be grumpy or have low energy, but kids can become hyper or disagreeable or have extremes in behavior.

Most kids' sleep requirements fall within a predictable range of hours based on their age, but each child is a unique individual with distinct sleep needs.

Help Them Label Emotions

Help kids get in the habit of saying what they're feeling and why— for example, "I'm mad because I have to clean my room while my friends are playing." Using words doesn't get a child out of doing a chore, but having the discussion can calm the situation. You're having a conversation instead of an argument. Praise your child for talking about it instead of slamming the door, for instance.

See That Kids Get a Lot of Physical Activity

Active play can really help kids who have big tempers. Encourage outside play and sports your child likes. Karate, wrestling, and running can be especially good for kids who are trying to get their tempers under control. But any activity that gets the heart pumping can help burn off energy and stress.

Encourage Kids to Take Control

Compare a temper to a puppy that hasn't yet learned to behave and that's running around all over the place getting into things. Puppies might not mean to be bad—but they need to be trained so that they can learn that there's no eating shoes, no jumping on people or certain furniture, etc. The point is that your child's temper—like a puppy—needs to be trained to learn when it's OK to play, how to use all that extra energy, and how to follow rules.

Recognize Successes

Many times these go unnoticed so be sure to comment on how well your child handled a difficult situation when you see positive behaviors.

Try to Be Flexible

Parenting can be a tiring experience, but try not to be too rigid. Hearing a constant chorus of "no" can be disheartening for kids. Sometimes, of course, "no" is absolutely the only answer—"no, you can't ride your bike without your helmet!" But other times, you might let the kids win one. For instance, if your child wants to keep the wiffle ball game going a little longer, maybe give it 15 more minutes.

Try to identify "at-risk" situations and be proactive. For example, if your child has difficulty with transitions, give warnings ahead of time. Similarly, if your kids have trouble turning off the television when asked, be clear how long they can watch TV or play video games and then set a 5-minute warning timer. Be sure to enforce the agreement.

As anyone who's been really angry knows, following sensible advice can be tough when emotions run high. Give your kids responsibility for getting under control, but be there to remind them how to do it.

Most kids can learn to get better at handling anger and frustration. But if your child often gets into fights and arguments with friends, siblings, and adults, additional help might be needed. Talk with the other adults in your child's life—teachers, school counselors, and coaches might be able to help, and your child's doctor can recommend a counselor or psychologist.

Chapter 46

Foster Care and Adoption

Chapter Contents

419

Section 46.1

Information for Foster Parents Considering Adoption

This section includes text excerpted from "Preparing and Supporting Foster Parents Who Adopt," Child Welfare Information Gateway, U.S. Department of Health and Human Services (HHS), January 2013.

Preparing and Supporting Foster Parents Who Adopt

Child welfare practitioners are increasingly aware of the importance of foster parents as permanency resources for children and youth in foster care. Many children in foster care who become available for adoption are adopted by their foster parents. In order to facilitate these types of adoption, professionals should be knowledgeable about the benefits, costs, and practice implications.

Trends in Foster Parent Adoption

Foster parents are the most important source of adoptive families for children in the child welfare system. According to the Adoption and Foster Care Analysis and Reporting System (AFCARS), in fiscal year 2011, 54 percent of children adopted from foster care were adopted by their foster parents. Data from the 2007 National Survey of Adoptive Parents (NSAP) and the 2007 National Survey of Children's Health (NSCH) show that among children adopted from foster care by nonrelatives, 8 out of 10 (80 percent) were adopted by their foster parents.

Foster parents were not always preferred candidates for adoptive parenthood. Earlier in child welfare practice, distinctions were made between foster parents, who were seen as temporary caregivers, and adoptive parents, who were specially matched with a particular child for permanent placement.

Additionally, if parents decided to discontinue foster parenting after they adopted, or if the number of children in the home after a child's adoption exceeded the number allowed by State policy, then the agency lost a foster home. The practice of discouraging adoption by foster parents continued through the mid-1970s, when two in three States either prohibited or warned against the practice. By the early 1980s the tide had turned, influenced by a combination of foster parent activism and permanency planning projects that demonstrated the benefits of foster parent adoption. The result was the passage of the Federal Adoption Assistance and Child Welfare Act of 1980, which supported foster parent adoption by making subsidies available for children adopted from foster care. It took a great deal of time—more than 30 years—and the passage of several Federal laws to shift practice toward acknowledging the important role foster parents play in achieving permanence for children and youth. At present, foster parents are recognized as valuable resources for waiting children. While 26 States give priority to a child's relatives when he or she enters out-of-home care, 28 States provide procedures for foster parents to adopt when their child becomes legally free for adoption.

Foster parent adoption is also the basis for two well-recognized practices in adoption, legal risk placements and concurrent planning. In legal risk placements, children whose situations indicate that parental rights will likely be terminated—legally freeing children and youth for adoption—are placed with foster parents who are willing to adopt. In concurrent planning, a practice supported by the Adoption and Safe Families Act (ASFA) of 1997, the permanency goal of reunification is supplemented by an alternative goal (often, adoption) to ensure that if reunification is not possible, the child has a clearly identified permanency option that can quickly be put in place.

Children and youth are often placed with foster families who would consider adoption should reunification with birth parents or other relatives become impossible, thus minimizing the number of placements children experience. For this model to work, these foster parents must be able to support both the reunification plan, as well as the plan for adoption. After the passage of ASFA, adoption from foster care increased 65 percent between 1997 and 2000. Additionally, foster parent adoption increased after ASFA's passage—28 percent between 1998 and 1999 alone.

The Fostering Connections to Success and Increasing Adoptions Act of 2008 also promotes foster parent adoption. This law included provisions aimed at increasing adoption from foster care. Among these were the requirements that States inform prospective adoptive parents, including foster parents, about the Federal adoption tax credit available to those who adopt a child with special needs. Other provisions included funds for Kinship Navigator programs, through new Family Connection grants, to help children in foster care locate relatives. The

National Resource Center for Permanency and Family Connections (NRCPFC) published an information packet titled Kinship Care and the Fostering Connections to Success and Increasing Adoptions Act of 2008 that provides facts and statistics on kinship care and the kinship care policies and provisions in the Fostering Connections Act.

Benefits of Foster Parent Adoption

Unlike most other types of adoption, children, youth, and foster parents involved in foster parent adoption have already spent time living as a family before the adoption is initiated and have had the opportunity to make some initial adjustments. In addition, research indicates that children waiting for adoption by their foster parents are less likely to experience disruption than children in nonrelative, nonfoster-parent adoption.

For children and youth, some of the other benefits include:

- A continuing and legally secure relationship with foster parents they know and trust

- An end to the uncertainty of foster care and, for many children, a positive psychological shift in their sense of identity, connection, and belonging

- The chance to remain in a familiar community, school, and neighborhood

- Tendency for shorter time to permanency than in other types of adoption

- Greater likelihood of maintaining an ongoing connection with the birth family than in families formed through matching

- Experienced parents to manage their needs (often including emotional and behavioral challenges due to trauma and complicated life histories)

- An established legal permanency for children and youth who would otherwise be wards of the court

For the adopting family, the advantages of adopting a child in their care include:

- Continuity of the relationship with the child or youth

- The opportunity to raise the child without oversight from an agency

- An established legal guardianship, becoming the sole decision-maker regarding school, religious practice, medical treatment, travel, discipline, and much more

- Often, both familiarity and a relationship with the child's birth family and greater knowledge of their child's background than in non-foster-parent adoption

- Access to continued support for the adoption of children with special needs, such as the adoption assistance subsidy

For the birth family, foster parent adoption sometimes means the birth parents know and can have a relationship with those who will be the permanent caregivers for their children. Foster parent adoptions are often open—an adoption arrangement in which identities are known and there is direct contact between birth families and adoptive families—either because a relationship developed between the birth and adoptive parents when the children were in care or because the children know their birth families' contact information and may contact them after adoption. More than one-third of all children who have been adopted (36 percent) had some postadoption contact with their birth families.

Foster parent adoption also provides an opportunity for siblings to stay together or remain connected. The Fostering Connections to Success and Increasing Adoptions Act of 2008 requires States to make reasonable efforts to maintain sibling connections in order to receive Federal funding. Since its passage in 2009-2011, 13 States passed statutes regarding sibling placement and visiting. Sibling placement and contact after permanency vary widely by State, however, and while it is possible that the percentage of sibling groups placed together has improved since the passage of the Fostering Connections Act, there are no current sibling studies sampling children placed after 2008. A number of barriers to placing siblings with the same foster family—including the size of the sibling group, age, varying needs for siblings, or siblings born to the birth family after other siblings entered care—may carry over into barriers to adoption of a sibling group by the same foster parents.

Child Welfare Information Gateway offers more information on the topics of open adoption and sibling issues in adoption from foster care.

For larger society, there are also benefits from foster parent adoption. These include:

- Reduced costs to government agencies when a child moves from foster care to adoption, since the administrative costs

423

of recruiting, training, and approving an adoptive family are reduced

- As with all adoptions from foster care, a decrease in the number of youth exiting foster care with no family, reducing risk for a host of problems, including homelessness, incarceration, and poverty

Costs of Foster Parent Adoption

Just as there are benefits, foster parents assume additional costs when they adopt.

- While families gain autonomy, they can lose the assistance of the agency and relationships with caseworkers.

- Families may receive fewer resources and supports, sometimes leaving them financially vulnerable.

- While foster/adoptive parents gain decision-making privileges, they become financially responsible for the child's welfare, as well as legally responsible for the child's actions.

Some of these costs to parents may be mitigated by adoption assistance and other post adoption services. According to a study, roughly 90 percent (88 percent) of children adopted with public agency involvement in 2009 received an adoption subsidy. It is important to educate foster parents about the availability of adoption subsidies and not assume that they've been provided with all the necessary information. Research shows that the Adoption Tax Credit is not widely used by families that adopt from foster care and that most tax credit dollars are used by families who adopt through intercountry adoption. Many families report not knowing that this tax credit exists.

Foster and adoptive families should be made aware of the nature of adoption subsidies. They are not merely maintenance payments; often they include services like counseling, Medicaid, and even respite or residential care in some States. Because adoption subsidies vary widely from State to State, it is also important to introduce parents to the fact that subsidies may be reduced over time.

Section 8 of the Children's Bureau's Child Welfare Policy Manual addresses the Adoption Assistance Program. Child Welfare Information Gateway's Adoption Assistance webpage provides resources for obtaining adoption assistance and other financial supports, including college scholarships, vocational education, and tuition waivers:

www.childwelfare.gov/adoption/preplacement/adoption_assistance.
cfm

Practice Implications with Children and Parents

Even though foster parents have the advantage of knowing and having cared for the children and youth they plan to adopt, they still need careful preparation and support. Research indicates that foster parents need and want more preparation and information than they typically or currently receive in making this important transition. Practices associated with moving families from foster care to adoption include assessment, preparation for adoption, facilitating an ongoing connection between the child and birth family, including the child's siblings (when it is in the child's best interests), and working with families who choose not to adopt. As with all adoption practice, policies vary greatly among States and agencies.

Assessment

Assessing the family's interest and ability to adopt is a crucial step. Workers should not assume that foster parents will choose to adopt, even if they have cared for a child for an extended period or have expressed interest in the past. Instead of asking parents, particularly those who are ambivalent, if they will adopt, another approach is to help them explore the benefits of adoption, while still addressing their concerns.

In reviewing the concerns of foster parents, the worker can explore the seriousness of each concern and determine what information or resources might reduce the parents' anxiety. This exercise may help parents realistically examine their fears and consider if they should proceed with adoption. If the worker helps the foster parents explore their feelings, fears, and hopes openly and honestly over time, the odds increase that the foster parents will commit to adopting or will be active in helping the child move to another permanent family. However, it is important to note that a foster parent should never be pushed to adopt a child or youth.

Foster parent interest in adoption may stem from their sincere desire to become the adoptive parents. It may also stem from strong feelings toward the child and discomfort with the idea of others raising the child, despite their own misgivings about adoption. It is important to help foster parents consider factors that may make it difficult for them to meet the child's needs now and in the future, due to the nature of adoption.

Indicators that the foster parents are good candidates to adopt include evidence of:

- A mutual emotional connection between children and parents, including signs of affection

- Understanding and accepting the child's behaviors, abilities, and challenges

- Commitment to keep siblings together whenever possible and, when not possible, encouraging and facilitating the ongoing communication between separated siblings

- Valuing the birth family (even when they have made serious mistakes as parents) and respecting and supporting the child's emotional connection to previous attachment figures, including siblings and other relatives or even previous foster parent relationships

- Competence in meeting the child's needs and advocating for needed resources

- Commitment to caring for the child now and in the future

Many agencies have specific assessment processes for determining whether adoption by a particular family is in the best interests of the child and for helping families come to a decision about their suitability for adoption. Those same processes are still relevant in cases of foster parent adoption. While the foster family may already have a completed home study, including background checks, the family should complete any remaining parts of the assessment specific to adoption. Agencies that have implemented a dual home study process that covers both foster care and adoption requirements initially will be able to process foster parent adoptions more quickly.

Preparation for Adoption

Once the parents (and the child, if old enough to consent to adoption) have committed to the adoption, the worker should help the family make the transition from fostering to adoption. Even though foster parents and children benefit from knowing each other, adoption is an adjustment for all persons involved. As with assessment, many agencies have standard procedures for helping families and children prepare for adoption. While some of the procedures may be unnecessary since the child has already been living in the home, the worker can facilitate other preparations.

For the family, these preparations may include:

- Providing full disclosure of information about the child and the birth family in writing, including explanations of the child's placement history and full medical history, as well as implications for parenting

- Preparing the family for the possibility of the child acting out feelings he or she may experience as a result of committing to adoption, after the adoption is formalized, such as testing the parents' boundaries to ensure their commitment is for the long term

- Preparing the family for less support from the child welfare system

- Preparing for the impact on other children in the family, particularly other foster children who are not being adopted

- Providing information on the legal steps in the adoption process

- Providing information and access to the adoption assistance payment (subsidy)

- Informing parents about the one-time, per child, Federal adoption tax credit

- Helping the family negotiate ongoing birth family contact, if in the child's best interest

- Providing parents with access to ongoing training, therapy, and/or other resources to prepare parents for the journey of adoption

For the child or youth, preparation may include:
For older children, involving them in the adoption decision

- Helping the child understand the differences between foster care and adoption and what those differences will mean on a day-to-day basis and in the future

- Assuring the child/youth about the types of feelings that may come up as a result of committing to adoption, such as grief, acceptance, loss, uncertainty, reassurance, identity formation, etc.

- With the family, helping the child review his or her history and put together a life book or life map that includes a visual presentation of the child's life and a chronology of the child's removals and placements and establishment of a forever family with the foster-adoptive parents

- Helping the child navigate the possible grief and the loss he or she might feel for birth family members and accept the addition of the adoptive family as a permanent family

- Helping the child to prepare for ongoing contact with the birth family if that is in his or her best interest and will occur in the future

A resource for workers and families is the Child Welfare Information Gateway factsheet Helping Your Foster Child Transition to Your Adopted Child.

Facilitating Ongoing Connection with the Birth Family

Children adopted by their foster parents often have deep emotional attachments to members of their original families, including siblings who may be placed elsewhere. Even children who were not well cared for in their birth families may experience profound loss at separation, which may deepen when they are adopted and/or when they learn they will never return to their biological family/home.

Foster parents are likely to have had contact or even relationships with their child's birth family. Workers and adopting parents, often with the help of therapists, need to assess what level of ongoing connection is in the child's best interests and how to develop a post adoption connection agreement that works well for everyone. Some States use mediation or family group decision-making to help develop such agreements. Post adoption connection does not necessarily mean contact, although it may.

Social Media and Adoption.

Facebook, Twitter, and other social media outlets have changed the landscape of adoption. Child Welfare Information Gateway's *Video Gallery* features digital stories told by children and youth waiting to be adopted and foster parents whose lives have been changed through adoption.

The Children's Bureau's *Adopt US Kids* provides several social media tools and resources for foster parents and child welfare professionals.

Although statistics are not yet available to document the number of adopted children or youth and their birth parents connecting via social networking sites, anecdotal evidence suggests that it is a growing trend. Evidence also suggests that adoptive families tend to ask for advice or help after they or the adopted child have already been in contact with the birth parents. With this in mind, it is suggested that preparation is needed for both parents and youth about the realities of birth family contact through social media, including safe and appropriate contact and use of these tools.

The 2011 issue of CW360° Child Welfare and Technology by the Center for Advanced Studies in Child Welfare (CASCW) reviews technology innovations to improve child welfare outcomes and considers current gaps in technological practice knowledge. One such gap is that of social media and networking and the use of technology by children and youth in foster care.

Adoption Star, a nonprofit child-placing agency, provides a list of tips and guidelines for adoptive and birth parents connecting online. Adoptions Together discussed the issue of social media's effect on the adoption field in its blog.

Families Who Do Not Adopt

Some parents may evaluate their situations and realistically conclude that adopting a particular child is not right for them or the child. If that is the decision foster parents make, and additional information and support do not allay their concerns, it is important to honor their decision and involve them in helping the child understand and transition to a new family. Specifically, the foster parents can help with:

- Not hindering the development of a new permanency plan for the child/youth

- Preparing the child for transition to a new family

- Helping the child grieve leaving the family and giving their blessing for the move

- Being an ongoing presence in the child's life, if this is in the child's best interests.

- Considering the possibility of providing respite care if needed, or even taking the child back into foster care in their home if the adoption disrupts

Caseworker Reservations

What if the family is willing to adopt the child or youth, but the worker has reservations? Despite good intentions, many initial foster placements are made quickly, without adequate time to assess the fit between family strengths and child needs. While the emotional connection between the child and family is one important consideration, workers must consider whether a foster parent adoption is the best long-term option for the child or youth. Older foster parents of young children, parents who have limited support systems, parents who are harshly critical of a child or the child's birth family or birth culture, and parents who exhibit limited ability to adapt to meet a child's needs are examples of situations workers need to assess with special care. On the other hand, it is important that workers do not allow personal biases to play a role in impeding the process for permanency through adoption.

Section 46.2

Sibling Issues in Foster Care and Adoption

This section includes text excerpted from "Sibling Issues in Foster Care and Adoption," Child Welfare Information Gateway, U.S. Department of Health and Human Services (HHS), January 2013.

Sibling Placements in Foster Care

Child welfare professionals can make a critical contribution to the well-being of children who enter care by preserving their connections with their brothers and sisters. Approximately two-thirds of children in foster care in the United States have a sibling also in care. For a variety of reasons, many of these siblings are not placed together initially or become separated over time. Foster youth describe this experience as "an extra punishment, a separate loss, and another pain that is not needed." This section will explore research, intervention strategies, and resources to assist professionals in preserving connections among siblings.

Defining a Sibling Relationship

The identification of siblings can be challenging, especially when children have lived in more than one family. Children's definitions of their siblings often differ from those of caseworkers or official legislative definitions. Children are less formal than adults in their view of who is a brother or sister. Research indicates that biological relatedness was not associated with young children's perceptions of closeness to siblings; being a full, half, or step-sibling did not influence their perception of closeness. Children in foster care may live with and develop ties to children with whom they may or may not have a biological relationship. In child welfare, the term "fictive kin" has been introduced to recognize types of relationships in a child's life where there is no legal or biological tie, but a strong, enduring bond exists.

There are many types of relationships that might be defined as sibling relationships:

- Full or half-siblings, including any children who were relinquished or removed at birth

- Step-siblings

- Adopted children in the same household, not biologically related

- Children born into the family and their foster/adopted siblings

- Other close relatives or nonrelatives living in the same kinship home

- Foster children in the same family

- Orphanage mates or group-home mates with a close, enduring relationship

- Children of the partner or former partner of the child's parent

- Individuals conceived from the same sperm or egg donor

While laws and policies may have restrictive definitions of siblings that typically require a biological parent in common, child- and family-centered practice respects cultural values and recognizes close, nonbiological relationships as a source of support to the child. In these cases, the child may be one of the best sources of information regarding who is considered a sibling.

Legal Framework for Protecting Sibling Connections

Even when professionals believe that maintaining sibling relationships is in children's best interests, laws and policies must be in place to support these connections, both in foster care and when permanency is achieved. It was not until the mid-1990s that State legislatures and courts initiated regulations regarding sibling placement and visitation, and in 2004 the Child and Family Services Reviews began to consider efforts to place siblings together. By 2005, sibling placement policies (28 States) and visitation statutes (32 States) had been established in over half the States.

State sibling statutes vary considerably in their definitions of sibling relationships, in the scope of activities they regulate, and in whether siblings have legal standing to file suit for access to each other. In 1993, California was one of the first States to pass legislation promoting sibling visitation for foster children, and several additional statutes have expanded legal protections of sibling relationships. The California Welfare and Institutions Code, Section 16002, is recognized by many as offering the strongest statutory protections for the needs of siblings in foster care and adoption among existing State statutes. It liberally defines a sibling as a child related to another person by blood, adoption, or affinity through a common legal or biological parent. California's law allows any person, including a dependent child, to petition the court to request sibling visitation, including post adoption sibling contact or placement with or near a sibling.

Fostering Connections Act

The Fostering Connections to Success and Increasing Adoptions Act of 2008 is the first Federal law to address the importance of keeping siblings together. This law requires States to make reasonable efforts to maintain sibling connections in order to receive Federal funding. The provisions of section 206 provide that reasonable efforts shall be made:

1. to place siblings removed from their home in the same foster care, kinship guardianship or adoptive placement, unless the State documents that such a joint placement would be contrary to the safety or well-being of any of the siblings; and

2. in the case of siblings removed from their home who are not so jointly placed, to provide for frequent visitation or other ongoing interaction between the siblings, unless that State documents that frequent visitation or other ongoing interaction would be contrary to the safety or well-being of any of the siblings.

While the Federal Government through the Fostering Connections Act has taken a leadership role in mandating reasonable efforts to maintain sibling relationships, it is up to the States to vigorously support these connections. Between 2009 and 2011, 13 States passed statutes regarding sibling placement and visitation, and many others already had such statutes. There is often a gap, however, between what is considered best practice or what the law requires and what happens in day-to-day practice. Ultimately, the State courts will help define reasonable efforts by their decisions as to whether the requirement has been met in specific cases.

Legal scholars assert that there is still a need to fortify statutory protections of siblings' rights to have contact after adoption. The Fostering Connections Act sends a clear message that sibling relationships are critically important to preserve, but it is unclear as to whether the reference to "adoptive placement" in the statute refers to the post adoption period as well. Mandelbaum recognizes the placement of this phrase after the term "kinship guardianship," which clearly is a permanent arrangement and can infer that "adoptive placement" also refers to the child's life in a permanent adoptive home.

Currently, only a minority of States provide a legal foundation for post adoption contact between siblings; seven States–Arkansas, Florida, Illinois (relative adoptions only), Massachusetts, Nevada, Maryland, and South Carolina allow a court to order post adoption contact without the consent of adoptive parents, and another 16 States allow for such a court order with the consent of adoptive parents.

State-by-State information regarding post adoption contact agreements can be found in Child Welfare Information Gateway's *Post adoption Contact Agreements between Birth and Adoptive Families.* These laws pertain not just to sibling contact but to contact with any birth family member.

Importance of Sibling Relationships

Sibling relationships are emotionally powerful and critically important not only in childhood but over the course of a lifetime. As children, siblings form a child's first peer group, and they typically spend more time with each other than with anyone else. Children learn social skills, particularly in sharing and managing conflict, from negotiating with brothers and sisters. Sibling relationships can provide a significant source of continuity throughout a child's lifetime and are likely to be the longest relationships that most people experience.

The nature and importance of sibling relationships vary for individuals, depending on their own circumstances and developmental stage. Typically, there is rivalry in the preschool years, variability in closeness during middle childhood (depending on the level of warmth in the relationship), and less sibling closeness in adolescence when teens are focused on peers. An extensive body of research addresses issues of birth order, gender, age spacing, and other influences on sibling relationships. Research has demonstrated that warmth in sibling relationships is associated with less loneliness, fewer behavior problems, and higher self-worth.

Marjut Kosonen studied the emotional support and help that siblings provide and found that when they needed help, children would first seek out their mothers but then turn to older siblings for support, even before they would go to their fathers. She also found that for isolated children (as is the case for many children in foster care), sibling support is especially crucial. For these children, an older sibling was often their only perceived source of help.

Sibling Relationships in Abusive or Neglectful Families

In many families involved with child welfare, sibling relationships take on more importance because they can provide the support and nurture that are not consistently provided by parents. For children entering care, siblings can serve as a buffer against the worst effects of harsh circumstances. While sibling relationships in particular families experiencing adverse situations do not always compensate for other deficits, research has validated that, for many children, sibling relationships do promote resilience. For example, a young child's secure attachment to an older sibling can diminish the impact of adverse circumstances such as parental mental illness, substance abuse, or loss. Adverse circumstances can magnify both the positive and negative qualities of sibling relationships. Some studies have found that the ties between siblings become closer as a result of helping each other through adversity, such a parental divorce.

A study of children's perspectives on their important relationships among 90 children ages 8 to 12 who were or were not in foster care concluded that the foster children's smaller networks of relationships with important persons made siblings proportionally more important. Nearly one-third of the related siblings named by foster children in this act were not known to their social workers—most were half- or steps-iblings. Kosonen's study also underscores the importance of obtaining children's perspectives on their family relationships. When siblings could not all be placed together, workers often decided to keep those closest in age together, resulting in placements that did not necessarily fit the preferences of the children.

Since children in foster care experience more losses of significant relationships, siblings are often their only source for continuity of important attachments. For children entering care, being with their brothers and sisters promotes a sense of safety and well-being, and being separated from them can trigger grief and anxiety. Therefore, it is especially important to protect these ties that offer support to children removed from their original families.

Benefits of Placing Siblings Together

For children entering care, being with their siblings can enhance their sense of safety and well-being and provide natural, mutual support. This benefit is in contrast to the traumatic consequences of separation, which may include additional loss, grief, and anxiety over their siblings' well-being. Siblings have a shared history, and maintaining their bond provides continuity of identity and belonging. The benefits of keeping brothers and sisters together are most clearly evidenced from the perspectives of youth themselves.

Children's Perspective

It is essential that professionals be able to understand children's experiences from the child's perspective in order to be able to grasp the critical importance of maintaining sibling connections whenever possible.

When youth in foster care unite to work toward protecting the rights of children entering out-of-home care, keeping brothers and sisters together is invariably near the top of their list; for example, a New England Youth Coalition joined with the New England Association of Child Welfare Commissioners and Directors in the summer of 2012 to develop a regional Siblings' Bill of Rights. Youth advocates in States across the country have sponsored similar efforts.

Studies that directly seek the perspective of foster children are relatively rare, but those that have done so consistently underscore the overwhelming importance of protecting sibling relationships. Folman, who interviewed 90 children (ages 8-14) about their memories of their initial removal, reported that many children did not know they were being separated from siblings until they were dropped off at different houses, nor did they know how to contact each other. In describing their distress at separation, she wrote, "All sense of family, of comfort, of familiarity and of belonging was gone and there was no one except strangers."

Not only is the support of siblings helpful in the immediate adjustment to the trauma of placement, but this contact continues to offer support to the child over the course of their time in care and into adulthood. Mary Herrick and Wendy Piccus are child welfare professionals who themselves spent considerable time in care. They poignantly described the central themes related to the value of sibling connections for children in foster care, illustrated by their own experiences.

For some siblings in care, their separation or infrequent visiting can cause their relationships to wither, sometimes to the point of permanent estrangement. Maintaining these relationships is important for the future as well as the present. Youth who age out of foster care report the value of sibling connections; for example, a Midwest study of over 600 foster alumni found that youth were most likely to identify a sibling as a family member they felt close to–59 percent felt very close and 23 percent somewhat close to a sibling. Moreover, a Texas study of adult foster alumni found that those who had greater access to their siblings and reported stronger relationships with them during childhood had higher levels of social support, self-esteem, and income, as well as stronger adult sibling relationships than those who did not.

Research on Outcomes of Placing Sibs Together

Research on sibling placement patterns has confronted methodological challenges and developed more sophisticated research designs; however, there are differences in findings across studies. When significant differences are found between siblings placed in different patterns, they typically favor siblings placed totally or partially with each other over those placed completely separately.

Joint sibling placements can increase the likelihood of achieving permanency. Several studies have found that placing siblings in the same foster home is associated with a significantly higher rate of family reunification. Leathers did not find such an association with reunification but did find that children placed with the same number of siblings consistently throughout foster care had greater chances for adoption or subsidized guardianship than those placed alone. Some studies find that children placed with their siblings also experience more stability and fewer disruptions in care than those who were separated.

Conversely, some studies have found that separated siblings in foster care or adoption are at higher risk for negative adjustment outcomes, including running away and higher levels of behavior problems, evidenced in some studies but not all. Another study found that girls separated from all of their siblings are at the greatest risk for poor mental health and socialization. Finally, a recent study based on the National Study of Child and Adolescent Well-Being did not find that separated sibs were reported to have more behavior problems but did find that teachers reported lower academic performance for separated siblings (either partially or totally) than for those placed together.

For agencies, placing siblings in the same home can streamline some processes such as visits by caseworkers. Also, caseworkers are relieved of the obligation to arrange and carry out visits among siblings if they are already living together. Communication between birth and foster families is also made more manageable when there is only one foster family involved.

Chapter 47

Parenting a Child Who Has Been Sexually Abused

Parenting a Sexually Abused Child

You may be a current or prospective foster or adoptive parent of a child with a known or suspected history of child sexual abuse. In some cases, you may not be certain that abuse has occurred, but you may have suspicions based on information you received or because of the child's behavior. You may feel confused, concerned, and unsure of the impact of prior child maltreatment, including sexual abuse.

It is important to understand that the term *sexual abuse* describes a wide range of experiences. Many factors affect how children react to abusive or neglectful experiences and how they recover. Most children who have been abused **do not** go on to abuse others, and many go on to live happy, healthy, successful lives. As parents, you will play an important role in your child's recovery from childhood sexual abuse.

This chapter discusses how you can help children in your care by educating yourself about child sexual abuse, establishing guidelines for safety and privacy in your family, and understanding when and how to seek help if you need it. Reading this alone will not guarantee that you will know what to do in every circumstance, but you can use

This chapter includes text excerpted from "Parenting a Child Who Has Been Sexually Abused: A Guide for Foster and Adoptive Parents," Child Welfare Information Gateway, U.S. Department of Health and Human Services (HHS), July 2013.

it as a resource for some of the potential challenges and rewards that lay ahead.

Educating Yourself

One of the most useful actions that kinship caregivers and foster and adoptive parents can take is equipping themselves with information. Parents of children who may have been sexually abused can learn about the definitions of child sexual abuse, behaviors associated with prior sexual abuse, and how sexual abuse affects children's trust of others. With this information in hand, it will be easier to recognize possible behaviors associated with past abuse and avoid taking them personally or feeling alarmed or uncertain if your child exhibits uncommon sexual behaviors. Most importantly, you will feel capable of responding to these behaviors in sensitive and informed ways that help both you and your child.

What Is Child Sexual Abuse?

The National Child Traumatic Stress Network (NCTSN) defines child sexual abuse as

"...any interaction between a child and an adult (or another child) in which the child is used for the sexual stimulation of the perpetrator or an observer. Sexual abuse can include both touching and nontouching behaviors. Touching behaviors may involve touching of the vagina, penis, breasts or buttocks, oral-genital contact, or sexual intercourse. Nontouching behaviors can include voyeurism (trying to look at a child's naked body), exhibitionism, or exposing the child to pornography. Abusers often do not use physical force but may use play, deception, threats, or other forms of coercion to engage children and maintain their silence. Abusers frequently employ persuasive and manipulative tactics to keep the child engaged. These tactics—referred to as 'grooming'—may include buying gifts or arranging special activities, which can further confuse the victim."

Child sexual abuse is defined in Federal law by the Child Abuse Prevention and Treatment Act as

"...the employment, use, persuasion, inducement, enticement, or coercion of any child to engage in, or assist any other person to engage in, any sexually explicit conduct or simulation of such conduct for the purpose of producing a visual depiction of such conduct; or the rape, and in cases of caretaker or interfamilial relationships, statutory rape, molestation, prostitution, or other form of sexual exploitation of children, or incest with children."

Within this Federal guideline, each State is responsible for establishing its own legal definition of child sexual abuse.

Signs of Sexual Abuse

If you are parenting a child who has been removed from his or her family, you may not know for sure whether or not the child in your care has been sexually abused. Child welfare agencies usually share all known information about your child's history with you; however, there may be no prior record of abuse, and many children do not disclose past abuse until they feel safe. For this reason, kinship caregivers or foster or adoptive parents are sometimes the first to learn that sexual abuse has occurred. Even when there is no documentation of prior abuse, you may suspect something happened because of your child's behavior.

There are no hard and fast rules about what constitutes normal sexual development and what behaviors might signal sexual abuse. Children show a range of sexual behaviors and sexual curiosity at each developmental level, and their curiosity, interest, and experimentation may occur gradually, based on their development. However, children who have been sexually abused may demonstrate behaviors that are unusual, excessive, aggressive, or explicit. There is no one specific sign or behavior that can be considered proof that sexual abuse has definitively occurred, but there are a number of signs that are suggestive of abuse. The following signs or symptoms may suggest the possibility of child sexual abuse:

- Explicit sexual knowledge beyond the child's developmental stage

- Sexual preoccupation indicated by language, drawings, or behaviors

- Inserting toys or other objects in genital openings

- Sexual behaviors with other children that seem unusual, aggressive, or unresponsive to limits or redirection

- Excessive masturbation, sometimes in public, not responsive to redirection or limits

- Pain, itching, redness, or bleeding in the genital areas

- Nightmares, trouble sleeping, or fear of the dark

- Sudden or extreme mood swings: rage, fear, anger, excessive crying, or withdrawal

- "Spacing out" or appearing to be in trance

- Loss of appetite, or difficulty eating or swallowing

- Cutting, burning, or other self-mutilating behaviors

- Unexplained avoidance of certain people, places, or activities

- An older child behaving like a much younger child: wetting the bed or sucking a thumb, for example

- Talking about a new, older friend

- Suddenly having money

This list of signs and symptoms is simply that: red flags designed to alert you to the fact that the child's behaviors may reflect an underlying problem. There are other possible explanations for some of these signs, and they need to be evaluated by a trained professional who specializes in child sexual abuse.

Healthy Sexual Development in Children

Children's sexual interest, curiosity, and behaviors develop gradually over time and may be influenced by many factors, including what children see and experience and the guidance they receive from parents and caretakers. The presence of sexual behavior is not in and of itself a conclusive sign that abuse has occurred.

Preschool (0 to 5 years)

Common:

- Sexual language relating to differences in body parts, bathroom talk, pregnancy, and birth

- Self-fondling at home and in public

- Showing and looking at private body parts

Uncommon:

- Discussion of sexual acts

- Sexual contact experiences with other children

- Masturbation unresponsive to redirection or limits

- Inserting objects in genital openings

School Age (6 to 12 years)

Common:

- Questions about menstruation, pregnancy, sexual behavior
- "Experimenting" with same-age children, including kissing, fondling, exhibitionism, and role-playing
- Masturbation at home or other private places

Uncommon

- Discussion of explicit sexual acts
- Asking adults or peers to participate in explicit sexual acts
- Masturbating in public or excessively to bleeding

Adolescence (13 to 16 years)

Common:

- Questions about decision-making, social relationships, and sexual customs
- Masturbation in private
- Experimenting between adolescents of the same age, including open-mouth kissing, fondling, and body rubbing
- Voyeuristic behaviors
- Sexual intercourse (more than half of 11th graders)
- Oral sex (approximately one-third of 15-17 year olds)

Uncommon

- Sexual interest in much younger children
- Aggression in touching others' genitals
- Asking adults to participate in explicit sexual acts
- The use of force, aggression, or drugs to obtain compliance

Factors Affecting the Impact of Sexual Abuse

If a professional has determined that a child in your care has been a victim of sexual abuse, or if you continue to suspect that the child in your care has been abused, it is important to understand how abusive experiences may affect children's behavior.

All children who have been sexually abused have had their physical and emotional boundaries violated or crossed in some way. Because of this, children may feel a lack of trust and safety with others. Children who have been abused may come to view the world as unsafe, and adults as manipulative and untrustworthy. As with other types of abuse or trauma, many factors influence how children think and feel about the abuse, how the abuse affects them, and how their recovery progresses. Some factors that can affect the impact of abuse or trauma include:

- The relationship of the abuser to the child and how much the abuse caused a betrayal of trust within an important interpersonal relationship

- How long the abuse occurred (chronicity)

- Whether the sexual abuse was extensive and there was penetration of some kind

- The age of the child (younger children are more vulnerable and less capable of facing these challenges alone)

- The abuser's use of "friendliness" or seduction and efforts to make the child a compliant participant

- The abuser's use of threats of harm or violence, including threats to pets, siblings, or parents

- The abuser's use of secrecy and threats to do harm or withdraw love and affection

- Gender of the abuser being the same as or different from the child (some children are less likely to report sexual activity with same gender after the fact, and those observing or assessing for abuse may have a stronger reaction to same-sex abuse than to abuse that is male-female)

- The child's emotional and social development at the time of the abuse

- The child's ability to cope with his or her emotional and physical responses to the abuse (for example, fear and arousal)

- How much responsibility the child feels for the abuse (and, for example, not telling right away, not stopping it somehow, etc.)

It is very important for children to understand that they are not to blame for the abuse they experienced. Your family's immediate

444

response to learning about the sexual abuse and ongoing acceptance of what the child has told you will play a critical role in your child's ability to recover and lead a healthy life.

Some parents may feel grave concern when children act out sexually with peers or younger children and may question why a child who has been abused, and suffered from that experience, could repeat it with someone else. Children who have experienced sexual abuse need an opportunity to process their own abuse in therapy or with a trusted trained adult to understand their thoughts and feelings and to have a chance to ask questions and achieve some kind of closure. Acting-out behaviors usually indicate that some traumatic impact of their abuse is still active and signals a need for additional attention. Responding in calm, informed ways while seeking appropriate professional help for children whose acting out persists will be important to resolving children's sexual behavior problems. The most important lesson is learning not to over- or under-respond to problem situations and finding just the right balance of guidance and empathic care.

If your child has a history of prior abuse, it's important to know that he or she may be vulnerable to acting out victim or victimizing behaviors. Some children may be more likely to be bullied or exploited, and others may be angry and aggressive towards others. You may need to pay special attention to protecting some children while setting firm limits on others. In addition, some children act out when memories of their own abuse are triggered. Triggers can happen unexpectedly, for example, by seeing someone who looks like the abuser or in a situation such as being alone in a public restroom, or by a variety of circumstances that occur in daily life. Other triggers might include the scent of a particular cologne or shampoo or the texture of a particular piece of clothing or blanket.

In addition, there are cultural differences among children with regard to their comfort level with physical proximity, physical affection, bathing and nudity practices, hygiene, and other factors that can lead to problem situations. There are many cultures in which parents never discuss sexuality directly with their children, or in which any type of sexual activity (for example, children touching themselves) can be viewed as unacceptable or punishable. Children may thus carry shame and guilt about their bodies.

Establishing Family Guidelines for Safety and Privacy

There are things you can do to help ensure that any child visiting or living in your home experiences a structured, safe, and nurturing environment. Some children who have been sexually abused may have a heightened sensitivity to certain situations. Making your home a comfortable place for children who have been sexually abused can mean changing some habits or patterns of family life. Incorporating some of these guidelines may also help reduce foster or adoptive parents' vulnerability to abuse allegations by children living with them. Consider whether the following tips may be helpful in your family's situation:

- **Make sure every family member's comfort level with touching, hugging, and kissing is respected.** Do not force touching on children who seem uncomfortable being touched. Encourage children to respect the comfort and privacy of others.

- **Be cautious with playful touch, such as play fighting and tickling.** These may be uncomfortable or scary reminders of sexual abuse to some children.

- **Help children learn the importance of privacy.** Remind children to knock before entering bathrooms and bedrooms, and encourage children to dress and bathe themselves if they are able. Teach children about privacy and respect by modeling this behavior and talking about it openly.

- **Keep adult sexuality private.** Teenage siblings may need reminders about what is permitted in your home when boyfriends and girlfriends are present. Adult caretakers will also need to pay special attention to intimacy and sexuality when young children with a history of sexual abuse are underfoot.

- **Be aware of and limit sexual messages received through the media.** Children who have experienced sexual abuse can find sexual content overstimulating or disturbing. It may be helpful to monitor music and music videos, as well as television programs, video games, and movies containing nudity, sexual activity, or sexual language. Limit access to grownup magazines and monitor children's Internet use. In addition, limit violent graphic or moving images in TV or video games.

- **Supervise and monitor children's play.** If you know that your child has a history of sexual abuse, it will be important to supervise and monitor his or her play with siblings or other children in your home. This means having children play within your view and not allowing long periods of time when children are unsupervised. Children may have learned about sexual abuse from others and may look for times to explore these activities with other children if left unsupervised. It will be important for parents and caretakers to be cautious but avoid feeling paranoid.

- **Prepare and develop comfort with language about sexual boundaries.** It will be important for you to be proactive in developing and practicing responses to children who exhibit sexual behavior problems. Many parents feel uncomfortable addressing the subject so they ignore or avoid direct discussions. For example, some parents are able to say, "Your private parts belong to you, and it's okay to touch them in private." Some parents hesitate to give this kind of permission, believing it's sinful behavior. In those cases, you might want to deliver different messages. When children have been abused, you can say, "Just like it was not okay for so-and-so to touch your private parts, it's not okay for you to touch other people's private parts." You might also give clear directives, "We don't use that language in this house," if it's offensive, or "I'd like you to use different words so that we can really hear what you're saying." Because there are so many differences in the messages parents want to convey to their children, it is useful to prepare ahead and be proactive.

If your child has touching problems (or any sexually aggressive behaviors), you may need to take additional steps to help ensure safety for your child as well as his or her peers. Consider how these tips may apply to your own situation:

- **With friends.** If your child has known issues with touching other children, you will need to ensure supervision when he or she is playing with friends, whether at your home or theirs. Sleepovers may not be a good idea when children have touching problems.

- **At school.** You may wish to inform your child's school of any inappropriate sexual behavior, to ensure an appropriate level of supervision. Often this information can be kept confidential by a school counselor or other personnel.

- **In the community.** Supervision becomes critical any time children with sexual behavior problems are with groups of children, for example, at day camp or after school programs.

Keep the lines of communication open, so children feel more comfortable turning to you with problems and talking with you about anything—not just sexual abuse. Remember, however, that sexual abuse is difficult for most children to disclose even to a trusted adult and that, ordinarily, children do not volunteer information about their sexual development.

Seeking Help

Responding to the needs of a child who has been sexually abused may involve the whole family and will likely have an impact on all family relationships. Mental health professionals (for example, counselors, therapists, or social workers) can help you and your family cope with reactions, thoughts, and feelings about the abuse. It is important to seek a behavioral health professional with a background in child development, child trauma, and sexual abuse. Before agreeing to work with a particular provider, ask questions about the person's background, experience, and approach to treating children.

Impact of Sexual Abuse on the Family

Being a kinship caregiver or a foster or adoptive parent to a child who has experienced sexual abuse can be stressful to marriages and relationships. Parenting in these situations may require some couples to be more open with each other and their children about sexuality in general and sexual problems specifically. If one parent is more involved in addressing the issue than another, the imbalance can create difficulties in the parental relationship. A couple's sexual relationship can also be affected, if sex begins to feel like a troubled area of the family's life. If and when these problems emerge, it is often helpful to get professional advice.

In addition, if one parent was more in favor of adopting, and the other parent merely complied, general stress can be added to the couple when children have a range of problem behaviors that require attention. Some parents develop resentful and angry or withdrawn feelings toward foster or adoptive children who take up a lot of time and energy (for example, children who need extra monitoring and supervision or transport to weekly therapy appointments)

Parents can also feel stress because the child's siblings (birth, foster, or adoptive) may be exposed to new or focused attention on sexuality that can be challenging for them. If one child is acting out sexually, you may need to talk with siblings about what they see, think, and feel, as well as how to respond. Children may also need to be coached on what (and how much) to say about their sibling's problems to their friends.

If your children see that you are actively managing the problem, they will feel more secure and will worry less.

When one child has been sexually abused, parents often become very protective of their other children. It is important to find a balance between reasonable worry and overprotectiveness. Useful strategies to prevent further abuse may include teaching children to stand up for themselves, talking with them about being in charge of their bodies, and fostering open communication with your children.

Counseling for Parents and Children

Talking with a mental health professional who specializes in child sexual abuse as soon as problems arise can help parents determine if their children's behavior is cause for concern. Specialists can also provide parents with guidance in responding to their children's difficulties and offer suggestions for how to talk with their children. A mental health professional may suggest special areas of attention in family life and offer specific suggestions for creating structured, safe, and nurturing environments.

To help a child who has been abused, many mental health professionals will begin with a thorough assessment to explore how the child functions in all areas of life. The specialist will want to know about:

- Past stressors (e.g., history of abuse, frequent moves, and other losses)

- Current stressors (e.g., a medical problem or learning disability)

- Emotional state (e.g., Is the child usually happy or anxious?)

- Coping strategies (e.g., Does the child withdraw or act out when angry or sad?)

- The child's friendships

- The child's strengths (e.g., Is the child creative, athletic, organized?)

- The child's communication skills

- The child's attachments to adults in his or her life

- How the child spends his or her time and how much time he or she spends with TV, Internet, video games, etc.

After a thorough assessment, the mental health professional will decide if the child and family could benefit from therapy. Not all children who have been abused require therapy. For those who do, the mental health professional will develop a plan tailored to the child and to the family's strengths and needs. This plan may include one or more of the following types of therapy:

- **Individual therapy.** The frequency and duration of therapy can vary tremendously. The style of therapy will depend on the child's age and the therapist's training. Some therapists use creative techniques (for example, art, play, and music therapy) to help children who are uncomfortable talking about their experiences. Other therapists use traditional talk therapy or a combination of approaches. All types of individual therapy that are evidence-based also include a component for family or parent engagement.

- **Group therapy.** Meeting in groups with other children who have been sexually abused or who have developed sexual behavior problems can help children understand themselves; feel less alone (by interacting with others who have had similar experiences); and learn new skills through role plays, discussion, games, and play. Group therapy for parents can also be extremely beneficial.

- **Family therapy.** Many therapists will see children and parents together to support positive parent-child communication and to guide parents in learning new skills that will help their children feel better and behave appropriately.

Whether or not family therapy is advised, it is vital for parents to stay involved in their child's therapy or other kinds of treatment. Skilled mental health professionals will always seek to involve the parents by asking for and sharing information.

Your Child Welfare Agency

If you are a kinship caregiver or foster parent, or if you are seeking to adopt a child, you may wish to talk with your social worker about what you discover about your child's history and any behaviors that worry you. Sharing your concerns will help your social worker help you and your family. If your child exhibits problem sexual behaviors toward other children, be aware that you may also be required to report these to child protective services in order to comply with mandated reporting laws in your jurisdiction.

Many adoptive parents also call their local child welfare agency to seek advice if their child shows troubling behaviors. Child welfare workers are often good sources of information, can offer advice, and are familiar with community resources. Adoption agencies may also be able to provide additional post adoption services or support to adoptive parents who find out about their child's history of sexual abuse after the adoption is finalized.

What to Look for in a Mental Health Professional

Finding a knowledgeable and experienced mental health professional is key to getting the help your family needs. Some communities have special programs for treating children who have been sexually abused, such as child protection teams and child advocacy centers. You may also find qualified specialists in your community through the organizations noted below.

- Child advocacy centers

- Rape crisis or sexual assault centers

- Local psychological or psychiatric association referral services

- Child abuse hotlines

- Information Gateway's *Selecting and Working With a Therapist Skilled in Adoption*

- Child protective services (CPS) agencies.

- The National Child Traumatic Stress Network maintains a list of its members that specialize in research and/or treatment

- Nonprofit service providers serving families of missing or exploited children

- University departments of social work, psychology, or psychiatry

- Crime victim assistance programs in the law enforcement agency or in the prosecutor's or district attorney's office

- Group private practices with a specialization in trauma services

- Family court services, including court-appointed special advocate (CASA) groups or guardians *ad litem*

- American Academy of Child & Adolescent Psychiatry

- American Psychological Association (APA)

Therapy for children who have been sexually abused is specialized work. When selecting a mental health professional, look for the following:

- An advanced degree in a recognized mental health specialty such as psychiatry (M.D.), psychology (Ph.D. or Psy.D.), social work (M.S.W.), counseling (L.P.C.), Marriage and Family Therapy (M.F.T.), or psychiatric nursing (R.N.)

- Licensure to practice as a mental health professional in your State (Some mental health services are provided by students under the supervision of licensed professionals.)

- Special training in child sexual abuse, including the dynamics of abuse, how it affects children and adults, and the use of goal-oriented treatment plans

- Knowledge about the legal issues involved in child sexual abuse, especially the laws about reporting child sexual victimization, procedures used by law enforcement and protective services, evidence collection, and expert testimony in your State

- A willingness to work in a coordinated fashion with other professionals involved in your family's care

Part Seven

Additional Help and Information

Chapter 48

Glossary of Terms Related to Child Abuse

abandonment: A situation in which the child has been left by the parent(s), the parent's identity or whereabouts are unknown, the child suffers serious harm, or the parent has failed to maintain contact with the child or to provide reasonable support for a specified period of time.

abusive head trauma: A term used to describe the constellation of signs and symptoms resulting from violent shaking or shaking and impacting of the head of an infant or small child.

adoption: The social, emotional, and legal process through which children who will not be raised by their birth parents become full and permanent legal members of another family while maintaining genetic and psychological connections to their birth family.

adoption services: Services or activities provided to assist in bringing about the adoption of a child.

adoptive parent: A person with the legal relation of parent to a child not related by birth, with the same mutual rights and obligations that exist between children and their birth parents.

alcohol abuse: Compulsive use of alcohol that is not of a temporary nature. Applies to infants addicted at birth, or who are victims of fetal

---

This glossary contains terms excerpted from documents produced by several sources deemed reliable.

alcohol syndrome, or who may suffer other disabilities due to the use of alcohol during pregnancy.

alcohol-related birth defects: Physical or cognitive deficits in a child that result from maternal alcohol consumption during pregnancy. This includes but is not limited to fetal alcohol syndrome.

alleged perpetrator: An individual who reports an alleged incident of child abuse or neglect in which he/she caused or knowingly allowed the maltreatment of a child.

assessment: The ongoing practice of informing decision-making by identifying, considering, and weighing factors that impact children, youth, and their families. Assessment occurs from the time children and families come to the attention of the child welfare system and continues until case closure.

behavior problem: Behavior of the child in the school and/or community that adversely affects socialization, learning, growth, and moral development. May include adjudicated or non-adjudicated behavior problems. Includes running away from home or a placement.

behavioral health: A state of mental/emotional being and/or choices and actions that affect wellness. Substance abuse and misuse, as well as serious psychological distress, suicide, and mental illness, are examples of some behavioral health problems.

biological parent: The birth mother or father of the child rather than the adoptive or foster parent or the stepparent.

birth mother: An individual's biological mother, after an adoption has occurred. Prior to an adoption decision and legal adoption, birth mother is referred to as a pregnant woman, or expectant mother.

birth parent: An individual's biological mother or father, after an adoption has occurred. Prior to an adoption decision and legal adoption, birth parents are referred to as a child's parents or expectant parents.

bonding: The process of developing lasting emotional ties with one's immediate caregivers; seen as the first and primary developmental achievement of a human being and central to a person's ability to relate to others throughout life.

caregiver: One who provides for the physical, emotional, and social needs of a dependent person. The term most often applies to parents or parent surrogates, child care and nursery workers, health-care specialists, and relatives caring for children, elderly, or ill family members.

case management: Coordination and monitoring of services on behalf of a client. In general, the role of the case manager does not involve the provision of direct services but the monitoring of services to assure that they are relevant to the client, delivered in a useful way, and effective in meeting the goals of the case plan. A key element of case management in child welfare is the ongoing assessment of the client's needs and progress in services.

child: A person less than 18 years of age or considered to be a minor under state law.

child abuse and neglect: Defined by the Child Abuse Prevention and Treatment Act (CAPTA) as any recent act or failure to act on the part of a parent or caretaker that results in death, serious physical or emotional harm, sexual abuse, or exploitation, or an act or failure to act that presents an imminent risk of serious harm. Child abuse and neglect are defined by federal and state laws.

Child Abuse Prevention and Treatment Act (CAPTA): The key Federal legislation addressing child abuse and neglect.

child protective services (CPS): The social services agency designated (in most states) to receive reports, conduct investigations and assessments, and provide intervention and treatment services to children and families in which child maltreatment has occurred. Frequently, this agency is located within larger public social service agencies, such as departments of social services.

child victim: A child for whom an incident of abuse or neglect has been substantiated or indicated by an investigation or assessment. A state may include some children with other dispositions as victims.

comprehensive family assessment: The ongoing practice of informing decision-making by identifying, considering, and weighing factors that impact children, youth, and their families. Assessment occurs from the time children and families come to the attention of the child welfare system (or before) and continues until case closure.

corporal punishment: Inflicting physical pain for the purpose of punishment in an effort to discipline a child.

counseling services: Beneficial activities that apply the therapeutic processes to personal, family, situational or occupational problems in order to bring about a positive resolution of the problem or improved individual or family functioning or circumstances.

court action: Legal action initiated by a representative of the CPS agency on behalf of the child. This includes, for instance, authorization

457

to place the child, filing for temporary custody, dependency, or termination of parental rights. It does not include criminal proceedings against a perpetrator.

court-appointed special advocate (CASA): A person, usually a volunteer appointed by the court, who serves to ensure that the needs and interests of a child in child protection judicial proceedings are fully protected.

custody: Refers to the legal right to make decisions about children, including where they live. Parents have legal custody of their children unless they voluntarily give custody to someone else or a court takes this right away and gives it to someone else. For instance, a court may give legal custody to a relative or to a child welfare agency. Whoever has legal custody can enroll the children in school, give permission for medical care, and give other legal consents.

cycle of abuse: A generational pattern of abusive behavior that can occur when children who have either experienced maltreatment or witnessed violence between their parents or caregivers learn violent behavior and learn to consider it appropriate.

developmental disability: A diverse group of severe chronic conditions caused by mental and/or physical impairments. People with developmental disabilities may have problems with major life activities such as language, mobility, learning, self-help, and independent living.

discipline: Training that develops self-control, self-sufficiency, and orderly conduct. Discipline is based on respect for an individual's capability and is not to be confused with punishment.

domestic violence: A pattern of assaultive and/or coercive behaviors, including physical, sexual, and psychological attacks, as well as economic coercion, that adults or adolescents use against their intimate partners. Intimate partners include spouses, sexual partners, parents, children, siblings, extended family members, and dating relationships.

drug abuse: Compulsive use of drugs that is not of a temporary nature. Applies to infants addicted at birth.

educational neglect: Failure to ensure that a child's educational needs are met. Such neglect may involve permitting chronic truancy, failure to enroll a child in school, or inattention to special education needs.

emotional maltreatment: Type of maltreatment that refers to acts or omissions, other than physical abuse or sexual abuse, that caused, or could have caused, conduct, cognitive, affective, or other mental disorders. Includes emotional neglect, psychological abuse, mental injury, etc. Frequently occurs as verbal abuse or excessive demands on a child's performance and may cause the child to have a negative self-image and disturbed behavior.

emotional neglect: Failure to provide adequate nurturing and affection or the refusal/delay in ensuring that a child receives needed treatment for emotional or behavioral problems. Emotional neglect may also involve exposure to chronic or extreme domestic violence.

family: A group of two or more persons related by birth, marriage, adoption, or emotional ties.

family preservation services: Short-term, family-focused, and community-based services designed to help families cope with significant stresses or problems that interfere with their ability to nurture their children. The goal of family preservation services (FPS) is to maintain children with their families or to reunify the family, whenever it can be done safely. These services are applicable to families at risk of disruption/out-of-home placement across systems and may be provided to different types of families—birth or biological families, kinship families, foster families, and adoptive families—to help them address major challenges, stabilize the family, and enhance family functioning.

fetal alcohol spectrum disorders (FASD): A group of conditions that can occur in a person whose mother drank alcohol during pregnancy. These effects can include physical problems and problems with behavior and learning. Often, a person with an FASD has a mix of these problems.

foster care: Twenty-four-hour substitute care for children placed away from their parents or guardians and for whom the state agency has placement and care responsibility. This includes, but is not limited to, family foster homes, foster homes of relatives, group homes, emergency shelters, residential facilities, child care institutions, and pre-adoptive homes regardless of whether the facility is licensed and whether payments are made by the state or local agency for the care of the child, or whether there is federal matching of any payments made.

foster children: Child who has been placed in the state's or county's legal custody because the child's custodial parents/guardians are unable to provide a safe family home due to abuse, neglect, or an inability to care for the child.

foster parent: Individual licensed to provide a home for orphaned, abused, neglected, delinquent or disabled children, usually with the approval of the government or a social service agency. May be a relative or a non-relative.

group home: Residence intended to meet the needs of children who are unable to live in a family setting and do not need a more intensive residential service. Homes normally house 4–12 children in a setting that offers the potential for the full use of community resources, including employment, health care, education, and recreational opportunities. Desired outcomes of group home programs include full incorporation of the child into the community, return of the child to his or her family or other permanent family, and/or acquisition by the child of the skills necessary for independent living.

guardian ad litem (GAL): A lawyer or layperson who represents a child in juvenile or family court. Usually this person considers the best interest of the child and may perform a variety of roles, including those of independent investigator, advocate, advisor, and guardian for the child. A layperson who serves in this role is sometimes known as a court-appointed special advocate (CASA).

guardianship: The transfer of parental responsibility and legal authority for a minor child to an adult caregiver who intends to provide permanent care for the child. This can be done without terminating the parental rights of the child's parents. Transferring legal responsibility removes the child from the child welfare system, allows the caregiver to make important decisions on the child's behalf, and establishes a long-term caregiver for the child. In subsidized guardianship, the guardian is provided with a monthly subsidy for the care and support of the child.

inadequate housing: A risk factor related to substandard, over-crowded, or unsafe housing conditions, including homelessness.

incest: Sexual intercourse between persons who are closely related by blood. In the United States, incest is prohibited by many state laws as well as cultural tradition.

intervention: An action intended to modify an outcome; a set of techniques and therapies practiced in counseling.

investigation: The gathering and assessment of objective information to determine if a child has been or is at risk of being maltreated. Generally includes face-to-face contact with the victim and results in a disposition as to whether the alleged report is substantiated or not.

juvenile and family court: Court that specializes in areas such as child maltreatment, domestic violence, juvenile delinquency, divorce, child custody, and child support. These courts were established in most states to resolve conflict and to otherwise intervene in the lives of families in a manner that promotes the best interest of children.

juvenile delinquency: A federal criminal violation committed prior to one's eighteenth birthday.

kinship care: Kinship care is the full time care, nurturing, and protection of a child by relatives, members of their tribe or clan, godparents, stepparents, or any adult who has a kinship bond with the child. This definition is designed to be inclusive and respectful of cultural values and ties of affection. It allows a child to grow to adulthood in a family environment.

learning disability: A disorder in basic psychological processes involved in understanding or using language, spoken or written, that may manifest itself in an imperfect ability to listen, think, speak, read, write, spell or use mathematical calculations. The term includes conditions such as perceptual disability, brain injury, minimal brain dysfunction, dyslexia, and developmental aphasia.

maltreatment: An act or failure to act by a parent, caretaker, or other person as defined under state law which results in physical abuse, neglect, medical neglect, sexual abuse, emotional abuse, or an act or failure to act which presents an imminent risk of serious harm to a child.

mandated reporter: Individuals required by state statutes to report suspected child abuse and neglect to the proper authorities (usually child protective services or law enforcement agencies). Mandated reporters typically include educators and other school personnel, health-care and mental health professionals, social workers, child care providers, and law enforcement officers or others who have frequent contact with children and families. Some states identify all citizens as mandated reporters.

medical neglect: A type of maltreatment caused by failure by the caretaker to provide for the appropriate health care of the child although financially able to do so, or offered financial or other means to do so.

mental health services: Beneficial activities which aim to overcome issues involving emotional disturbance or maladaptive behavior adversely affecting socialization, learning, or development. Usually provided by public or private mental health agencies and includes both residential and non-residential activities.

nurturance: Behaviors and activities that further the growth and development of another person, family, group, or community.

out-of-home care: Also called foster care, including family foster care, kinship care, treatment foster care, and residential and group care. Out-of-home care encompasses the placements and services provided to children and families when children must be removed from their homes because of child safety concerns, as a result of serious parent-child conflict, or to treat serious physical or behavioral health conditions that cannot be addressed within the family. (See Out-of-Home Care).

parent: The birth mother/father, adoptive mother/father, or step mother/father of the child.

parent-child interaction therapy (PCIT): A family-centered treatment approach proven effective for abused and at-risk children ages 2 to 12 and their biological or foster caregivers. A key activity is the therapist's role in coaching the parent to interact more positively with the child.

parental rights: The legal rights and corresponding legal obligations that go along with being the parent of a child.

perpetrator: The person who has been determined to have caused or knowingly allowed the maltreatment of the child.

physical abuse: Child abuse that results in physical injury to a child. This may include, burning, hitting, punching, shaking, kicking, beating, or otherwise harming a child. Although an injury resulting from physical abuse is not accidental, the parent or caregiver may not have intended to hurt the child. The injury may have resulted from severe discipline, including injurious spanking, or physical punishment that is inappropriate to the child's age or condition. The injury may be the result of a single episode or of repeated episodes and can range in severity from minor marks and bruising to death.

physical neglect: Failure to provide for a child's basic survival needs, such as nutrition, clothing, shelter, hygiene, and medical care. Physical neglect may also involve inadequate supervision of a child and other forms of reckless disregard of the child's safety and welfare.

prenatal substance exposure: Fetal exposure to maternal drug and alcohol use that can significantly increase the risk for developmental and neurological disabilities in the child. The effects can cause severe neurological damage and growth retardation in the substance-exposed newborn.

preventive services: Beneficial activities aimed at preventing child abuse and neglect. Such activities may be directed at specific populations identified as being at increased risk of becoming abusive and may be designed to increase the strength and stability of families, to increase parents' confidence and competence in their parenting abilities, and to afford children a stable and supportive environment.

protective custody: A form of custody required to remove a child from his or her home and place in out-of-home care. Law enforcement may place a child in protective custody based on an independent determination that the child's health, safety, and welfare is jeopardized.

protective factor: Strengths and resources that appear to mediate or serve as a buffer against risk factors that contribute to maltreatment. These factors may strengthen the parent-child relationships, ability to cope with stress, and capacity to provide for children. Protective factors include nurturing and attachment, knowledge of parenting and of child and youth development, parental resilience, social connections, and concrete supports for parents.

relinquishment: Voluntary termination or release of all parental rights and duties that legally frees a child to be adopted. This is sometimes referred to as a surrender or as making an adoption plan for one's child.

resilience: The ability to adapt well to adversity, trauma, tragedy, threats, or even significant sources of stress. Parental resilience is considered a protective factor in child abuse and neglect prevention. Resilience in children enables them to thrive, mature, and increase competence in the midst of adverse circumstances. Resilience can be fostered and developed in children as it involves behaviors, thoughts, and actions that can be learned over time and is impacted by positive and healthy relationships with parents, caregivers, and other adults.

respite care: Child care offered for designated periods of time to allow a caregiver to tend to other family members; alleviate a work, job, health, or housing crisis; or take a break from the stress of caring for a seriously ill child. Respite for foster and adoptive parents is a preventive measure that enhances quality of care for the child, gives the caregiver a deserved and necessary break, and ensures healthy and stable placements for children.

risk: In child welfare, the likelihood that a child will be maltreated in the future. A risk assessment is a measure of the likelihood that a child will be maltreated in the future, frequently through the use of checklists, matrices, scales, and other methods of measurement.

risk factor: Behaviors and conditions present in the child, parent, or family that will likely contribute to child maltreatment occurring in the future. Major risk factors include substance abuse, domestic/family violence, and mental health problems.

safe haven: When applied to legislation, refers to the policy in which a parent can relinquish a child, usually a newborn, to lawfully designated places such as a hospital. When a child is surrendered in this way, the parent is protected from criminal prosecution. The scope and specifications of the rule vary widely across the states.

safety plan: A casework document developed when it is determined that a child is in imminent or potential risk of serious harm. In the safety plan, the caseworker targets the factors that are causing or contributing to the risk of imminent serious harm to the child and identifies, along with the family, the interventions that will control the safety factors and assure the child's protection.

sexual abuse: According to the Child Abuse Prevention and Treatment Act (CAPTA), the employment, use, persuasion, inducement, enticement, or coercion of any child to engage in, or assist any other person to engage in, any sexually explicit conduct or simulation of such conduct for the purpose of producing a visual depiction of such conduct; or the rape, and in cases of caretaker or interfamilial relationships, statutory rape, molestation, prostitution, or other form of sexual exploitation of children, or incest with children.

shaken baby syndrome: The collection of signs and symptoms resulting from the violent shaking of an infant or small child. The consequences of less severe cases may not be brought to the attention of medical professionals and may never be diagnosed. In severe cases that usually result in death or severe neurological consequences, the child usually becomes immediately unconscious and suffers rapidly escalating, life-threatening central nervous system dysfunction.

sibling abuse: The physical, emotional, or sexual maltreatment of a child by a brother or sister.

substance abuse services: Beneficial activities designed to deter, reduce, or eliminate substance abuse or chemical dependency.

substantiated: An investigation disposition concluding that the allegation of child maltreatment or risk of maltreatment was supported or founded by state law or state policy. A child protective services determination means that credible evidence exists that child abuse or neglect has occurred.

Temporary Assistance for Needy Families (TANF): A program that provides assistance and work opportunities to needy families by granting states the federal funds and wide flexibility to develop and implement their own welfare programs. The focus of the program is to help move recipients into work and to turn welfare into a program of temporary assistance.

unsubstantiated: Not substantiated. An investigation disposition that determines that there is not sufficient evidence under state law or policy to conclude that a child has been maltreated or is at risk of maltreatment. A child protective services determination means that credible evidence does not exist that child abuse or neglect has occurred.

visitation: Scheduled contact among a child in out-of-home care and his or her family members. The purpose of visitation is to maintain family attachments, reduce the sense of abandonment that children may experience during placement, and prepare for permanency.

well-being: The result of meeting a child's educational, emotional, and physical and mental health needs. Well-being is achieved when families have the capacity to provide for the needs of their children or when families are receiving the support and services needed to adequately meet the needs of their children.

youth development: A process that prepares young people to meet the challenges of adolescence and adulthood through a coordinated, progressive series of activities and experiences that help them to become socially, morally, emotionally, physically, and cognitively competent.

Chapter 49

Where to Report Child Abuse

The chapter includes a list of state contact numbers for specific agencies designated to receive and investigate reports of suspected child abuse and neglect.

Alabama
Phone: 334-242-9500
Website: dhr.alabama.gov/services/Child_Protective_Services/Abuse_Neglect_Reporting.aspx
Additional information: Visit the website above for information on reporting or call Childhelp (800-422-4453) for assistance.

Alaska
Toll-Free: 800-478-4444
Website: dhss.alaska.gov/ocs/Pages/default.aspx

Arizona
Toll-Free: 888-SOS-CHILD (888-767-2445)
Website: dcs.az.gov/report-child-abuse-or-neglect

Information in this chapter was compiled from resources listed in "Related Organizations: State Child Abuse and Neglect Reporting Numbers," Child Welfare Information Gateway (www.childwelfare.gov) and other sources deemed reliable. All contact information was verified in May 2016.

Arkansas
Toll-Free: 800-482-5964
Website: humanservices.arkansas.gov/dcfs/Pages/
ChildProtectiveServices.aspx

California
Website: www.dss.cahwnet.gov/cdssweb/PG20.htm
Additional information: Visit the website above for information on reporting or call Childhelp (800-422-4453) for assistance.

Colorado
Phone: 303-866-5932
Website: www.colorado.gov/apps/cdhs/rral/volumeDetails.jsf
Additional information: Visit the website above for information on reporting or call Childhelp (800-833-9844) for assistance.

Connecticut
Toll-Free: 800-842-2288
Toll-Free TDD: 800-624-5518
Website: www.ct.gov/dcf/site/default.asp

Delaware
Toll-Free: 800-292-9582
Website: kids.delaware.gov/services/crisis.shtml

District of Columbia
Phone: 202-671-SAFE (202-671-7233)
Website: cfsa.dc.gov/service/report-child-abuse-and-neglect

Florida
Toll-Free: 800-96-ABUSE (800-962-2873)
Website: www.dcf.state.fl.us/abuse

Georgia
Website: dfcs.dhs.georgia.gov/child-abuse-neglect
Additional information: Visit the website above for information on reporting or call Childhelp (800-422-4453) for assistance.

Hawaii
Phone: 808-832-5300
Website: humanservices.hawaii.gov

Idaho
Toll-Free: 800-926-2588
TDD: 208-332-7205
Website: healthandwelfare.idaho.gov/Children/AbuseNeglect/
ChildProtectionContactPhoneNumbers/tabid/475/Default.aspx

Illinois
Toll-Free: 800-25-ABUSE (800-252-2873)
Phone: 217-785-4020
Website: www.state.il.us/dcfs/child/index.shtml

Indiana
Toll-Free: 800-800-5556
Website: www.in.gov/dcs/protection/dfcchi.html

Iowa
Toll-Free: 800-362-2178
Website: dhs.iowa.gov/report-abuse-and-fraud

Kansas
Toll-Free: 800-922-5330
Website: www.dcf.ks.gov/Pages/Default.aspx

Kentucky
Toll-Free: 877-KYSAFE1 (877-597-2331)
Website: chfs.ky.gov/dcbs/dpp/childsafety.htm

Louisiana
Toll-Free: 855-4LA-KIDS (855-452-5437)
Website: dss.louisiana.gov/index.
cfm?md=pagebuilder&tmp=home&pid=109

Maine
Toll-Free: 800-452-1999
Toll-Free TTY: 800-963-9490
Website: www.maine.gov/dhhs/ocfs/hotlines.htm

Maryland
Website: www.dhr.state.md.us/blog/?page_id=3957w

Additional information: Visit the website above for information on reporting or call Childhelp (800-422-4453) for assistance.

Massachusetts
Toll-Free: 800-792-5200
Website: www.mass.gov/eohhs/gov/departments/dcf/
child-abuse-neglect/

Michigan
Toll-Free: 855-444-3911
Website: www.michigan.gov/mdhhs/0,5885,7-339-
73971_7119_50648_7193---,00.html

Minnesota
Website: mn.gov/dhs/people-we-serve/children-and-families/services/
child-protection/index.jsp
Additional information: Visit the website above for information on reporting or call Childhelp (800-422-4453) for assistance.

Mississippi
Toll-Free: 800-222-8000
Phone: 601-432-4570
Website: www.mdhs.state.ms.us/report-child-abuseneglect/

Missouri
Toll-Free: 800-392-3738
Phone: 573-751-3448
Website: dss.mo.gov/cd/can.htm

Montana
Toll-Free: 866-820-5437
Website: www.dphhs.mt.gov/cfsd/index.shtml

Nebraska
Toll-Free: 800-652-1999
Website: dhhs.ne.gov/children_family_services/Pages/children_
family_services.aspx

Nevada
Toll-Free: 800-992-5757
Phone: 702-399-0081
Website: dcfs.nv.gov/Programs/CWS/CPS/CPS/

New Hampshire
Toll-Free: 800-894-5533
Phone: 603-271-6562
Toll-Free TDD: 800-735-2964
Fax: 603-271-6565 (Report Child Abuse Fax)
Website: www.dhhs.state.nh.us/dcyf/cps/contact.htm

New Jersey
Toll-Free: 877-NJ ABUSE (877-652-2873)
Toll-Free TDD/TTY: 800-835-5510
Website: www.nj.gov/dcf/about/divisions/dcpp/

New Mexico
Toll-Free: 855-333-SAFE (855-333-7233)
Website: cyfd.org/child-abuse-neglect

New York
Toll-Free: 800-342-3720
Phone: 518-473-7793
Toll-Free TDD/TTY: 800-638-5163
Website: www.ocfs.state.ny.us/main/cps

North Carolina
Website: www2.ncdhhs.gov/dss/cps/
Additional information: Visit the website above for information on reporting or call Childhelp (800-422-4453) for assistance.

North Dakota
Website: www.nd.gov/dhs/services/childfamily/cps/#reporting
Additional information: Visit the website above for information on reporting or call Childhelp (800-422-4453) for assistance.

Ohio
Website: jfs.ohio.gov/ocf/childprotectiveservices.stm
Additional information: Contact the county Public Children Services Agency or call Childhelp (800-422-4453) for assistance.

Oklahoma
Toll-Free: 800-522-3511
Website: www.okdhs.org/services/cps/Pages/default.aspx

Oregon
Website: www.oregon.gov/DHS/CHILDREN/CHILD-ABUSE/Pages/index.aspx

471

Additional information: Visit the website above for information on reporting or call Childhelp (800-422-4453) for assistance.

Pennsylvania
Toll-Free: 800-932-0313
Toll-Free TDD: 866-872-1677
Website: keepkidssafe.pa.gov/laws/index.htm

Puerto Rico
Toll-Free: 800-981-8333
Phone: 787-749-1333
Website (Spanish): www2.pr.gov/agencias/secretariado/Directorio/Pages/emergencia.aspx

Rhode Island
Toll-Free: 800-RI-CHILD (800-742-4453)
Website: www.dcyf.ri.gov/child_welfare/index.php

South Carolina
Phone: 803-898-7318
Website: dss.sc.gov/content/customers/protection/cps/ index.aspx
Additional information: Visit the website above for information on reporting or call Childhelp (800-422-4453) for assistance.

South Dakota
Website: dss.sd.gov/childprotection/
Additional information: Visit the website above for information on reporting or call Childhelp (800-422-4453) for assistance.

Tennessee
Toll-Free: 877-237-0004 or 877-54ABUSE (877-542-2873)
Website: www.tn.gov/dcs/article/report-child-abuse

Texas, Department of Family and Protective Services
Toll-Free: 800-252-5400
Toll-Free TTY: 800-735-2989
Website: www.dfps.state.tx.us/child_protection/

Utah
Toll-Free: 855-323-3237
Website: dcfs.utah.gov/

Vermont
Toll-Free: 800-649-5285
Website: dcf.vermont.gov/prevention

Virginia
Toll-Free: 800-552-7096
Phone: 804-786-8536
Website: www.dss.virginia.gov/family/cps/index.html

Washington
Toll-Free: 800-562-5624 or 866-END-HARM (866-363-4276)
Toll-Free TTY: 800-624-6186
Website: www1.dshs.wa.gov/ca/safety/abuseReport.asp?2

West Virginia
Toll-Free: 800-352-6513
Website: www.wvdhhr.org/report.asp

Wisconsin
Website: dcf.wisconsin.gov/children/CPS/cpswimap.htm
Additional information: Visit the website above for information on reporting or call Childhelp (800-422-4453) for assistance.

Wyoming
Website: dfsweb.wyo.gov/social-services/child-protective-services
Additional information: Visit the website above for information on reporting or call Childhelp (800-422-4453) for assistance.

Chapter 50

Directory of Organizations Dedicated to Promoting Healthy Families

Adult Survivors of Child Abuse
The Morris Center
P.O. Box 14477
San Francisco, CA 94114
Website: www.ascasupport.org
E-mail: info@ascasupport.com

Advocates for Youth
2000 M St. N.W., Ste. 750
Washington, DC 20036
Phone: 202-419-3420
Fax: 202-419-1448
Website: www.
advocatesforyouth.org

American Academy of Pediatrics
141 N.W. Point Blvd.
Elk Grove Village
IL 60007-1098
Toll-Free: 800-433-9016
Phone: 847-434-4000
Fax: 847-434-8000
Website: aap.org
E-mail: commun@aap.org

Resources in this chapter were compiled from several sources deemed reliable; all contact information was verified and updated in May 2016.

American Humane Association
1400 16th St. N.W., Ste. 360
Washington, DC 20036
Toll-Free: 800-227-4645
Phone: 303-792-9900
Fax: 303-792-5333
Website: www.americanhumane
.org
E-mail: info@americanhumane
.org

American Professional Society on the Abuse of Children
350 Poplar Ave.
Elmhurst, IL 60126
Toll-Free: 877-402-7722
Phone: 630-941-1235
Fax: 630-359-4274
Website: www.apsac.org
E-mail: apsac@apsac.org

Association for Play Therapy
3198 Willow Ave., Ste. 110
Clovis, CA 93612
Phone: 559-294-2128
Fax: 559-294-2129
Website: www.a4pt.org
E-mail: info@a4pt.org

Association for the Treatment of Sexual Abusers
4900 S.W. Griffith Dr., Ste. 274
Beaverton, OR 97005
Phone: 503-643-1023
Fax: 503-643-5084
Website: www.atsa.com
E-mail: atsa@atsa.com

Australian Institute of Family Studies
Level 20 S. Tower
485 La Trobe St.
Melbourne, Victoria 3000
Australia
Phone: +61 3 9214 7888
Fax: +61 3 9214 7839
Website: www.aifs.gov.au
E-mail: oma@act.gov.au

AVANCE, Inc.
National Headquarters, 118 N.
Medina
San Antonio, TX 78207
Phone: 210-270-4630
Fax: 210-270-4636
Website: www.avance.org
E-mail: info@avance.org

Center for Effective Discipline
327 Groveport Pike
Canal Winchester, OH 43110
Phone: 614-834-7946
Fax: 614-321-6308
Website: www.stophitting.org
E-mail: Info@StopHitting.org

Center for Violence and Injury Prevention
Washington University in St. Louis
CB 1007, 700 Rosedale Ave.
St. Louis, MO 63112
Phone: 314-935-8129
Fax: 858-966-8535
Website: cvip.wustl.edu/Pages/
Home.aspx
E-mail: bcvip@wustl.edu

Chadwick Center for Children and Families
3020 Children's Way, MC 5017
San Diego, CA 92123
Phone: 858-966-5814
Website: www.ChadwickCenter
.org
E-mail: chadwickcenter@rchsd.org

Chapel Hill Training-Outreach Project, Inc.
800 Eastowne Dr., Ste. 105
Chapel Hill, NC 27514
Phone: 919-490-5577
TDD: 919-490-5577
Fax: 919-490-4905
Website: chtop.org
E-mail: val@
coloradorespitecoalition.org

Child Abuse Prevention Network
Website: www.child-abuse.com

Child AbuseWatch.NET
One Child International, Inc.
590 S.W. 9th Terr., Ste. 2
Pompano Beach, FL 33069
Website (English): www
.abusewatch.net
E-mail: info@abusewatch.net

Child Lures Prevention
5166 Shelburne Rd.
Shelburne, VT 05482
Toll-Free: 800-552-2197
Phone: 802-985-8458
Fax: 802-985-8418
Website: www.
childluresprevention.com
E-mail: info@
childluresprevention.com

Child Molestation Research and Prevention Institute
2515 Santa Clara Ave., Ste. 208
Alameda, CA 94501
Phone: 510-740-1410
Website: www.
childmolestationprevention.org
E-mail: contact@
childmolestationprevention.org

Child Safe
St. Vincent's Center/Catholic
Charities
2600 Pot Spring Rd.
Timonium, MD 21093
Phone: 410-252-4000
Website: www
.childsafeeducation.com
E-mail: childsafe@
catholiccharities-md.org

Child Welfare Information Gateway
Children's Bureau/ACYF
1250 Maryland Ave. S.W.
Eighth Fl.
Washington, DC 20024
Toll-Free: 800-394-3366
Fax: 703-225-2357
Website: www.childwelfare.gov
E-mail: info@childwelfare.gov

Child Welfare League of America
1726 M St. N.W., Ste. 500
Washington, DC 20036
Phone: 202-688-4200
Fax: 202-833-1689
Website: www.cwla.org
E-mail: memberservices@cwla
.org

Childhelp USA
15757 N. 78th St., Ste. B
Scottsdale, AZ 85260
Toll-Free: 800-4-A-CHILD
(800-422-4453)
Phone: 480-922-8212
Toll-Free TDD: 800-2-A-CHILD
(800-222-4453)
Fax: 480-922-7061
Website: www.childhelp.org
E-mail: khackley@childhelp.org

Children Without a Voice USA
P.O. Box 4351
Alpharetta, GA 30023
Website: www.
childrenwithoutavoiceusa.org
E-mail: email@
childrenwithoutavoiceusa.org

Circle of Parents
2100 S. Marshall Blvd., Ste. 305
Chicago, IL 60623
Phone: 773-257-0111
Fax: 773-277-0715
Website: www.circleofparents
.org
E-mail: circleofparents@pcav
.org.

Committee for Children
2815 Second Ave., Ste. 400
Seattle, WA 98121
Toll-Free: 800-634-4449
Fax: 206-438-6765
Website: www.cfchildren.org
E-mail: clientsupport@
cfchildren.org

Cooperative Extension System, United States Department of Agriculture
National Institute of Food and
Agriculture
1400 Independence Ave. S.W.
Stop 2201
Washington, DC 20250-2201
Phone: 202-720-4423
Website: nifa.usda.gov/
Extension
E-mail: webcomments@csrees.
usda.gov

Court Appointed Special Advocates for Children
100 W.Harrison St., N. Tower
Ste. 500
Seattle, WA 98119
Toll-Free: 800-628-3233
Website: www.casaforchildren
.org
E-mail: executiveoffice@
casaforchildren.org

Crime Victims' Institute, College of Criminal Justice
Sam Houston State University
P.O. Box 2180
Huntsville, TX 77341-2180
Phone: 936-294-3100
Fax: 936-294-4296
Website: www.
crimevictimsinstitute.org
E-mail: crimevictims@shsu.edu

Darkness to Light
7 Radcliffe St., Ste. 200
Charleston, SC 29403
Toll-Free: 866-FOR-LIGHT
(866-367-5444)
Phone: 843-965-5444
Fax: 843-965-5449
Website: www.d2l.org/
E-mail: FacilitatorSupport@
D2L.org

Doris Duke Charitable
Foundation
650 Fifth Ave., 19th Fl.
New York, NY 10019
Phone: 212-974-7000
Fax: 212-974-7590
Website: www.ddcf.org
E-mail: webmaster@ddcf.org

Every Child Matters
Education Fund
1023 15th St. N.W., Ste. 401
Washington, DC 20005
Phone: 202-223-8177
Fax: 202-223-8499
Website: www.
everychildmatters.org
E-mail: info@everychildmatters
.org

FaithTrust Institute
2900 Eastlake Ave. E., Ste. 200
Seattle, WA 98102
Toll-Free: 877-860-2255
Phone: 206-634-1903
Fax: 206-634-0115
Website: www.
faithtrustinstitute.org
E-mail: info@faithtrustinstitute
.org

Family Life Development
Center
Cornell University
Beebe Hall
Ithaca, NY 14853-4401
Phone: 607-255-7794
Fax: 607-255-8562
Website: www.human.cornell.
edu/fldc
E-mail: fldc@cornell.edu

Fight Crime: Invest in Kids
1212 New York Ave N.W.
Ste. 300
Washington, DC 20005
Phone: 202-776-0027
Fax: 202-776-0110
Website: www.fightcrime.org
E-mail: info@fightcrime.org

Freddie Mac Foundation
8250 Jones Branch Dr.
MS A40
McLean, VA 22102-3110
Phone: 703-918-8888
Fax: 703-918-8895
Website: www.
freddiemacfoundation.org
E-mail: freddiemac_foundation@
freddiemac.com

Future of Children
267 Wallace Hall
Princeton University
Princeton, NJ 08544
Phone: 609-258-5894
Website: www.princeton.edu/
futureofchildren
E-mail: foc@princeton.edu

General Federation of Women's Clubs
1734 N St. N.W.
Washington, DC 20036-2990
Toll-Free: 800-443-4392
Phone: 202-347-3168
Fax: 202-835-0246
Website: www.gfwc.org
E-mail: gfwc@gfwc.org

Healthy Families America
200 S. Wabash, 10th Fl.
Chicago, IL 60604
Phone: 312-663-3520
Fax: 312-939-8962
Website:
healthyfamiliesamerica.org
E-mail: lcashion@
preventchildabuse.org

International Center for Assault Prevention (ICAP)
107 Gilbreth Pkwy, Ste. 200
Mullica Hill, NJ 08062
Toll-Free: 800-258-3189
Phone: 856-582-7000
Fax: 856-582-3588
Website: www.internationalcap.
org
E-mail: childassaultprevention@
gmail.com

International Initiative to End Child Labor
1016 S. Wayne St., Ste. 702
Arlington, VA 22204
Phone/Fax: 703-920-0435
Website: www.endchildlabor.org
E-mail: IIECL@endchildlabor
.org

International Society for Prevention of Child Abuse and Neglect
13123 E. 16th Ave., B390
Aurora, CO 80045-7106
Phone: 303-864-5220
Fax: 303-864-5222
Website: www.ispcan.org
E-mail: ispcan@ispcan.org

Jacob Wetterling Resource Center
2324 University Ave. W, Ste. 105
St. Paul, MN 55114
Toll-Free: 800-325-HOPE
(800-325-4673)
Phone: 651-714-4673
Fax: 651-714-9098
Website: www.
gundersenhealth.org/ncptc/
jacob-wetterling-resource-center
E-mail: volunteer-jwrc@
gundersenhealth.org

Kempe Foundation for the Prevention and Treatment of Child Abuse and Neglect
Anschutz Medical Campus, Gary Pavilion
13123 E. 16th Ave., B390
Aurora, CO 80045
Phone: 303-864-5250
Website (English): www.kempe
.org
E-mail: questions@kempe.org

Kidpower Teenpower Fullpower International
P.O. Box 1212
Santa Cruz, CA 95061
Toll-Free: 800-467-6997
Website: www.kidpower.org
E-mail: safety@kidpower.org

Liberty House
2685 4th St. NE
Salem, OR 97301
Phone: 503-540-0288
Website: libertyhousecenter.org
E-mail: kwolfer@
libertyhousecenter.org

Massachusetts Children's Trust Fund
55 Court St., 4th Fl.
Boston, MA 02108
Toll-Free: 888-775-4KID
(800-775-4543;
Massachusetts only)
Phone: 617-727-8957
Fax: 617-727-8997
Website (English): www
.onetoughjob.org
E-mail: info@mctf.org

Maternal Infant Health Outreach Worker Program
Center for Community Health
Solutions
Vanderbilt University, Stn. 17
Nashville, TN 37232-8180
Phone: 615-322-4184
Fax: 615-343-0325
Website: www.mihow.org
E-mail: mihow@vanderbilt.edu

National Alliance of Children's Trust and Prevention Funds
P.O. Box 15206
Seattle, WA 98115
Phone: 206-526-1221
Fax: 206-526-0220
Website: www.ctfalliance.org
E-mail: info@ctfalliance.org

National Association of State Mental Health Program Directors
66 Canal Center Plaza, Ste. 302
Alexandria, VA 22314
Phone: 703-739-9333
Fax: 703-548-9517
Website: www.nasmhpd.org

National Center for Mental Health Promotion and Youth Violence Prevention
Education Development
Center, Inc.
43 Foundry Ave.
Waltham, MA 02453
Toll-Free: 877-217-3595
Fax: 617-969-5951
Website: www.promoteprevent
.org
E-mail: info@promoteprevent.org

National Center for Missing and Exploited Children
Charles B. Wang International Children's Bldg.
699 Prince St.
Alexandria, VA 22314-3175
Toll-Free: 800-THE-LOST
(800-843-5678)
Phone: 703-224-2150
Fax: 703-224-2122
Website: www.missingkids.com
E-mail: RLeonard@ncmec.org

National Center on Shaken Baby Syndrome
1433 N. Hwy 89, Ste. 110
Farmington, UT 84025
Phone: 801-447-9360
Fax: 801-447-9364
Website: www.dontshake.org
E-mail: mail@dontshake.org

National Child Protection Training Center
Winona State University Campus
Maxwell Hall, 2nd Fl.
Winona, MN 55987
Phone: 507-457-2890
Fax: 507-457-2899
Website: www
.gundersenhealth.org/ncptc/
jacob-wetterling-resource-center
E-mail: trainings@ncptc-jwrc.org

National Children's Advocacy Center
210 Pratt Ave.
Huntsville, AL 35801
Phone: 256-533-KIDS
(256-533-5437)
Fax: 256-534-6883
Website: www.nationalcac.org
E-mail: intervention@
nationalcac.org

National Children's Alliance
516 C St. NE
Washington, DC 20002
Toll-Free: 800-239-9950
Phone: 202-548-0090
Fax: 202-548-0099
Website: www.
nationalchildrensalliance.org
E-mail: mgadmin@nca-online
.org

National Coalition to Prevent Child Sexual Abuse and Exploitation
Website: www.preventtogether
.org
E-mail: PreventTogether@gmail
.com

National Council on Child Abuse and Family Violence
1025 Connecticut Ave. N.W.,
Ste. 1000
Washington, DC 20036
Phone: 202-429-6695
Fax: 202-521-3479
Website: www.nccafv.org
E-mail: info@nccafv.org

National Indian Child Welfare Association
5100 S.W. Macadam Ave., Ste. 300
Portland, OR 97239
Phone: 503-222-4044
Fax: 503-222-4007
Website: www.nicwa.org
E-mail: info@nicwa.org

National Parent Helpline
250 W.First St.
Ste. 250
Claremont, CA 91711
Toll-Free: 855-4-A-PARENT (855-427-2736)
Phone: 909-621-6184
Website: www. nationalparenthelpline.org
E-mail: info@ nationalparenthelpline.org

NetSafeKids, Computer Science and Telecommunications Board
The National Academies
500 Fifth St. N.W.
Washington, DC 20001
Phone: 202-334-2605
Fax: 202-334-2318
Website: www.nap.edu/ netsafekids
E-mail: cstb@nas.edu

Office for Victims of Crime
U.S. Department of Justice
810 Seventh St. N.W., Eighth Fl.
Washington, DC 20531
Phone: 202-307-5983
Fax: 202-514-6383
Website: www.ovc.gov
E-mail: itverp@ojp.usdoj.gov

Parents Anonymous, Inc.
250 W.First St.
Ste. 250
Claremont, CA 91711
Phone: 909-236-5757
Fax: 909-236-5758
Website: www. parentsanonymous.org
E-mail: Parentsanonymous@ parentsanonymous.org

Parents for Megan's Law and the Crime Victims Center
Toll-Free: 888-ASK-PFML (888-275-7365)
Phone: 631-689-2672
Website (English): www. parentsformeganslaw.org/ welcome.jsp
E-mail: pfmeganslaw@aol.com

Prevent Child Abuse America
228 S. Wabash Ave., 10th Fl.
Chicago, IL 60604
Phone: 312-663-3520
Fax: 312-939-8962
Website: www. preventchildabuse.org
E-mail: mailbox@ preventchildabuse.org

Rape, Abuse and Incest National Network (RAINN)
2000 L St. N.W., Ste. 406
Washington, DC 20036
Toll-Free: 800-656-HOPE (800-656-4673)
Phone: 202-544-3064
Fax: 202-544-3556
Website: www.rainn.org
E-mail: info@rainn.org

Safe4Athletes
P.O. Box 650
Santa Monica, CA 90406
Phone: 855-SAFE-4-AA
(855-723-3422)
Website: safe4athletes.org
E-mail: info@safe4athletes.org

Safe Child Program
Coalition for Children, Inc.
P.O. Box 6304
Denver, CO 80206
Phone: 303-320-6328
Fax: 303-809-6328
Website: www.safechild.org
E-mail: info@safechild.org

Safer Society Foundation, Inc.
P.O. Box 340
Brandon, VT 05733-0340
Phone: 802-247-3132
Fax: 802-247-4233
Website: www.safersociety.org
E-mail: info@safersociety.org

Sexuality Information and Education Council of the United States (SIECUS)
90 John St., Ste. 402
New York, NY 10038
Phone: 212-819-9770
Fax: 212-819-9776
Website: www.siecus.org
E-mail: kromines@siecus.org

Stop It Now!
351 Pleasant St., Ste. B-319
Northampton, MA 01060
Toll-Free: 888-PREVENT
(888-773-8368)
Phone: 413-587-3500
Fax: 413-587-3505
Website: www.StopItNow.org
E-mail: info@stopitnow.org

Substance Abuse and Mental Health Services Administration
SAMHSA's Health Information Network
P.O. Box 2345
Rockville, MD 20847-2345
Toll-Free: 877-SAMHSA-7
(877-726-4727)
Phone: 240-221-4036
Toll-Free TTY: 800-487-4889
Fax: 240-221-4292
Website: store.samhsa.gov
E-mail: SAMHSAInfo@samhsa.hhs.gov

Survivors of Incest Anonymous
World Service Office
P.O. Box 190
Benson, MD 21018-9998
Phone: 410-893-3322
Website: www.siawso.org
E-mail: GatheringInfo@siawso.org

Wind and Fire Missions Base
(Formerly Center to Restore
Trafficked and Exploited
Children)
P.O. Box 126
Hiawatha, IA 52233
Phone: 319-294-5307
Fax: 319-892-0203
Website: wfmmissionsbase.org
E-mail: info@windandfire.org

Witness Justice
P.O. Box 2516
Rockville, MD 20847-2516
Phone: 301-846-9110
Website: witnessjustice.org
E-mail: info@witnessjustice.org

Index

Index

489